PROBLEMS, ISSUES & CONCEPTS IN THERAPEUTIC RECREATION

Ronald P. Reynolds
Virginia Commonwealth University

and

Gerald S. O'Morrow
Radford University

Prentice-Hall, Inc., Englewood Cliffs, NJ 07632

GALLAUDET UNIVERSITY LIBRARY
WASHINGTON, D.C. 20002

Library of Congress Cataloging in Publication Data

Reynolds, Ronald P., 1947-
   Problems, issues & concepts in therapeutic
recreation.

   Bibliography: p.
   Includes index.
   1. Recreational therapy. I. O'Morrow, Gerald S.
II. Title. III. Title: Problems, issues, and concepts
in therapeutic recreation.
RM736.7.R48 1985   615.8′5153′023   84-18075
ISBN 0-13-717430-6

Editorial/production supervision and
   interior design: Helen Maertens and Sylvia Moore
Cover design: Lundgren Graphics, Ltd.
Manufacturing buyer: Harry P. Baisley

© 1985 by Prentice-Hall, Inc., Englewood Cliffs, New Jersey 07632

All rights reserved. No part of this book may be
reproduced, in any form or by any means,
without permission in writing from the publisher.

Printed in the United States of America

10 9 8 7 6 5 4 3 2 1

ISBN 0-13-717430-6 01

Prentice-Hall International, Inc., *London*
Prentice-Hall of Australia Pty. Limited, *Sydney*
Editora Prentice-Hall do Brasil, Ltda., *Rio de Janeiro*
Prentice-Hall Canada Inc., *Toronto*
Prentice-Hall of India Private Limited, *New Delhi*
Prentice-Hall of Japan, Inc., *Tokyo*
Prentice-Hall of Southeast Asia Pte. Ltd., *Singapore*
Whitehall Books Limited, *Wellington, New Zealand*

GALLAUDET UNIVERSITY LIBRARY
WASHINGTON, D.C. 20002

615.8
R4p
1985

This book is dedicated to Diane Reynolds and Mary O'Morrow,
who provided the assistance and support necessary for its completion.

023240

CONTENTS

PREFACE

Recreation has been recognized and extolled as an important element in the prevention and amelioration of disabling conditions for centuries. However, despite this acknowledgment of the general benefits that might accrue from participation in leisure activities, the notion of "therapeutic recreation" as an area of service and as a distinct helping profession is scarcely four decades old.

In contemplating the future of this young field, there is every indication that the demand for therapeutic recreation service and a resulting need for professional development will increase sharply over the next several years. Improved diagnostic techniques, highly sophisticated medical procedures, and new medications will prolong the lives of thousands of individuals. There is also a growing recognition on the part of society that leisure services are a *right* of disabled persons and that leisure needs *must* be addressed in the implementation of any comprehensive program of rehabilitation.

In light of these factors, members of the profession face several important short- and long-term issues concerning the future direction of the field. The authors of this volume have attempted to outline these salient problems and to provide the reader with information which may be used as a basis to develop informed opinions. Each topical area has been defined and delineated by providing an historical account of its evolution and emergence to its present status. Particular attention has been paid to articulating various points of controversy and summarizing the views of individuals in the discipline who have addressed these concerns over the years. In this process, the authors have been careful to ensure that all available perspectives on each issue have been presented accurately. Current reference sources, contemporary professional documents, and actual case-study examples are utilized in a manner designed to assist the reader in formulating a personal position on each topic. In this fashion, therapeutic recreation specialists may develop and refine their individual values and attitudes related to professional standards, preparation, certification, technologies, ethics, and other issues inherent in a vibrant and dynamic field.

ACKNOWLEDGMENTS

Many people are directly and indirectly involved in the development of ideas for and the making of a textbook. In the process, grateful acknowledgment is due many individuals for various comments, advice, and information. The authors are particularly indebted to Lee E. Meyer for reviewing Chapter 2; to Marcia Jean Carter for reviewing Chapter 4; and to Gerald S. Fain for his suggestions concerning Chapter 5, specifically the section on Ethics.

We would like to extend our thanks for the gratuitous assistance received from the respective library staffs at Virginia Commonwealth University and Radford University. We also thank the authors, editors, and publishers who granted permission for their work to be reprinted herein. Lastly, our thanks to the production staff of Prentice-Hall, Inc. for accepting the idea of this book, as well as for their assistance and editing.

In the final analysis, it is hard to see how this publication could have been brought to fruition without the assistance of Mrs. Linda Rothweiler and Mrs. Janet Favale Turner for their effort in typing the initial drafts. Finally, no small measure of thanks is again given to Mrs. Turner, who put so much patient, untiring effort into the preparation of the final manuscript.

CHAPTER ONE
INTRODUCTION

BACKGROUND, PURPOSE, AND ASSUMPTIONS

As one of the youngest and most rapidly developing of the helping professions, the field of therapeutic recreation stands at a critical stage of development. Scarcely four decades after its beginning, its members are currently facing some of the greatest challenges which may ever confront our profession. Indeed, the decisions concerning the discipline's professional direction made during the next five years will impact on the working lives of its members far into the next century.

This book was conceived of, and developed in response to, the "real-life" issues that therapeutic recreation personnel are now seeking to resolve. Part of the impetus for its development was the need to structure materials and discussion for college courses involving both the emerging and the practicing therapeutic recreation specialist. Consequently, it is designed to provide information and insights of direct use to members of the profession when they are:

— Articulating the mission of our field to other health care professions, organizations, and agencies
— Seeking to upgrade the status of therapeutic recreation service within a given job setting
— Contemplating the various credentialling options currently available

— Complying with standards of practice in clinical and community settings
— Selecting or completing professional preparation programs
— Improving direct service to clients
— Undertaking research or evaluation activities

The reader is cautioned that this is not an "introduction to therapeutic recreation" text. It assumes that the reader has a basic working knowledge of the field of therapeutic recreation and a genuine interest and concern for the issues discussed. Practitioners and students with practicum or previous work experience would probably be most able to benefit from the material. Therefore, the text is appropriate for both classroom and continuing-education workshop settings.

As with any work attempting to deal with contemporary issues, this text provides a "stop-action" picture of conditions and situations as they existed shortly before publication. Therefore, while considering these issues, the reader is cautioned regarding the need to monitor developments which may have occurred after the time of printing. Several suggestions are made in the final chapter concerning this process.

In a sense, the text deals with both "knowns" and "unknowns." The reader is therefore again cautioned that, in many instances, there are no right or wrong answers to problems discussed here; there may be many possible solutions to specific issues. Also, because of the newness of the field, the final resolution of certain problems may realistically take months and years. Rather than feeling frustrated, it is hoped that the reader will appreciate his or her opportunity to participate in the process of shaping the profession.

Every attempt has been made to provide an adequate historical overview of each issue addressed in the text. It was felt that such background information is necessary to insure that readers can fully understand, and make informed decisions, concerning the topics presented. The authors have made every effort to substantiate the accuracy of the references used and the interpretation of the documents consulted. They welcome any corrections or additions from members of their profession. Considerable attention has been paid to defining terms and explaining the origin of contemporary terminology in the field, particularly in the early chapters. This was done in many cases to illustrate the evolution of the issue or problem at hand. The reader is urged to consider this rationale when assimilating the information presented. In many cases, one person's position has been quoted in reference to more than one issue. Similarly, the reader may note the occasional use of a specific reference in more than one location throughout the text.

In researching this text, the authors have drawn heavily from disciplines and other sources outside the field of therapeutic recreation. This approach was taken for three important reasons. *First*, in certain instances, our field has modeled itself after others in its move toward professionalization. *Second*, in certain chapters, the main objective was to show the relation which our profession has to allied health care and other fields. *Third*, it was felt that drawing upon outside, yet related, literature would provide additional depth to the text. Indeed, the authors learned much from this practice. The larger recreation and parks field, likewise, has not been overlooked. In fact, many issues related to accreditation, professional preparation, and defining the field could not have been discussed without drawing heavily from the broader field of recreation.

A final disclaimer is in order. While the authors have held many positions within the organizational structure of the National Therapeutic Recreation Society, and have drawn heavily on the documents and publications of this body, the opinions and interpretations expressed in this book are the authors' and not those of the Society.

CONCEPTUAL OVERVIEW

Before proceeding to the description of the major topical areas, a word is in order about the organizational scheme of the text and the relevance of each issue to the reader. The book is divided into eight chapters (excluding the introductory and final chapters), each of which deals with a contemporary issue or problem. In the treatment of the various areas of study, the field of therapeutic recreation is presented in the broader context of society, with particular attention being paid to legislative and economic trends. The following is a brief outline of the major issues and trends contained within the text:

Chapter 2: "The Status of Therapeutic Recreation as a Profession" asks the questions: How far have we advanced in our efforts to achieve professional status and recognition? What future measures should we employ to ensure our rightful position within the health care professional hierarchy?

Chapter 3: "The Challenge of Defining Therapeutic Recreation as a Profession" outlines the pros and cons of adopting various models or approaches to service as our reason for being and challenges readers to clarify and defend their own philosophies of therapeutic recreation.

Chapter 4: "Credentialling—Which Path?" asks the reader to weigh the relative merits of the various credentialling processes described and to consider the ramifications of each. This is seen as directly affecting the practice of therapeutic recreation service.

Chapter 5: "The Development and Implementation of Professional Standards" discusses the development of regulations which shape the everyday activities of therapeutic recreation specialists, allowing readers to reflect upon the impact of these standards in association with therapeutic recreation standards in their agencies.

Chapter 6: "The Dilemma of Professional Preparation" confronts the reader with questions concerning the content of pre- and in-service training programs and the desirability of having standardized courses of academic study.

Chapter 7: "The Normalization-Integration Issue" urges readers to reflect upon their own attitudes and approaches regarding direct client service. Common practices in therapeutic recreation, such as special events, skill upgrading programs, and "special" activities, are questioned.

Chapter 8: "Scientific Inquiry: The Foundation for Professional Development" surveys readers as to their own use of research and evaluation. It then polls readers as to their specific suggestions concerning strategies to improve communication between producers and consumers of knowledge.

Chapter 9: "Therapeutic Techniques: Issues and Trends" inquires: Are we duplicating services provided by other professions? and Are techniques such as leisure counseling rightfully (and exclusively) ours?

As to the order of the chapters, many combinations were possible. However, the authors decided upon the present sequence. Chapter 2 (on status) overviews some of the general concerns faced by therapeutic recreation specialists over the years and sets the tone for the more specific discussion of concerns related to defining the field, credentialling, standards, and professional preparation (Chapters 3–6). Chapters 7–9 (on normalization, research, and techniques) deal with problems inherent in the practice of therapeutic recreation which, in fact, may be outgrowths of the preceding professional issues. Although the issues are presented separately, the reader is cautioned that they are highly interrelated and that the direction chosen in solving one problem could strongly influence the stance taken in other situations. For example, if one chose a particular model of therapeutic recreation service as a personal philosophy, this model might then dictate which organizational affiliations, forms of credentialling, standards of practice, content of professional preparation, types of client services, and areas of research would be favored.

Although each chapter is devoted to a major problem or topic, the reader is alerted to the fact that, in reality, there may be many subissues within each broad area of inquiry which must be dealt with. For example, before examining the standards and regulations imposed by external organizations, it may well be necessary to resolve fundamental issues concerning our own philosophical position and professional ethics.

In developing each issue, we have emphasized the achievement of a balance in airing the consumer, practitioner, and educator perspectives of the problem. Likewise, various settings, disabilities, and philosophies of service have been included. Nevertheless, imbalances may occur. The reader is therefore cautioned to identify inequities which might exist relative to certain issues and to take these into account when formulating opinions.

Finally, the reader will note that the chapters vary in organization. For example, some follow a chronological exposure of the issue, while others compare and contrast varying points of view or techniques. The learning tasks and study guide questions also appear in different locations from chapter to chapter. In each case, the authors feel that the chosen schema best represents or illustrates the particular issue and facilitates its discussion and debate.

SUGGESTED APPROACHES
FOR LEARNING

As indicated, the primary purpose of this text is to provide a common basis of information and a focal point for discussion of contemporary issues in therapeutic recreation. Although the chapters vary in format, each presents an historical overview of the issue, a basic discussion of the implications and relevance of the topic, an exploratory pros-and-cons treatise of the issue, a suggested learning plan(s), and an annotated bibliography. When utilizing the text in a classroom setting, it is suggested that Chapters 1–3 be read in sequence, to assure that a core of knowledge exists prior to undertaking the more specialized issues which follow. After the initial chapters have been assimilated, the group may want to devise an alternative order of presentation. Due to the large amount of information, the responsibility for presenting units and leading discussions may be distributed among co-learners in the educational setting. Furthermore, selected study guide questions and learning tasks should be chosen for classroom use or shared among students and instructors. It is hoped that these exercises will be added to and modified by their users to suit their needs. For example, settings, clients, and conditions could easily be altered to meet the learning requirements of participants. Although the articles in the annotated bibliography are excellent references for term and position papers, learners are encouraged to go beyond these sources into the existing literature. Indeed, many of the resources cited have excellent references for this purpose. When actually discussing an issue, it may be helpful to invite other therapeutic recreation practitioners or members of other professions such as the creative arts, occupational therapy, counseling, rehabilitation services, and adapted physical education to attend selected meetings. Disabled consumers are also invaluable resource persons who can provide insights into many of the problems outlined.

With this prospectus, the reader is invited to react to the issues presented in subsequent chapters in an honest, open, and thoughtful manner. Only in this fashion can our personal and professional development be continued.

CHAPTER TWO
THE STATUS
OF THERAPEUTIC
RECREATION
AS A PROFESSION

Like living organisms, professions grow and develop throughout their existence. The way they emerge over time is influenced by many factors. Professions are born of a need in the society to have available certain services that require specialized knowledge and skills. They are nurtured by the public's approval of these services. They flourish or wither depending on the society's need for these services, the profession's ability to satisfy this need, and the flexibility of the profession in adapting to a society's changes.

In the United States the professions are not always sharply distinguished from other vocations or occupations. Moreover, in such a dynamic social order, the occupational pattern undergoes rapid changes, and the status of various occupations shifts from time to time. What was yesterday known merely as an occupation may tomorrow be so developed as to take on the earmarks of a full-fledged profession. Furthermore, new services, professional in character, are continually being devised and refined, as witness, for example, the development of therapeutic recreation.

FACTORS SHAPING
THERAPEUTIC RECREATION

Since the turn of this century, many factors have contributed to the evolution and shaping of therapeutic recreation as a service field, an occupation, and an emerging profession. Men and women as individuals with a high sense of personal commitment and responsibility and men and women in organized groups with a common goal have brought about the events that were woven together to form the background of what today is called *therapeutic recreation.*

The most striking characteristic of our present society is change. The speed and the amount of this change affect all aspects of our lives—physical, emotional, social, and economic. We seem to be in transition, moving from an abandoned past toward a future we are as yet unable to comprehend. The goals of our time are complex and technical. Therapeutic recreation, along with other professional services to society, is not self-contained but modifies and is modified by its social setting. Many of the issues that confront therapeutic recreation are only reflections of issues that face many other groups, for instance, increased health discipline specializations, increased involvement of the federal government in health and welfare legislation, and increased cost of health services. Similarly, many of the changes that seem to be unique to therapeutic recreation have resulted, wholly or in part, from forces that have their origins outside of therapeutic recreation, and they represent the ways in which therapeutic recreation has reacted to the conditions created by these forces.

Periods of war and peace have influenced the demand for therapeutic recreators and their services. The provision of health services has changed radically as a result of increased knowledge and the use of newer technological devices. Changing societal problems or changing perceptions of problems have had an impact on identifying client needs and on the demand for varied services. Variations in the way Americans view health have exerted a profound impact on the provision of health services. Shifts in the settings in which health care is provided, the types of services offered, and the particular helping techniques have also changed over time. These and a host of other influences have expanded and modified the role of the therapeutic recreator in our society.

This chapter is guided by yet another means of addressing the development of therapeutic recreation and the issue of emerging professional status. Therapeutic recreation requires community or society approval to maximize the quality of services provided. Without this approval, the services that can be provided are restricted. Although the term *profession* commonly carries implicit connotations, the concept of profession helps to explain the development of therapeutic recreation. This chapter uses the professionalization of therapeutic recreation as a vehicle for understanding its historical evolution.

THE NATURE
OF PROFESSIONALISM

To have one's occupational status accepted as a professional or to have one's occupational conduct judged as professional is highly regarded in all postindustrial societies and in at least the modernizing sectors of others.[1]

[1] Wilbert E. Moore, *The Professions: Roles and Rules* (New York: Russell Sage Foundation, 1970), p. 3.

If professions are so highly regarded, what is the definition of a profession? Dictionaries initially provide some help in understanding the concept. In *Webster's Third New International Dictionary* a profession is defined as:

> A calling requiring specialized knowledge and often long and intensive preparation including instruction in skills and methods as well as in the scientific, historical, or scholarly principles underlying such skills and methods, maintaining by force of organization or concerted opinion high standards of achievement and conduct, and committing its members to continued study and to a kind of work which has for its prime purpose the rendering of a public service.[2]

Another definition is found in the *International Dictionary of Education*, which states that a profession is:

> An evaluative term describing the most prestigious *occupations* which may be termed professions if they carry out an essential social service, are founded on systematic *knowledge*, require lengthy academic and practical training, have high autonomy, a code of ethics, and generate in-service growth.[3]

The *New Dictionary of the Social Sciences* makes reference to a study by Geoffrey Millerson, who cited the following characteristics most frequently enumerated by twenty-one individuals:

1. A profession involves a skill based on theoretical knowledge.
2. The skill requires training and education.
3. The professional must demonstrate competence by passing a test.
4. Integrity is maintained by adherence to a code of conduct.
5. The service is for the public good.
6. The profession is organized.[4]

Lastly, the most recent *Encyclopedia of Careers and Vocational Guidance* makes reference to the term *professional* within the professional, managerial, and technical occupations thus: "highly formalized extensive training . . . requiring some type of licensing before practice."[5]

As one considers professions, one needs to keep in mind that they evolved from the vocations of ancient times. Lawyers, clergy, and physicians, the earliest recognized members of vocations, were initiated into their vocations by undergoing

[2] Philip Babcock Gove, ed. in chief, *Webster's Third New International Dictionary of the English Language* (Springfield, Mass.: G & C Merriam Company, Publishers, 1971), p. 1811.

[3] G. Terry Page and J. B. Thomas, eds., *The International Directory of Education* (New York: Nichols Publishing Company, 1977), p. 273.

[4] G. Duncan Mitchell, ed., *New Dictionary of the Social Sciences* (New York: Aldine Publishing Company, 1979), p. 149.

[5] "Professional, Managerial, and Technical Occupations," *Encyclopedia of Careers and Vocational Guidance,* 4th ed., ed. William E. Hopke (Chicago: Doubleday & Co., Inc., J. G. Ferguson Publishing Company, 1978), I, p. 1.

a type of apprenticeship training. As knowledge increased, however, a greater need for teachers arose. In many instances, groups of scientists and practitioners formed schools where education took on the character of an apprenticeship. Instruction was individual, and students assisted practitioners. As the professions grew and greater numbers of students enrolled in training programs, the system of individual instruction disappeared. Today, in less limited fashion, a profession is identified as an occupation usually involving specialized preparation on the level of higher education and governed by its own code of ethics.

The rise of professions has been associated with the emergence of social problems and of resultant specializations. The sequence of events in this process begins with the recognition by the community or society of a difficult and extensive problem. Then, as untrained personnel deal with the problem, a differentiation of procedures emerges, and apprenticeships are instituted and skills are transmitted. The theoretical and applied body of knowledge basic to the procedures is formulated, and the program of education becomes prolonged so that the theory and skills may be learned. Although the members of a profession continue to work as individuals, group consciousness evolves, and social groups with activities based on professional interests are formed. When people begin to pay directly or indirectly for services, codes and standards are developed for controlling and defining client or consumer relationships. These codes are concerned with the establishment of formal rules and informal practices of behavior expected of the members of the profession. Methods of enforcing these standards are established. Further, the professional group or association reserves the right to enforce, by its own means, discipline and ethical standards, thus preserving the independence of its members in the practice of the profession. Although this sequence of events appears to follow an orderly progression, in reality, such progression is uneven. Power struggles and status strivings common to all occupations explain deviations from the sequence.[6]

The public expects high-quality service from members of a profession, believing that professional men and women should possess considerable knowledge and high ideals. Professional people are accorded a high status in our society. Over the years, members of the professions have been dedicated both to a particular course of service and to establishing and maintaining the prestige of the profession. Professionals felt that they had a responsibility and were more motivated to promote the cause they were serving than to achieve financial success. Many worked long hours for small pay and little appreciation. Although the training in a body of abstract knowledge was specified and prolonged, people were not deterred from pursuing the professions. In this regard Goode stated, "No occupation becomes a profession without a struggle. . . . The emotion-laden identification of men with their occupation, their dependence on it for much of the daily meaning of their lives, causes them to defend it vigorously and to advance its cause when possible."[7]

[6] Harold L. Wilensky, "The Professionalization of Everyone?" *American Journal of Sociology,* 120, no. 2 (1964), 141–46.

[7] William J. Goode, "Encroachment, Charlatanism, and the Emerging Professions: Psychology, Sociology, and Medicine," *American Sociological Review,* 25, no. 12 (1960), 902.

The criteria of professionalization have been expressed by many writers.[8] The consensus of these writers seems to indicate that the following are the essential criteria of any profession: (1) It requires an organized body of specialized knowledge; (2) it necessitates special and sometimes protracted study and training of an intellectual and technical nature, capable of being transmitted through a required educational discipline; (3) it demands a high degree of individual responsibility and competence; (4) it has the provision of a necessary and skilled service as its basic purpose; (5) it represents an organized activity involving a plurality of persons performing a similar function according to shared norms; (6) it tends toward self-organization for the promotion of standards of professional competence and the advancement of professional self-interest; and (7) it is expected to demonstrate, as a primary obligation, a responsiveness to the public interest and welfare.

The criteria of a profession, according to William Shephard, are:

1. A profession must satisfy an indispensable social need and be based upon well-established and socially accepted scientific principles.
2. It must demand adequate preprofessional and cultural training.
3. It must demand the possession of a body of specialized and systematized knowledge.
4. It must give evidence of needed skills which the public does not possess; that is, skills which are partly native and partly acquired.
5. It must have developed a scientific technique which is the result of tested experience.
6. It must require the exercise of discretion and judgment as to time and manner of the performance of duty. This is in contrast to the kind of work which is subject to immediate direction and supervision.
7. It must be a type of beneficial work, the result of which is not subject to standardization in terms of unit performance or time element.
8. It must have a group consciousness designed to extend scientific knowledge in technical language.
9. It must have sufficient self-impelling power to retain its members throughout life. It must not be used as a mere stepping-stone to other occupations.
10. It must recognize its obligations to society by insisting that its members live up to an established code of ethics.[9]

A substantial field of sociological inquiry has been devoted to the definition and description of the nature of professions during the twentieth century. One approach to this study has been to examine medicine, law, the ministry, and higher education to identify the fundamental elements of professions such as specialized skill and training, minimum fees or salaries, formation of professional associations, and codes of ethical behavior governing professional practice. Occupational groups

[8] Professionalization criteria can be found in works cited in the Footnotes (nos. 1, 6, 7, 8, 10, 11, 14, 33, and 51, the Annotated Bibliography (authors Barber, Goode, Greenwood, Hughes, Moore, and Wilensky) and the Bibliography (authors Bledstein; Etzioni; Ferguson; Goode; Gross and Osterman; Hall; Marston; and Vollmer and Mills) at the end of this chapter.

[9] William Shephard, "The Professionalization of Public Health," *American Journal of Public Health and the Nation's Health,"* 38 (January 1948), p. 146.

could then be evaluated to determine whether they meet these criteria. Using this approach, an occupational group could be classified in one of two categories: professional or nonprofessional.[10]

More recently, the prevalent approach to the study of professions has been to identify their attributes, then to evaluate occupational groups by the degree to which they possess these qualities. The most professional would be the occupation which achieves each of the attributes to the greatest extent. In this manner a relative degree of professionalism can be determined for each occupation.[11] Moore, for example, identified the primary characteristics or attributes of professions as a full-time occupation, a commitment to a calling, an indentification with peers, a specified training or education, a service orientation, and an autonomy restrained by responsibility.[12] Using such criteria, it is possible to identify each occupational group (note that the criteria rule out volunteers) on a scale of professionalism.

In more general terms, a profession includes three elements that reflect the obligations and responsibilities of both the professional and the consumer served.

First, the professional is required to possess both a general and a specialized body of knowledge that can be used to benefit the consumer. Because a professional serves consumers in sensitive areas of their lives, he or she must have considerable latitude in making judgments. The professional must therefore possess a general knowledge of human functioning in order to place this specialty in context. At the same time, the community expects the professional to have particular technical competencies not generally held by the public; for example, the therapeutic recreator, in working with a physically disabled consumer, must not only know what activity to use for success but must also consider the consumer's ability to participate and must recognize fears about participation. Thus it is evident that the professional is much more than a technician. It is necessary for this individual to have acquired both the general and specialized knowledge and the skill to prepare for practice.

As Goode has pointed out, members of a profession are bound together by common identity, values, and language. The "distinctive focus" of these bonds is the "possession of some specific skill or cluster of skills".[13] In other words, a professional is one who possesses competence in some area shared only by the other members of one's own profession. It is this unique competence which determines the relations of professionals to the larger society.

Second, because it is considered inefficient for everyone in the population to complete the extensive education required in this process, society grants professional sanction or authority to a few people who have this preparation. These

---

[10] A. M. Carr-Saunders and P. A. Wilson, *The Professions* (Oxford, England: Clarendon Press, 1933), pp. 3–31.

[11] Ernest Greenwood, "Attributes of a Profession," *Social Work*, 2, no. 7 (1957), 47.

[12] Moore, *The Professions*, pp. 5–6.

[13] William J. Goode, "Community Within a Community: The Professions," *American Sociological Review*, 22, no. 7 (1957), 194–200.

professionals are accorded the exclusive right to make judgments and to give advice in the areas of their specialties.

Last, when the right to judge practice is relinquished, the public expects professionals to prevent abuses that may accrue from that monopoly. Everett C. Hughes indicated that the motto of the professions must be *credat emptor* ("buyer trust"), as opposed to the motto of the marketplace, *caveat emptor* ("buyer beware").[14] In short, the consumer's inherent vulnerability is intensified in the helping services, which deal in areas where the unwitting public could potentially be harmed by the actions of the professional. To offer protection, professions have developed codes of ethics and established bodies to investigate situations where abuses of this monopoly are alleged. For many professions, additional protection is afforded the consumer through certification or registration of members by their respected professional organization board or state licensing of members.

Professions, then, serve a vital function by sanctioning particular occupational groups to provide specialized services in sensitive areas of human life. In the United States, professions have emerged as occupational groups with high status. But where does therapeutic recreation fit among the professions, if at all?

THERAPEUTIC RECREATION AS A PROFESSION: HISTORICAL PERSPECTIVE

Therapeutic recreation has devoted considerable energy and time to the attempt to achieve professional status. Although it is not possible to present all the details of the emergence of therapeutic recreation as a service and practice or the history of the field's organizational evolution itself, it is useful to examine some aspects of the historical development of the field. The evolution of therapeutic recreation, as you will note, has been uneven, but, at the same time, its development has been similar to other health-related professions.

Before World War II

The origins of therapeutic recreation are obscure. There is no indication that any form of organized recreation service programs for the ill and disabled existed prior to the nineteenth century. Although some evidence exists that activities of a recreational nature were used in caring for the ill and disabled in ancient times, it appears that such practices were associated more with natural remedies and religion. In the periods that followed ancient civilizations, only brief mention is made in historical texts of the use of recreation activities with the ill and disabled. Where reference to such practice is made, it suggests that such activities were used only to distract individuals from their problems. The growth of social concern and responsi-

---

[14] Everett C. Hughes, "Professions," *Daedalus,* 92 (Fall 1963), p. 657.

bility in the eighteenth century, and more so in the nineteenth century, resulted in a humane concern for the care and treatment of the mentally ill and the mentally retarded. As a result, recreational activities were introduced into some institutions for the mentally ill not only for their diversional qualities, but also for their therapeutic value as an adjunct to treatment.[15]

Time and circumstances often provide the opportunity for action. Military strife has always created havoc and horror, but, without such conflict, the beginnings of organized recreation service to the ill and disabled might not have occurred.

Shortly after the entry of the United States into World War I, the American Red Cross initiated the provision of recreation service to military personnel in hospitals and convalescent centers overseas and stateside. Later these services, which were considered diversional as well as therapeutic, were introduced into public health service hospitals by the Red Cross. When the Veterans Bureau assumed responsibility for treatment and rehabilitation of ex-servicemen, Red Cross recreation staff were assigned to these hospitals. It probably can be said with some reservation that the establishment of recreation services in military and veterans' hospitals greatly affected the future of recreation services to all disabled persons.

Another significant recreation service development prior to World War II was the initiation of such services to the mentally retarded. The White House Conference on Child Health and Protection in 1930 brought about a new concern for the rights and needs of the mentally retarded. This new attitude, according to Witt:

> . . . led to programs based on the individual needs and differences of the participants; further, the institutional recreation program of the 1920's and early 1930's . . . began, by the late 1930's, to assume the form of a free-play recreation program. Research into the play patterns of the mentally retarded fostered a recognition of the types of recreation programs necessary to meet both the structure of community living and the confines of institutionalization.[16]

One other significant development in this period of time was the establishment of the Playground Association of America (PAA) in 1906. The professional roots of the park and recreation movement may be found in the social reforms and concerns of the late 1800s and early 1900s; specifically, in a determination to provide opportunity for meaningful recreational activities for all people. The rationale for the

---

[15] Virginia Frye, "Historical Sketch of Recreation in the Medical Setting," *Recreation in Treatment Centers*, 1 (1962), pp. 40–43; Norman Dain, *Concepts of Insanity in the United States 1789–1865* (New Brunswick, N.J.: Rutgers University Press, 1964), pp. 117–19; Elliott M. Avedon, *Therapeutic Recreation Service: An Applied Behavioral Science Approach* (Englewood Cliffs, N.J.: Prentice-Hall, Inc., 1974), pp. 9–11; Jack Meislen, "The Role of Physical Medicine and Rehabilitation in Psychiatry: A Historical Approach," in *Rehabilitation Medicine and Psychiatry,* ed. Jack Meislen (Springfield, Ill: Charles C Thomas Publisher, 1976), pp. 9–21; Lee E. Meyer, "Recreation and the Mentally Ill," in *Recreation and Special Populations,* 2nd ed., eds. Thomas A. Stein and H. Douglas Sessoms (Boston: Holbrook Press, Inc., 1977), pp. 142-45; Gerald S. O'Morrow, *Therapeutic Recreation: A Helping Profession,* 2nd ed. (Reston, Va., Reston Publishing Company, 1980), pp. 84–91.

[16] Peter A. Witt, "A History of Recreation for the Mentally Retarded," personal copy, n.d.

inclusion of this movement here is that the formation of the PAA was the direct result of a desire on the part of early municipal recreators to integrate disadvantaged persons into community life through recreation.[17]

The beginning of organized therapeutic recreation service can thus be characterized as a response to the social concerns of the early twentieth century. The first paid hospital recreator positions were jobs in long-term care institutions. Beginning as diversional activities, provided on a sporadic basis, and directed by volunteers, recreation services gradually became more formalized and eventually received public support. To deal with this trend toward organized recreation service, paid hospital recreators were employed to further direct and develop these services in federal and state institutions.

After World War II (to 1970)

The period from World War II to the late 1960s might best be characterized at the beginning as a time of continued expansion of services and later as a time when hospital recreators moved toward some professional unity. In fact, this period was indeed rich in the development of new service possibilities, in concern for new problem areas and new client and consumer groups, and in the use of old methods or practices in new ways. In considering this period we will focus on three factors which appear to have contributed to the early development of therapeutic recreation as an occupation and as an emerging profession; namely, shifting concepts in health care service, provisions of therapeutic recreation service and practice, and organizational development.

Shifting Health Care.   The community's interest in matters of health has always been accelerated by war. Even when the acute war need is past, that interest is found to be at a higher level in all matters of health than at the beginning of the war. Many communities since World War II have increased the size and scope of existing health facilities or have built additional ones with the aid of funds from both voluntary and governmental sources. The bulk of the middle-class American population is covered by some form of health insurance. Mass media bombards the population with information and misinformation about health, illness, and services. All of these factors contribute to an increase in the utilization of existing health facilities. When health is seen as a right, rather than a privilege, then society assumes an obligation to provide this service to its members. Associated with this concept is the demand on the part of the public for quality service, regardless of ability to pay for it.

The hospital is a diagnostic, therapeutic, preventive, rehabilitative, and educational institution, as well as one carrying on the traditional functions of providing health facilities and services. As medicine became more specialized, and with the

---

[17] Arthur Williams, "An Organization Is Born," in *Notes on History and Theory,* Cited in Jay B. Nash, *Recreation: Pertinent Readings—Guideposts to the Future* (Dubuque, Iowa: William C. Brown, Co., Publishers, 1965), p. 18.

expansion of preventive, psychiatric, and rehabilitative services, a need or demand was created for workers with special education in the fields allied to medicine, specifically, allied health professions. As a result, the federal government assumed an increasing share of the cost of both professional and technical education through direct scholarship aid and indirect subsidization of students and schools via projects and demonstration grants and loans. Likewise, some state departments of both public and mental health initiated scholarship aid programs through legislative funding.

Coupled with the demand for allied health workers was the need for different types of health care facilities as a result of changes in the patterns of illness. For example, instead of hospitals or institutions for communicable diseases, more facilities were constructed for the short-term and extended care of the mentally ill and retarded, the physically disabled, and the chronically ill.

These vast changes had a significant effect on therapeutic recreation. In 1963 the Office of Vocational Rehabilitation (now the Rehabilitation Services Administration) of the then Department of Health, Education and Welfare (now the Department of Health and Human Services and the Department of Education respectively), initiated a traineeship program in the area of recreation for the ill and handicapped. This was the first recognition by a federal agency of the importance of recreation services to ill and disabled individuals. These programs laid the foundation for the growth and development of specialized training in the area. Subsequent legislation in the 1960s and into the 1970s continued to support the value of therapeutic recreation service: the Education for the Handicapped Act of 1967 (PL 90-170, Title V, Physical Education and Recreation for the Handicapped Child); the Architectural Barriers Act of 1968 (PL 90-480); the Nationwide Outdoor Recreation Plan of 1963 (within PL 88-29); the Rehabilitation Act of 1973 (PL 93-112, specifically Titles II, III, and V, Sections 502 and 504); the Rehabilitation Act Amendment of 1974 (PL 93-516); the Education of All Handicapped Children Act of 1975 (PL 94-142); and the Rehabilitation Act and Developmental Disabilities Amendments of 1978 (PL 95-602).

Services and Practices.   As a result of federal legislation which deeply affected our system of health care following World War II, there came an increasing acceleration and expansion of recreation services in all types of health care facilities well into the mid-century. Recreation services became common in state psychiatric hospitals, residential facilities for the mentally retarded, local mental health and mental retardation centers, extended care facilities, and rehabilitation centers. In addition, there was an increasing demand for hospital recreation workers, an upgrading of personnel practices, and an eventual recognition of the recreation service function and its workers as important members of the health team.

By the end of the 1950s, attention was being given in special schools and general medical hospitals to clients with specific conditions or problems such as alcoholics, substance abusers, persons with orthopedic and cardiovascular conditions, the visually and hearing impaired, and others. Moreover, a national voluntary registration plan had been in effect since 1953, which set minimum standards of qualification and identified those who met the standards. This registration program also affected employment policies of various public and private agencies and institutions.

As noted, in spite of recreation service expansion into a variety of health care settings during the mid-century, hospital recreation workers struggled for recognition and acceptance as members of health teams. There was a tendency for physicians and other allied health personnel to still consider recreation service to be diversional in nature and to question its therapeutic value. This problem was resolved to some degree, beginning in 1948, when several significant statements concerning the role of recreation in the treatment process were extended by prominent physicians and psychiatrists,[18] the American Psychiatric Association,[19] and the American Medical Association (AMA).[20] In 1961 the AMA designated recreation service as an allied health field. This acknowledgment, as detailed elsewhere, was the result of "recreation's contribution to the promotion of health, the prevention of illness or further disability, the treatment of illness, and the rehabilitation of persons with physical, psychological, mental or social disabilities.[21]

Another development during this period that further stimulated the acceptance of hospital recreation workers occurred in the educational arena. Initially, the training of hospital recreation personnel was provided through staff development or in-service training programs within the various employing agencies. Following World War II there was an increase in the number of recreation curricula in colleges and universities. Some of these institutions of higher learning initiated graduate study in hospital recreation in the early 1950s. The Standards and Training Committee, Hospital Recreation Section of the American Recreation Society, in 1953 made recommendations concerning the educational preparation of hospital recreation workers. It is of interest to note here that the first national conference on college training of recreation leaders, conducted at the University of Minnesota in 1937, recognized "Recreation Therapy" as a specialization.[22] To further develop the

[18] William Menninger and Isabelle McCall, cited in Lee E. Meyer, "Recreation and the Mentally Ill," p. 147; Alexander Reid Martin, "Professional Attitudes and Practices" in *Recreation for the Mentally Ill*, ed. B. E. Phillips (Washington, D.C.; American Association for Health, Physical Education, and Recreation, 1958), pp. 13–18; Robert H. Felix, Preface to *Recreation in Treatment Centers*, I (1962), 3; Joseph B. Wolffe, "Recreation, Medicine and the Humanities," in *The Doctors and Recreation in the Hospital Setting* (Raleigh, N.C.; North Carolina Recreation Commission, January 1962), pp. 14–21; Paul Haun, *Recreation: A Medical Viewpoint* (New York: Columbia University, Teachers College Press, Bureau of Publication, 1965).

[19] Daniel Blain and Pat Vosburgh, *Recreation Trends in North American Mental Institutions* (Washington, D.C.; American Psychiatric Association, 1952).

[20] American Medical Association, *Proceedings of the Committee to Study the Relationship of Medicine with Health Professions and Services* (Chicago, 1960).

[21] O'Morrow, *Therapeutic Recreation: A Helping Profession, 2nd ed.*, p. 111.

[22] University of Minnesota and Work Progress Administration, *Report on the First College Conference on Training Recreation Leaders* (Minneapolis, Minn.: University of Minnesota, 1937), pp. 25–26. From a professionalization perspective, professional association formation usually precedes university-based training of individuals for the specific profession (Wilensky, "The Professionalization of Everyone?" p. 145).

quality of hospital recreation workers, institutes in hospital recreation were held on various campuses during the 1950s and into the 1960s. In this regard, the University of North Carolina made a rich contribution with the publication of papers and proceedings from their institutes (Southern Regional).

Another developing stream during this period was community recreation ser vices to the ill and disabled. This concern for recreational experiences for the ill and disabled in the community was based on the concept that the total recreation interest pattern of individuals and their participation in the expression of those interests during leisure constitute a part of daily living. In our society a deep appreciation of the dignity of man, freedom of choice, equal opportunity for all, and the right to leisure has become synonymous with our way of life. Recreative experiences connote freedom; they encourage self-expression, initiative, self-leadership. Participation in recreation is an expression of the process of democratic living.

In the early 1950s a small number of cities established special centers to offer recreation services to the physically and mentally disabled. Likewise, a number of municipal recreation departments in major cities appointed or employed specialists with a recreation service background in working with the ill and disabled to initiate and develop recreation service programs for special groups. For the most part, these programs were for the mentally retarded, as a result of the vital concern of parents for the well-being of their retarded children. Although there was a concern for the ill and disabled in the community, it was not until the mid-1960s that a definite trend toward the provision of such services was established.

By the 1960s and thereafter, hospital recreators sought to identify a distinctive method of practice that would distinguish their area of service from other helping professions such as occupational therapy, physical therapy, and corrective therapy. In addition to this effort, two other matters were of concern; namely, terminology, or what to call this emerging profession, and educational preparation. These issues were directly and indirectly associated with a study by Silson, Cohen, and Hill concerned with organized recreation programs in hospitals and the personnel who conducted them.[23] These concerns eventuated in a significant conference in 1961 which discussed terminology, identified problems and trends, considered the role and function of the specialist in recreation service to the ill and disabled, and proposed appropriate knowledges and skills to serve as the fundamentals of practice and need to be included within the graduate curriculum.[24] Educational preparation in hospital recreation at this point was found primarily at the graduate level.

As a result of this conference within two years the term *therapeutic recreation* was adopted to identify the field, in lieu of such terms as *Recreation for the Ill and Handicapped, Hospital Recreation, Recreational Therapy, Medical Recreation,* and *Institutional Recreation.* For more than thirty years workers had sought a

[23] John E. Silson, Elliott M. Cohen, and Beatrice H. Hill, *Recreation in Hospitals: Report of a Study of Organized Recreation Programs in Hospitals and the Personnel Conducting Them* (New York: National Recreation Association, 1959).

[24] *Therapeutic Recreation Curriculum Development Conference,* February 1961 (New York: Comeback, Inc., n.d.).

common title which would reflect a description of their services and field. Titles, as noted, have ranged from the philosophical to the practical. As a result, there was general agreement that growth and development of needed services was restricted. The reason given for a change in terminology at that time was stated by MacLean.

> First, the term itself places the emphasis not on therapy but on recreation, thus avoiding conflict with those who feel that to prescribe recreation is contradictory to the implication of freedom of choice, the voluntary aspect of recreation.
>
> Second, the term is more inclusive than one which would indicate only institutional care, since many ill and handicapped are not hospitalized.
>
> Third, the term has not been employed to designate special sections of any of the professional or service organizations and, therefore, its use would not present seeming deference to any particular vested interests.
>
> Fourth, it is less cumbersome terminology than the possibly more descriptive title of *recreation for the ill and handicapped.*[25]

A number of other important developments occurred in the middle and late 1960s. One such significant activity was in the area of approach to practice. The therapeutic recreation specialist is concerned with helping the ill and disabled function more effectively as they interact with some part of the environment. Avedon described this focus of practice in this way:

> Recreation must be thought of as a service within the rehabilitation process that can be deliberately structured to enable the person with disability to function in society at his maximum degree of efficiency and independence. To do this, programs of recreation must include a continuum of experiences and services in which the disabled are progressively assisted to function as independently and self-sufficiently as they possibly can.[26]

This concept of *continuum and process* was the first attempt to develop a descriptive guide to practice with the ill and disabled. It was also the first attempt to offer an adequate theoretical base for therapeutic recreation practice. Nevertheless, the argument of "treatment" or "clinical" versus "end unto itself" or nontreatment-nonclinical continued to persist, and therapeutic recreation continued to define its practice according to settings.

As attitudes toward the disabled in society shifted during the 1960s, more and more municipal recreation departments began to offer recreation services to disabled people of all ages who were not under medical supervision. Likewise, as the result of the social upheaval and civil disturbances that occurred during this period, recreation services for the socioeconomically disadvantaged and for minority group members developed.

Recreation services in adult and juvenile correctional settings also expanded

[25] Janet R. MacLean, "Therapeutic Recreation Curriculums," *Recreation in Treatment Centers,* 2 (1963), 23–24.

[26] Elliott M. Avedon, "The Function of Recreation Service in the Rehabilitation Process," *Rehabilitation Literature,* 27, no. 8 (1966), 227.

during this time. In fact, the recreation standards of service developed in 1960 by the American Correctional Association were elaborated upon and expanded by the Task Force on Corrections of the President's Commission on Law Enforcement and Administration of Justice in 1967.

Employment patterns in all fields are subject to fluctuations in supply and demand. As a result of the acceptance and continued expansion of therapeutic recreation services in health and community settings, a shortage of qualified personnel developed. This problem resulted in a rapid growth in the number of colleges and universities offering curricula in therapeutic recreation. At the same time that senior institutions were developing programs of study, many junior college institutions initiated programs to provide technical training for positions related to therapeutic recreation in the late 1960s.

Other developments which gave impetus to the service and practice of therapeutic recreation during this period were the strengthening of certification requirements and the increasing research efforts resulting from federal funding. On the horizon was the accreditation of recreation curricula including the specialized area of therapeutic recreation.

Organizational Development.   As recreation services expanded in the 1940s in the community sector and in other private and voluntary agencies, as well as in settlement houses, institutions, and hospitals, various recreation professional and service organizations developed. The growing importance and acceptance of recreation service to the ill and disabled, primarily in hospital and institutional settings, and the concern to embrace the general betterment of those providing these services were spotlighted when hospital recreation personnel established the Hospital Recreation Section of the American Recreation Society (HRS-ARS) in 1949. The name *Hospital Recreation Section* is indicative of the delivery of recreation services at this point; persons providing recreation service in hospitals wanted their specialization termed *Hospital Recreation.* Such specialization labeling is not unusual; it is found in the professional developmental periods of nursing, social work, and other regarded professions of today.

An important contribution of the HRS, as related to this chapter, was the publication of *Basic Concepts of Hospital Recreation* in 1953. This publication was the result of a study committee created to consider the concept of recreation and its applicability and place in various health settings and to review the opinions of physicians concerning recreation and the role of the hospital recreation worker.[27] In essence, the study dealt with services and practices. Its historical significance lies in the fact that this study and publication were the first attempts to create a philosophical foundation for recreation services in hospitals and institutions serving the ill and disabled.

In the years that followed, two additional organizations were formed—the

---

[27] Hospital Recreation Society, *Basic Concepts of Hospital Recreation* (Washington, D.C.; American Recreation Society, 1953), p. 2.

Recreation Therapy Section of the American Association for Health, Physical Education, and Recreation (now called the American Alliance for Health, Physical Education, Recreation, and Dance) in 1952 and the National Association of Recreation Therapists in 1953. Although these organizations differed in philosophies and approaches to service, they did contribute to the further development of the concepts and interests of hospital recreation through the Council for the Advancement of Hospital Recreation. This overall concern for recreation personnel in health care settings led to the establishment of a voluntary registration program called the National Voluntary Registration of Hospital Recreation Personnel. In subsequent years this program was recognized by various federal, state, and local agencies.

In the early 1960s the question arose of whether to unite all recreation professional and service organizations regardless of specialization and interest area. By 1966 this became a reality under the organizational umbrella of the National Recreation and Park Association (NRPA). To meet the needs and interests of the various organizations that had merged, branches were established. It became clear that the requirements of those organizations concerned with recreation for the ill and disabled would be better served through one organization, the National Therapeutic Recreation Society (NTRS), formed in October, 1966.

From the turn of the twentieth century to the late 1960s, therapeutic recreation displayed the typical pattern of an emerging profession: moving from unorganized services involving part-time workers to organized services using full-time paid workers; shifting from voluntary, sponsored services to governmental and voluntary agency support; establishing measures of professional behavior; devising a national certification plan; strengthening control of the professional organization; providing for university-based programs of study; acquiring governmental (federal) funding to support research and training; conducting public education campaigns to seek support and recognition; and engaging in conflict with elements both inside and outside the occupational group over the "turf" of the profession. More important, however, was that by the end of this period therapeutic recreation was firmly established as an *occupation*.

Professional Emergence to 1980

The 1970s were a time of great activity and introspection. Controversy thrived among practitioners, educators, and students over issues related to philosophy, education, certification, personnel and service standards, and professionalism. The publications, *Therapeutic Recreation Annual, Therapeutic Recreation Journal,* and proceedings from therapeutic recreation institutes, were filled with articles such as:

"The Meaning of Therapeutic Recreation" (1970)
"Therapeutic Recreation as a Profession: A Status Report" (1970)
"Therapeutic Recreation and the 1970's: Challenge or Progress" (1970)
"Toward a New Philosophy of Therapeutic Recreation" (1971)

"An Alternative to the Therapeutic Model in Therapeutic Recreation" (1973)

"Therapeutic Recreation: A Behavioral Rationale" (1973)

"The Challenge of Professionalism in Therapeutic Recreation (1974)

"Therapeutic Recreation: Stagnation in a Time of Change" (1975)

"Therapeutic Recreation: The Outmodel Label" (1977)

"National Therapeutic Recreation Society: The First Twelve Years" (1978)

"A Rejoinder to the Twelve-Year History of the National Therapeutic Recreation Society" (1978)[28]

The issues raised in these articles were the result of increasing attempts to find a clear conception of service and practice within an ideology that would embrace both the breadth and depth of therapeutic recreation. Perhaps the diveristy of settings (hospital, institution, and community), specific clients (mentally ill, mentally retarded, visually impaired, and the like), and methods of practice (therapy, treatment, and diversional), or, to be even more general, the emerging nature of therapeutic recreation, interfered with the development of a widely acceptable philosophical statement in the early 1970s. To compound the problem in many health care agencies and institutions, therapeutic recreation was not the primary discipline, as opposed to municipal recreation agencies wherein the mission was to provide generic services to all people. Still further, there was the apparent inability, in theory and practice, to bridge the gap between health care and community settings. As Humphrey commented in this regard:

> The common error in efforts directed toward philosophical formulations is failure to relate philosophy to current practice. Philosophical formulations inevitably are oriented to a conceptual ideal, which is a most appropriate orientation, but of equal need are philosophical formulations based upon an analysis of current practice. A failure to integrate the two in conceptualization and implementation of projected efforts, whether immediate or long range, creates a performance gap which leaves a discipline in the awkward position of masterfully administering a functional void. In essence, a

[28] Edith L. Ball, "The Meaning of Therapeutic Recreation," *Therapeutic Recreation Journal,* 4, no. 1 (1970), 17–18; William A. Hillman, "Therapeutic Recreation as a Profession: A Status Report," *Therapeutic Recreation Annual,* 7 (1970), 1–7; Fred Humphrey, "Therapeutic Recreation and the 1970's: Challenge or Progress?" *Therapeutic Recreation Annual,* 7 (1970), 8–13. Gerald S. O'Morrow, "Toward a New Philosophy of Therapeutic Recreation," in *Expanding Horizons in Therapeutic Recreation I,* ed. Jerry D. Kelley (Champaign, Ill.: University of Illinois, Office of Recreation and Park Resources, 1971), pp. 13–18. Herbert Rusalem "An Alternative to the Therapeutic Model in Therapeutic Recreation," *Therapeutic Recreation Journal,* 7, no. 1 (1973), 8–15. Professional Development Committee, Therapeutic Section, Wisconsin Park and Recreation Association, "Therapeutic Recreation: A Behavioral Rationale," *Therapeutic Recreation Journal,* 7, no. 3 (1973), 35–38. David C. Park, "The Challenge of Professionalism in Therapeutic Recreation," in *Expanding Horizons in Therapeutic Recreation II,* ed. Jerry D. Kelley (Champaign, Ill: Univerisity of Illinois, Office of Recreation and Park Resources, 1974), pp. 65–72. Gary Robb, "Therapeutic Recreation: Stagnation in a Time of Change," *Therapeutic Recreation Journal,* 9, no. 2 (1975), 47–53. Peter A. Witt, "Therapeutic Recreation: The Outmoded Label," *Therapeutic Recreation Journal,* 11, no. 2 (1977), 39–41. David Austin and Benjamin K. Hunnicutt, "National Therapeutic Recreation Society: The First Twelve Years," *Therapeutic Recreation Journal,* 12, no. 3 (1978), 4–14. Benjamin K. Hunnicutt, "A Rejoinder to the Twelve-Year History of the National Therapeutic Recreation Society," *Therapeutic Recreation Journal,* 12, no. 3 (1978), 15–19.

philosophical statement must be developmental and thus have a valid and functional tie to the present state of the art.[29]

Whatever the reasons for the difficulty, the absence of a philosophical stance hindered the growth and development of therapeutic recreation. A clear and acceptable philosophy statement or position would help therapeutic recreators make maximum contribution of their professional skills by clearly indentifying their practice arena and would enhance development of the necessary knowledge and skills for providing services.

An initial step toward formulating a philosophical statement had already been taken in mid-1969 at the Southern Regional Institute on Therapeutic Recreation. During the institute, a small group of participants drafted a position statement. This paper was then circulated and responded to by those attending the annual conference of the NTRS (1969 Congress for Recreation and Parks). Later, Frye[30] and Ball[31] published papers on the philosophy of therapeutic recreation. And, in 1970, Indiana State University sponsored an invitational work-study conference on the topic.

But momentum from these efforts was lost for several years as the NTRS and its members pursued other matters in their quest for professionalism: attaining higher visibility in community service to the ill and disabled as well as with external agencies and organizations (i.e., Joint Commission on Accreditation of Hospitals, American Nursing Home Association, and the like); developing standards for delivery of services in association with the Joint Commission on Accreditation of Hospitals working with the U.S. Public Health Service in strengthening regulations relating to therapeutic recreation services in intermediate and extended care facilities; revising and upgrading registration standards; and implementing educational competencies within the accreditation process, to name a few. As Park commented on the twenty-fifth anniversary of the existence of an organization in the therapeutic recreation field:

> Professionalism has been and continues to be a concern of the field of therapeutic recreation. . . . As a profession we have begun to take pride in ourselves as a professional body; we believe that we have a unique and valuable service to perform; and we are beginning to assert ourselves on behalf of the people we serve. This is an important step toward assuming full responsibility as a member of a professional team that provides services to the ill, disabled, or handicapped.
>
> . . . During the first twenty-five years of our development, we have grown a great deal and have experienced significant changes. We began as a profession that was almost exclusively hospital oriented, but we have since developed and declared a broader interpretation of therapeutic recreation. We have recognized the needs of all disabled individuals regardless of where they may reside, including such new areas as nursing homes, day care centers, and penal institutions. We were a profession that was split by semantics and even, to a degree, by philosophy. We now agree that therapeutic

[29] Humphrey, "Therapeutic Recreation and the 1970's," p. 11.

[30] Virginia Frye, "A Philosophy Statement on Therapeutic Recreation Service," *Therapeutic Recreation Journal,* 3, no. 4 (1969), 11–14.

[31] Ball, "The Meaning of Therapeutic Recreation."

recreation is a process which is applicable in many different types of settings. Finally, we began as a profession that included several separate professional groups, but now there is one strong central organization that is becoming instrumental in bringing about acceptance and the realization that therapeutic recreation is a significant part of the rehabilitation process.[32]

Between 1977 and 1980, the NTRS embarked upon an extensive self-evaluation of issues critical to its professionalization including credentialling, accreditation, personnel and program standards, governance structure, legislation, and a definition and philosophical statement of therapeutic recreation. Of all issues, the latter two created the greatest interest among the members. This would be natural because, without the development of a definition and mission statement at this point which clearly identified parameters, functions, and processes of therapeutic recreation, further professionalization of therapeutic recreation would have been hindered. According to Kleingartner, "The inability of many occupations to define their mission, obtain agreement on the occupational objectives that require attention, and retain their identity as relatively homogeneous occupational catergories is undoubtedly an important factor in shaping the character of emerging professions."[33]

The importance of this statement is found in an investigation of views of recreation professionals toward therapeutic recreation and its professionalization by Meyer in 1978.[34] His study focused on elements within therapeutic recreation that may affect the " 'direction and pace' " of therapeutic recreation professionalization efforts. Specifically, the purpose of the study was to "determine the extent of agreement and disagreement among professional recreation leaders regarding the nature, purpose, and delimitations of therapeutic recreation and the actions necessary to pursue professionalization."[35] He used a three-round Policy Delphi technique consisting of a two-part questionnaire—the first centering on the views of leaders toward therapeutic recreation, and the second on views of leaders toward actions necessary for professionalization—and involving thirty-six leaders from three branches of the NRPA—American Park and Recreation Society (APRS), Society of Park and Recreation Educators (SPRE), and NTRS. He found:

1. . . . extensive nonagreement and disagreement among recreation professionals, in general, and therapeutic recreators, in particular, regarding a definition of therapeutic recreation.

2. [Regarding actions for professionalization] . . . extensive nonagreement and disagree-

[32] Park, "The Challenge of Professionalism," pp. 63–64.

[33] Archie Kleingartner, *Professionalism and Salaried Worker Organization* (Madison, Wis.: University of Wisconsin Press, 1967), p. 23.

[34] Lee E. Meyer, "An Analysis of Views of Recreation Professionals Toward Therapeutic Recreation and Its Professionalization" (Unpublished Doctoral dissertation, University of North Carolina at Chapel Hill, 1978).

[35] *Ibid.,* p. 148

ment between general recreators and therapeutic recreators, but a high level of agreement between therapeutic recreation practitioners and therapeutic recreation educators.

3. Conditions existed between general recreation leaders and the therapeutic recreation leaders and among the therapeutic recreation leaders which could present barriers to the professionalization of therapeutic recreation.[36]

The implications of this study, according to Meyer, were: (1) Lack of agreement regarding the definitions of therapeutic recreation and educational preparation represent obstacles to the pursuit of professionalism, and these differences need to be identified and resolved before progress toward professionalization can take place; (2) disagreement among general recreation leaders and therapeutic recreation leaders may suggest barriers to professionalism of therapeutic recreation; (3) lack of agreement among the three professional branches concerning goal priority leads to conflict and frustrates professionalization efforts; (4) failure to clarify mission and purpose and to determine training needs on the part of therapeutic recreation leaders may prevent achievement of goals of professionalism and attributes associated with advanced stages of professionalization.[37]

In 1977, the NTRS Voluntary Registration Program was revised. In 1980, the NTRS Registration Board requested the approval of a new plan with two levels of registration, a professional level and a paraprofessional level, instead of the six registration levels in the 1977 revision. Simultaneously, within NTRS there was movement toward the establishment of an independent body outside of NTRS to address the credentialling needs of therapeutic recreators.

Other action deserving of mention during the late 1970s involved the revision of professional standards. Although initial work in revising program and personnel standards relative to clinical and residential facilities began in 1976, the final document was not completed until 1979. This finished document set general standards for therapeutic recreation services in ten different types of clinical and residential settings.[38] In 1980 this document was divided into two documents, one concerned with standards of practice for therapeutic recreation service,[39] and the other focused on administration of therapeutic recreation service in clinical and residential settings.[40] Simultaneously with these activities, standards for recreation programs and services relative to special populations in the community sector were developed and approved in 1978.[41] Subsequently, these standards were approved by the APRS's

[36] *Ibid.*, pp. 150–53.

[37] *Ibid.*, pp. 154–57.

[38] Judith Goldstein and Glen E. Van Andel, *National Therapeutic Recreation Society Guidelines for Therapeutic Recreation Service in Clinical and Residential Facilities* (Arlington, Va.: National Recreation and Park Association, 1979).

[39] National Therapeutic Recreation Society, *Standards of Practice for Therapeutic Recreation Service* (Alexandria, Va.: National Recreation and Park Association, 1980).

[40] National Therapeutic Recreation Society Standards Committee, *Guidelines for Administration of Therapeutic Recreation Service in Clinical and Residential Facilities* (Alexandria, Va.: National Recreation and Park Association, 1982).

[41] Jacquelyn Vaughan and Robert Winslow, eds., *Guidelines for Community-Based Recreation Programs for Special Populations* (Alexandria, Va.: National Recreation and Park Association, 1979).

board of directors.

We have noted earlier that those providing therapeutic recreation service to special populations had been concerned about educational preparation and training since the inception of the HRS–ARS. In the years thereafter, therapeutic recreation practitioners and educators worked jointly within the committee structure of NTRS and through specially designed education conferences and workshops to develop and recommend educational competencies necessary for service and practice. Of special note was the 1978 *Accreditation Committee Report*, which considered and investigated a number of critical issues associated with the status of therapeutic recreation curricula, educational competencies, faculty, and accreditation procedures.[42]

In the mid-1970s a curriculum accreditation program was inaugurated by the NRPA. By 1976 the NTRS had approved minimal competencies needed for practice. These competencies were incorporated into the *Standards and Evaluative Criteria for Recreation, Leisure Services, and Resources Curricula . . .* in 1977.[43] In 1979 the National Council on Accreditation (NCA), with NTRS input, proposed comprehensive revisions in their accreditation standards. By 1980 NCA was embarked on a major review and revision of accreditation standards.

Although educational competencies were developed for accreditation purposes, there was in reality no specific research to support the therapeutic recreation accreditation standards. In order to be recognized as a profession, a given occupation must be identified by a standard body of knowledge. A study conducted in 1978 by Peterson and Connolly to determine the content of professional programs of study found a lack of standardization in therapeutic recreation curriculum courses.[44] These authors stated that "Well-trained, competent entry level personnel are essential in any profession. . . . Continued focus on the development and maintenance of quality professional preparation programs is critical at this point in the professionalization of therapeutic recreation.[45]

Even though therapeutic recreation emerged as an occupation during this period, its growth toward professional status after World War II was uneven. The rapid development of therapeutic recreation created a situation in which efforts to conceptualize service and practice within a philosophical statement occurred after therapeutic recreation had been providing services for some years. But at the same time it was a period characterized by movement toward professionalization; consol-

[42] Carol Ann Peterson, *Accreditation Committee Report* (Report submitted to the National Therapeutic Recreation Society Board of Directors and Past Presidents Council, September 30, 1978, personal copy).

[43] National Council on Accreditation, *Standards and Evaluative Criteria for Recreation, Leisure Services, and Resources Curricula Baccalaureate and Masters Degree Program* (Arlington, Va.: National Recreation and Park Association, March 1977), pp. 11–12.

[44] Carol Ann Peterson and Peg Connolly, "Professional Preparation in Therapeutic Recreation," *Therapeutic Recreation Journal*, 15, no. 2 (1981), 41.

[45] *Ibid.*, p. 45.

idation of three occupational groups into a single organization, development of prescribed training programs, establishment of program and personnel standards, and other related activities.

THERAPEUTIC RECREATION
AS A PROFESSION:
CURRENT STATUS

In May, 1982, a philosophical position statement was adopted by the NTRS membership and the NTRS board of directors.[46] One is cautioned, however, that this adoption of a philosophical position did not necessarily mean that therapeutic recreation had become a profession. In fact, the statement of one's mission is in reality an ongoing process of defining and redefining; "professionalism is a matter of degree."[47] However, this statement represented another step in the professionalization process; it was the achievement of a particular characteristic or attribute.

Although a position statement was adopted, the reader is alerted to the low membership response to the four positions considered and to the lack of unanimous agreement among members about the positions. Admittedly, the statement does provide guidelines for the present for measures to be taken by NTRS. Further, the declaration not only informs the public of the mission of NTRS, but also indicates to the membership what action it is to take regarding the effective discharge of their roles. However, if one is allowed to speculate, the low response to the various positions, coupled with the lack of agreement regarding the position adopted, would appear to indicate that divergent views among the membership are present which have and will have their effect on continued professionalization efforts.

A most recent significant development within the therapeutic recreation field has been the proposal for the establishment of a new national therapeutic recreation organization. The disenchantment of educators and practitioners with the inability of the NRPA to be all things to all people (disappointment on the part of some members of NTRS with the effectiveness of NRPA/NTRS to advance the state of the therapeutic recreation profession, coupled with the fact that NTRS expectations as a branch within NRPA apparently could not be fully realized) appears to have contributed to the creation of this new organization. In Kansas City in October, 1983, interested educators and practitioners met to define and clarify the purpose, mission, and scope of the potential new organization, tentatively called the American Therapeutic Recreation Association.

Other matters which focused on professionalization emerged including the establishment in October, 1981 of the National Council for Therapeutic Recreation

---

[46] National Therapeutic Recreation Society, "Philosophical Position Statement of the National Therapeutic Recreation Society," May 1982.

[47] Bernard Barber, "Some Problems in the Sociology of Professions," *Daedalus,* 92 (Fall 1963), 671.

Certification and the approval of the two-level certification plan. In the same year the National Council on Accreditation adopted revised standards including expanded therapeutic recreation competencies. Also in this year, the Joint Commission on Accreditation of Hospitals incorporated therapeutic recreation as one of the activity services within their Consolidated Standards. Such recognition by JCAH represented a step forward in professional practice and prestige.

Also during this period, from a legislative funding perspective, recreation services to special populations have fared quite well, thereby reflecting continued recognition of therapeutic recreation. As a result of the amendments to the Rehabilitation Act of 1978 (PL 95–602), with reference to Sections 311 and 316, approximately $7 million have been allocated through the two sections to various agencies to make recreation facilities and programs accessible to handicapped individuals. Further, another $2 million was projected through Section 316 for allocation in 1984. This type of legislative support, along with support from the Special Education Program (Office of Special Education and Rehabilitation Services), in personnel preparation and research will certainly continue to contribute to the growth and development of therapeutic recreation as a service field and to its professionalization.

In bringing this chapter to a close, let us consider the professionalization process and sequencing according to Goode, while keeping in mind the progress of therapeutic recreation toward professionalization. Goode identified two sets of characteristics; one, core characteristics and the other, derivative characteristics. Core characteristics consist of "a prolonged specialized training in a body of abstract knowledge, and a collectivity or service orientation."[48] As an occupation becomes more professionalized, it acquires characteristics which are derivatives of the core characteristics, namely:

1. The profession determines its own standards of education and training.
2. The student professional goes through a more far-reaching adult socialization experience than the learner in other occupations.
3. Professional practice is often legally recognized by some form of licensure.
4. Licensing and admission boards are manned by members of the profession.
5. Most legislation concerned with the profession is shaped by that profession.
6. The occupation gains in income, power, and prestige ranking, and can demand higher caliber students.
7. The practitioner is relatively free of lay evaluation and control.
8. The norms of practice enforced by the profession are more stringent than legal controls.
9. Members are more strongly identified and affiliated with the profession than are members of other occupations with theirs.
10. The profession is more likely to be a terminal occupation. Members do not care to leave it, and a higher proportion assert that if they had it to do over again, they would again choose that type of work.[49]

[48] Goode, "Encroachment, Charlatanism, and the Emerging Professions," p. 903.
[49] *Ibid.*

SUMMARY

This chapter has attempted, through an examination of the historical development of therapeutic recreation, to touch upon those efforts which characterize the development of professionalism as related to therapeutic recreation. Although there have been significant advances and declines since 1976, one is very cautious in saying that therapeutic recreation has arrived as one of the professions as opposed to being an occupation. Although therapeutic recreation has followed in a loose fashion the "natural history" of professionalism as described by Wilensky (becoming a full-time occupation, establishing training schools, forming an occupational association, seeking legal protection, and establishing a code of ethics),[50] it is the degree to which the various characteristics or attributes are sought and achieved on a scale of professionalism that is important.

At the present stage of development, therapeutic recreation falls lower on the scale of professions than do the older ones such as medicine, law, and the ministry. Etzioni, for example, used *semi-profession* to describe the positions on the professional scale of teaching and nursing. He indicated that the term is not used in a derogatory sense but describes the fact that "their training is shorter, their status is less legitimated, their right to privileged communication less established, there is less of a specialized body of knowledge, and they have less autonomy from supervision or societal control than 'the' professions."[51] Howsam, likewise, used the term *semiprofession* to refer to education, but from a different perspective.

> A semiprofession does not have the necessary authority to warrant status as a profession. . . . A profession typically has control of and responsibility for its knowledge and expertise—which causes the individual practitioner to be accountable to *the profession*. The professional who is a member of a semiprofession, however, is directly accountable to *his and her employer.*"[52]

It is perhaps inevitable that, in a period of attempting to reach professional status, there would be conflict about the professionalization of therapeutic recreation; its mission, service, and practice. The potential establishment of a new organization (American Therapeutic Recreation Association) may produce a duplication of effort and weaken the effectiveness of each organization. Such action, on the other hand, reflects the continued evolution of becoming a profession, as noted earlier in this chapter. Perhaps such a movement is an attempt to seek greater exclusiveness or more extensive specialization, which is a tendency of emerging professions according to many investigators who have studied the process of professionalization. It is apparent, however, that therapeutic recreation as an emerging

---

[50] Wilensky, "The Professionalization of Everyone?" pp. 142–46.

[51] Amatai Etzioni, *The Semi-Professions and Their Organization* (New York: The Free Press, 1969), p. v.

[52] R. Howsam, cited in Harold W. Heller, "Special Educators: Status and Prospects," *Exceptional Education Quarterly* (February 1982), pp. 84–85.

profession is undergoing fundamental changes which may eventually make it more responsive to consumers of therapeutic recreation service. Whatever the problem or conflict may be, it is by no means unusual for an occupational group as it strives for professionalism. According to Kleingartner:

> An occupation aspiring to professional identification will encounter resistance both from without and from within. The clarity with which the boundaries of the occupation are defined, the training and background of its members, the context in which the work is performed, and the leadership of the occupation are only a few of the many factors that will affect the direction and pace of occupational development. We cannot assume that all members of an occupation share a common system of values and expectations developed around the bonds of colleagueship.[53]

In closing, how much has been achieved in each of those attributes sought by therapeutic recreation? A philosophical position statement has been adopted; however, having a document is not the same as having a common philosophy. Further, the low response of the membership to the *Alternative Positions and Their Implications to Professionalism*,[54] coupled with the lack of total agreement regarding Position C (Treatment/Education/Recreation), which eventually, with minor revisions, become the philosophical stance of the society, would appear to indicate that divergent views among the membership are present which have and will have their effect on continued professionalization efforts. A code of ethics exists, but on paper only. Even though our body of knowledge has expanded, there is, on the other hand, a lack of consensus about the specifics of this base. This lack of agreement is due to the fact that, as an occupational group, we still have different views of who we are and what we do. Such views may have resulted in the low response to the philosophical position statements. Our research efforts appear to be very minimal, while our programs of study, specifically content areas, are vague and without validation. The remaining years of the 1980s will therefore be a critical period in our attempt to resolve the issue of professional status.

STUDY GUIDE QUESTIONS

1. Would you consider therapeutic recreation an occupation or a profession in 1970? In 1980? At present? Why or why not?
2. Some individuals in the therapeutic recreation service field are suggesting that therapeutic recreation is a profession. How would you defend that position? How might you oppose it?
3. Examine the issues discussed for the last fifteen years in the *Therapeutic Recreation Journal* on the "professional status of therapeutic recreation." Review these articles and use them as a basis for discussion.
4. At the 1915 meeting of the National Conference on Charities and Corrections, Dr. Abraham Flexner spelled out six characteristics of professions:

[53] Kleingartner, *Professionalism and Salaried Worker Organization*, p. 29.

[54] National Therapeutic Recreation Society, *Alternative Positions and Their Implications to Professionalism* (Alexandria, Va.: National Recreation and Park Association, 1981).

    a. Professions are essentially intellectual operations with large individual responsibility.

    b. They derive their raw material from science and learning.

    c. This material is worked up to a practical and clear-cut end.

    d. Professions possess an educationally communicable technique.

    e. They tend to self-organization.

    f. They become increasingly altruistic in motivation.[55]

    Evaluate these criteria in relation to therapeutic recreation. To what degree have they been met by therapeutic recreation to date?

5. Review the major philosophical perspectives outlined in the next chapter and identify potential implications of each perspective for the professionalization of therapeutic recreation as discussed in this chapter.

6. The following factors are usually associated with professionalization. How would you prioritize them in relation to therapeutic recreation professionalization? Provide a justification for your priority.

    a. Governance structure

    b. Federal support

    c. Training and education

    d. Registration, certification, licensure

    e. Public education

    f. Research

    g. Credibility in service and goals

    h. Mission and goals

7. There are different meanings given to the word *profession* by various occupational groups. Locate as many of these different definitions as you can. Compare each, and debate the pros and cons of each.

8. Trace the major influences to date on the development of a philosophical statement.

9. Two principal characteristics of a profession are an extended period of training and an orientation toward service to the community. Compare these characteristics, as applied to therapeutic recreation, with the

    a. Profession of elementary and secondary school teachers

    b. Profession of medicine

    c. Profession of law

10. What conflicts within the therapeutic recreation movement to 1980 may have hindered its advancement and development toward professionalization?

11. Considering the professionalization process and sequencing according to Goode, how does therapeutic recreation fare?

12. How would you respond to the statement that ''Professionalization is a matter of degree'' in reference to therapeutic recreation?

13. In 1957 Ernest Greenwood identified five critical attributes of professions which, depending on the degree to which they have been accomplished, determine the relative degree of professionalism of any occupational group. These attributes are as follows:

    a. A systematic body of theory

    b. Professional authority

    c. Sanction of the community

    d. A regulative code of ethics

    e. A professional culture[56]

---

[55] Cited in Ralph E. Pumphrey and Muriel W. Pumphrey, eds., *The Heritage of American Social Work* (New York: Columbia University Press, 1961), p. 301.

[56] Greenwood, "Attributes of a Profession."

Relate the development of therapeutic recreation to each of these five criteria.

14. Interview several therapeutic recreators in practice in your area as to whether they consider themselves professionals. If so, why; if not, why?

15. Write a paper elaborating on the meaning of therapeutic recreation as a profession to you.

16. What factors since the turn of the century, from your perspective, have contributed to the shaping of therapeutic recreation?

17. Therapeutic recreation requires community sanction to maximize the quality of service provided. Does therapeutic recreation have this sanction? If so, where was it obtained? If no, how should it be obtained?

18. Perhaps the most critical question for therapeutic recreation in the 1980s is to what degree it will continue to allow the desire for professional status to serve as a dominant force in the development of service and practice. Develop the approach you would take to meet this challenge.

ANNOTATED BIBLIOGRAPHY

AMERICAN RECREATION SOCIETY, *Basic Concepts of Hospital Recreation*. Washington, D.C.: American Recreation Society, Hospital Recreation Section 1953. The result of a study soliciting ideas from physicians and hospital recreators about the definition of recreation, its application in hospital settings, and the function of physicians in determining activities for groups and individual patients. Findings resulted in the "Statement of Tenet, Hospital Recreation Section."

AUSTIN, DAVID, and BENJAMIN K. HUNNICUTT, "National Therapeutic Recreation Society: The First Twelve Years," *Therapeutic Recreation Journal*, 12, no. 3 (1978), 4–14. As the title implies, offers a brief overview of therapeutic recreation professionalization efforts.

BARBER, BERNARD, "Some Problems in the Sociology of the Professions," in *The Professions in America*, pp. 15–34, ed. Kenneth S. Lynn. Boston: Houghton Mifflin Company, 1965. Considers some of the central problems of the structure and functioning of the professions. Specifically, six problems are discussed: social concerns, definition, role of professional schools, emerging professions, professional roles and organization, and professionals and politics.

GOODE, WILLIAM J., "Encroachment, Charlatanism, and the Emerging Professions: Psychology, Sociology, and Medicine," *American Sociological Review*, 25, no. 12 (1960), 902–14. Reviews the patterns and process of professionalization with attention to the development of psychology, sociology, and medicine.

GREENWOOD, ERNEST, "Attributes of a Profession," *Social Work*, 2, no. 7 (July 1957), 45–55. A discussion of those attributes contributing to professionalization and their implications for social work, many of the implications being relevant to therapeutic recreation today.

HILLMAN, WILLIAM A., "Therapeutic Recreation as a Profession: A Status Report," *Therapeutic Recreation Annual*, 7 (1970), 1–7. Highlights some significant aspects of the challenges of professionalization to be confronted during the 1970s by the practitioner and the NTRS.

HUGHES, EVERETT C., "Professions," *Daedalus*, 92 (Fall 1963), 655–68. Also, reprinted in *The Professions in America*, pp. 1–14, ed. Kenneth S. Lynn. Boston: Houghton Mifflin Company, 1965. Discusses the concepts of professions; what they mean, changes relative to them, and how society views them.

HUMPHREY, FRED, "Therapeutic Recreation and the 1970s: Challenge or Progress?" *Thera-*

peutic Recreation Annual, 7 (1970), 8–13. Addresses the need to consider therapeutic recreation a process incorporating the concept of recreative experiences being potentially therapeutic for all, regardless of setting. Advocates development of a philosophical statement which reflects the present state of the art.

HUNNICUTT, BENJAMIN K., "A Rejoinder to the Twelve-Year History of the National Therapeutic Recreation Society," *Therapeutic Recreation Journal*, 12, no. 3 (1978), 15–19. A personal reaction to the Austin and Hunnicutt article above, specifically, items or concerns that were left out.

JAMES, ANN, "Historical Perspective: The Therapy Debate," *Therapeutic Recreation Journal*, 14, no. 1 (1980), 13–16. Offers an historical perspective of the debate among American Red Cross personnel and other recreation specialists concerning the concept of recreation as therapy from 1918 through the 1940s.

LORD, JOHN, PEGGY HUTCHISON, AND FRED VANDERBECK, "Narrowing the Options: The Power of Professionalism in Daily Life and Leisure," pp. 228–45, in *Recreation and Leisure: Issues in an Era of Change*, eds. Thomas L. Goodale and Peter A. Witt. State College, Pa.: Venture Publishing, 1980. Argues that professionalism may hinder the development of play in individuals because, as individuals, we more or less become dependent on professions that provide a service.

MEYER, LEE E., "An Analysis of Views of Recreation Professionals Toward Therapeutic Recreation and Its Professionalization." (Unpublished Doctoral dissertation, University of North Carolina at Chapel Hill, 1978). A study to determine the extent of agreement and disagreement among professional recreation leaders regarding the nature, purpose, and delimitations of therapeutic recreation and the actions necessary to pursue professionalization.

MOORE, WILBERT E., *The Professions: Roles and Rules*. New York: Russell Sage Foundation, 1970. Explores the development of professionalism; professional roles in relation to client, peers, employer, and administrator, to name a few; and social responsibilities of professions. Extensive bibliography on professions and professionalization.

PETERSON, CAROL A., "Pride and Progress in Professionalism," pp. 1–9, in *Expanding Horizons in Therapeutic Recreation VIII*, ed. Gerald Hitzhusen. Columbia, Mo.: University of Missouri, Department of Recreation, 1981. Considers the importance of being a professional and the progress made to date, suggesting steps students and therapeutic recreation specialists must take to gain further professional status.

ROBB, GARY M., "President's Message," *Therapeutic Recreation Journal*, 12, no. 2 (1978), 3–4. Based on an address given at the 1978 Mid-West Symposium on Therapeutic Recreation. Focuses on a number of issues, but spotlights the concept of whether we are therapists first and recreators second or the reverse. Concludes that there needs to be a refocus of purpose by NTRS.

———, "Therapeutic Recreation: Stagnation in a Time of Change," *Therapeutic Recreation Journal*, 9, no. 2 (1975), 47–53. Reflects a personal concern for NTRS and the fact that its membership has failed to reach desired goals during the 1970s, and points out that to do so the membership must become more aggressive. Also outlines some goals that have yet to be reached or accomplished.

SESSOMS, H. DOUGLAS, "Therapeutic Recreation Service: The Past and Challenging Present," in *Extra Perspectives: Concepts in Therapeutic Recreation*, pp. 1–14, eds. Larry L. Neal and Christopher R. Edginton. Eugene, Oreg.: University of Oregon, Center of Leisure Studies, 1982. Provides an historical review of therapeutic recreation service, asks questions about the role and uniqueness of therapeutic recreation, and indicates the challenges facing therapeutic recreation.

THORSTENSON, WILLIAM, "Beyond Professionalism," in *Recreation and Leisure: Issues in an Era of Change*, pp. 269–79, eds. Thomas L. Goodale and Peter A. Witt. State

College, Pa.: Venture Publishing, 1980. Discusses whether practitioners in park and recreation service "want to or should join" in the pursuit toward professionalism.

WILENSKY, HAROLD L., "The Professionalization of Everyone?" *American Journal of Sociology*, 120, no. 2 (1964), 141–46. Examines the process and degree of professionalization, with a brief historical look at various occupations. Also considers newer structural forms now emerging relative to professionalization.

Articles specifically concerned with the development of therapeutic recreation philosophical positions or statements are also quoted in the following chapter.

BIBLIOGRAPHY

BLEDSTEIN, BURTON J., *The Culture of Professionalism.* New York: W. W. Norton and Company, Inc., 1976.

BRIGGS, JOHN F., and ALBERT J. SHAFTER, "Two Administrators Look at Mental Health, Professionalism, and Activity Therapy," pp. 33–42, in *Expanding Horizons in Therapeutic Recreation I,* ed. Jerry D. Kelley, Champaign, Ill.: University of Illinois, Department of Recreation and Park Administration, 1971.

EDGINTON, CHRISTOPHER R., "Consumerism and Professionalization," *Parks and Recreation,* 11, no. 9 (1976), 41–42, 83–86.

ETZIONI, AMATAI, ed., *The Semi-Professions and Their Organization.* New York: The Free Press, 1969.

FERGUSON, C. M., "Professions, Professionals and Motivation," *Journal of the American Dietetic Association,* 53, no. 10 (1968), 197–201.

GOLDSTEIN, JUDITH E. and DAVID M. COMPTON, "Therapeutic Recreation," *Parks and Recreation,* 11, no. 7 (1976), 28–34, 95–98.

GOODE, WILLIAM J., "Community within a Community: The Professions," *American Sociological Review,* 22, no. 7 (1957), 194–200.

GROSS, RONALD, and PAUL OSTERMAN, *The New Professionals.* New York: Simon & Schuster, Inc., 1972.

HALL, RICHARD H., "Professionalization and Bureaucratization," *American Sociological Review,* 35, no. 2 (1968), 99–104.

HARTSOE, CHARLES, "Recreation: A Profession in Transition," *Parks and Recreation,* 8, no. 7 (1973), 33–34, 59–60.

HENKEL, DONALD, Professionalism," *Parks and Recreation,* 11, no. 7 (1976), 52–54.

HUMPHREY, FRED, "An Analysis of Goal Congruency in a Diverse Membership Normative Organization" (Unpublished Doctoral dissertation, Pennsylvania State University, 1973).

LUBOVE, ROY, *The Professional Altruist.* Cambridge, Mass.: Harvard University Press, 1965.

MARSTON, JAMES, "Hallmarks of a Profession," *Public Relations Journal,* 28, no. 7 (1968), 8–10.

MEYER, HAROLD D., "The Need for Unity by Recreators Serving the Ill and Disabled," *Recreation in Treatment Centers,* 4 (September 1965), 5, 7.

MEYER, LEE E., "Philosophy and Curriculum" in *Directions in Health, Physical Education, and Recreation—Therapeutic Recreation Curriculum: Philosophy, Strategy, and Concepts,* Monograph Series 1, pp. 9–12, ed. David R. Austin. Bloomington, Ind.: Indiana University School of Health, Physical Education, and Recreation, 1980.

NAVAR, NANCY, "A Study of the Professionalization of Therapeutic Recreation in the State of Michigan" *Therapeutic Recreation Journal,* 15, no. 2 (1981), 50–56.

O'MORROW, GERALD S., "Complimentary Functions and Responsibilities," in *Expanding Horizons in Therapeutic Recreation IV,* pp. 11–16, eds. Gerald L. Hitzhusen, Gerald O'Morrow, and John Oliver. Columbia, Mo.: Department of Recreation and Park Administration, University of Missouri, 1977.

PETERSON, CAROL A., "Therapeutic Recreation in the Eighties: Excellence, Existence or Extinction," *National Therapeutic Recreation Society Newsletter,* 6, no. 1 (1981), 3–5.

ROBB, GARY M., "Letter to the Editor," *Therapeutic Recreation Journal,* 12, no. 1 (1978), 5–6.

ROWTHORN, ANNE W., "A History of the Evolution and Development of Therapeutic Recreation Services for Special Populations in the United States from 1918 to 1977," (Unpublished Doctoral dissertation, New York University, 1978).

——, "An Open Letter to Peter Witt," *Therapeutic Recreation Journal,* 12, no. 1 (1978), 7–8.

SESSOMS, H. DOUGLAS, "Our Body of Knowledge: Myth or Reality?" *Parks and Recreation,* 10, no. 11 (1975), 30–31, 38.

SHIVERS, JAY S., "New Understanding of Therapeutic Recreational Services and a Look at the Future," *Recreation in Treatment Centers,* 6 (May 1969), 21–23.

——, "Why Not Recreational Therapy," *Leisurability,* 4, no. 4 (1977), 4–10.

VOLLMER, HOWARD M., and DONALD L. MILLS, *Professionalization.* Englewood Cliffs, N.J.: Prentice-Hall, Inc., 1966.

CHAPTER THREE
THE CHALLENGE OF DEFINING THERAPEUTIC RECREATION AS A PROFESSION

No single issue could be more important or require more urgent attention from the profession of therapeutic recreation than the development of a well-defined occupational philosophy. The creation and adoption of such an ideology is, in fact, central to resolving the subsequent issues in this text relating to our relationship to other disciplines and areas of service; the credentialling paths we choose via registration, certification, and licensure; the development of professional standards of service; our academic preparation and training; our relationships with clients; the research directions we pursue; and the techniques and technologies we employ.

To illustrate the crossroads at which the field of therapeutic recreation finds itself in respect to embracing a philosophical position regarding its service parameters, the following notion of paradigm as presented by Kuhn will prove useful.[1] According to this author, a paradigm includes the shared values and beliefs of the members of a professional community. Paradigms progress through three basic stages: the pre-paradigm period, in which intradisciplinary conflict and debate occurs relative to rival paradigms; the paradigm period, in which values and beliefs are accepted, and professional problems and avenues for solution are agreed upon; and the postparadigm period, in which scientific method proceeds to develop a body

[1] T. S. Kuhn, *The Structure of Scientific Revolutions* (Chicago, Ill.: University of Chicago Press, 1970).

of knowledge. Considering the events of the past three decades, it would appear that the field of therapeutic recreation has functioned largely at a pre-paradigm stage and struggled mightily toward a consensus concerning the basic values and beliefs surrounding our occupational orientation to service. The need for the development of a unified position has been articulated by Martin.

> It is almost self-evident that a philosophical overview unifying the approaches and techniques of the therapeutic recreation field would be quite useful. Less certain, but a definite possibility is that while horizontal progress in terms of the number of facilities incorporating therapeutic recreation services may continue, vertical development of the quality and the effectiveness of this service will be continually curtailed, if attention is not focused on unifying component aspects of the service continuum.[2]

Meyer agreed with this need and listed several recent developments which have made the generation of a unified philosophical overview a particularly urgent matter for therapeutic recreation professionals today, including:

— A rapid increase in pre-service training of therapeutic recreators without accompanying training standards and accreditation programs
— An increase in demand for community-based leisure services for disabled people
— An expansion of the role of non-therapeutic recreation personnel in providing leisure services to disabled persons
— A greater demand for individualized treatment programs in health care/rehabilitation agencies and a concern for higher standards of service and evidence of program efficacy in these facilities
— An extension of the concepts of "therapy" and "treatment" beyond traditional "medical" intervention.[3]

Recent events indicate that the field of therapeutic recreation appears to have reached a general consensus concerning the adoption of a unified philosophical position statement. In short, we may have progressed through the "nonparadigm" stage of development as a profession. However, this process has not been a smooth one. Vigorous debate has taken place since the mid 1940s regarding many subissues inherent in defining a complex profession. As in any philosophical debate of this nature, positions have been misunderstood and modified. Compromises have also taken place in the give and take which accompanies the discussion process. Most importantly, the *implications* of our philosophical position with respect to other professional issues have not yet been delineated and will not be ultimately known for several years!

This chapter traces from an historical perspective the development of our quest for a common philosophical orientation to service. Particular attention is paid

---

[2] Fred Martin, "Therapeutic Recreation Practice: A Philosophic Overview," *Leisurability*, 1, no. 1 (1974), 23.

[3] Lee E. Meyer, "Philosophical Alternatives and the Professionalization of Therapeutic Recreation" (Paper submitted as part of the Philosophical Statement Task Force to the National Therapeutic Recreation Society, May, 1980), p. 2.

to identifying elements of controversy which have appeared at various stages of this process. Study guide questions appear at three locations within the chapter to assist the reader to thoroughly understand the complex issue of defining our professional identity. The first set follows an overview of the field's efforts to reach a unified position at its pre-paradigm stage. These questions challenge the reader to reflect upon the historical developments which have led to current approaches to conceptualizing our occupation. The second series appears in a discussion of four alternative philosophical statements which were recently developed by our professional society. This exercise will assist the reader to understand the process involved in the development of our current philosophical position and the differences inherent in each of the ideologies which might have potentially represented the field. The final set of questions follows the philosophical position which was adopted by the NTRS. In responding to these inquiries, the reader is asked to examine the future implications and ramifications of this document.

PRE-PARADIGM
CONTROVERSY

Meyer categorized occupational developments related to recreation and disabled persons into two broad periods which existed before the creation of the NTRS in 1966.[4] He termed the first of these eras, 1880 through the 1930s, the *recreation-in-hospitals* period. Rising out of humanitarian concerns for hospitalized individuals, and influenced by emerging values concerning the benefits of play and recreation, this "preprofessional" stage viewed recreation in hospitals as being basically the same as recreation in community settings. The second, or "professional," period, late 1930s to mid-1960s, saw three diverse orientations develop. Two of these, the *hospital recreation* perspective and the *recreational therapy* perspective, differed sharply concerning the fundamental purpose or role of recreation in medical settings. Hospital recreation viewed the recreative experience as the major objective of the hospital recreator. This experience, while having therapeutic benefits, was essentially the same as that achieved in community settings. Recreational therapy differed from hospital recreation in four fundamental ways.[5] *First,* activities were seen as treatment tools. *Second,* the recreative experience was not of major concern. *Third,* there was little recognition of our affiliation with the organized recreation movement. *Fourth,* the approach stressed concern with illness and treatment of disease. The remaining occupational orientation to service, *recreation for ill and handicapped,* reflected a community-setting orientation. As Meyer noted, the term *therapeutic recreation* was first used as a concept to unify the perspectives of hospital recreation, recreational therapy, and recreation for the ill and handicapped. It should be noted that a significant controversy took place within the Amer-

[4] *Ibid.*

[5] *Ibid.*, p. 10.

ican Red Cross in the mid to late 1940s which reflected the dispute between proponents of the recreation in hospitals and recreational therapy positions. James pointed out that the Red Cross espoused a "treatment" orientation in its recreational services from their inception in 1918 to shortly after World War II.[6] She cited the following quotes from the Red Cross and other sources regarding the purpose of recreation to support this contention:

> . . . to give the patients such diversion and training as will contribute to recovery.[7]
> . . . to (serve) as a tool . . . to re-educate the patient in normal, healthy pursuits in order that he may effect a speedier mental and physical recovery.[8]
> There must be some element which will provide for individual growth and development beyond the mere acquisition of activity skill. . . . There must be constant change and adjustment in meeting the needs of patients. Thus our progress in the development of a hospital recreation program in the days ahead will make a real contribution to the recognition of the therapeutic value of recreation.[9]

Interestingly, this treatment-oriented philosophy was reversed in 1948. The following passage illustrates a sharp shift to the recreation-in-hospitals position:

> The purpose of the recreation program in the hospital is the same as that of any recreation program in any setting, namely to provide opportunities for individuals to do the things of their choice, in their leisure time, for the satisfaction derived from the doing. . . . Hospital recreation leaders are not therapists whose primary purpose is treatment, and they should not be asked to participate in providing treatment.[10]

James suggested that this turnabout in ideology might have resulted from logistical factors, such as budget and staff reductions, rather than from ideological influences. Nevertheless, it is symptomatic of the basic controversy which would permeate the professional era of therapeutic recreation from 1966 to the present.

CONTROVERSY IN THE PARADIGM ERA

The merger of the National Association of Recreational Therapists, the Hospital Recreation Section of the American Recreation Society, and members of the Recreation Therapy Section of the American Alliance for Health, Physical Education, and Recreation, and Dance into the Council for the Advancement of Hospital Recreation

---

[6] Ann James, "Historical Perspective: The Therapy Debate," *Therapeutic Recreation Journal*, 14, no. 1 (1980), 13–16.

[7] American Red Cross, *Manual of Red Cross Camp Service: ARC 307*, Record Group 200, (Washington, D.C.: National Archives, 1919), p. 44.

[8] P. L. McCready, "Social Work Components of a Hospital Recreation Program," File 616, Record Group 200 Mimeographed, (Washington, D.C.: National Archives, 1944), p. 1.

[9] C. Nice, "Recreation in Military Hospitals," *Recreation*, 37, (July 1943), 204.

[10] *Ibid.*

in 1953, and eventually into the National Therapeutic Recreation Society (NTRS) in 1966, did little to still the earlier debate over philosophical orientations to service. While the term *therapeutic recreation* had largely replaced *recreation therapy* as a descriptive term by the mid-1960s,[11] substantial controversy remained concerning the philosophical orientation of the field. A significant portion of the *Therapeutic Recreation Journal,* the official publication of the NTRS, was devoted to this controversy in 1967 and 1968. The fourth-quarter, 1967 issue, in fact devoted four of seven articles (including an editorial) to this subject. A summary of these writings follows. In a guest editorial, Ira J. Hutchison, Jr., executive secretary of the NTRS, lobbied strongly for a broad and in-depth view of the field's service areas. Taking exception to the position that "the therapeutic recreation profession is primarily one that deals with overt pathology or breakdowns and gaps in the normal socio-recreative patterns of individuals in an institution of one kind or another," he stated:

> Most of us do know better and are aware of the broad comprehensive effectiveness of therapeutic recreation in a variety of areas other than that of the clinical or institutional setting. Therapeutic recreation is being more commonly recognized as a member of that group of professions that can effectively assist in the common effort to create an optimum social environment within which all citizens can find meaning and satisfaction. We are becoming increasingly active, singularly, and in concert with other health-oriented professions, in the areas of preventive, supportive, and remedial services.[12]

Three pages later, in the same issue of the *Journal,* Dr. Jack Goodzeit presented a diametrically opposed view of the nature of therapeutic recreation. Far from viewing the words as broad and encompassing, he proposed that the term be applied to only a specific treatment process. Commenting upon the relationship between the concepts of therapy and recreation, he felt that:

> Therapy means treatment. That is, the utilization of specific or general processes that lead to the amelioration of disease or disability. The random, non-directive exposure to recreative process whose objective is fun, cannot be termed therapeutic. A therapy

---

[11] According to E. M. Avedon, in his paper "A Critical Analysis of the National Therapeutic Recreation Society Position Statement," 1970 the first reference to the term *"therapeutic recreation"* appeared in the *Annals of the American Academy of Political and Social Science* (September 1957, pp. 87–91) in an article by Verna Rensvold, Beatrice Hill, Elizabeth Roggs, and Martin Meyer entitled "Therapeutic Recreation." The second reference appeared in *Hospital Management* (April 1960, pp. 1–2) in a series of articles by Dr. Howard A. Rusk. The third major reference to the term was made in a document published by Comeback, Inc. (1962) entitled *Therapeutic Recreation Curriculum Development Conference Report.* In 1963 reference was made to the term in the textbook *Recreation in American Life,* by Reynold E. Carlson, Janet R. MacLean, and Theodore R. Deppe (Belmont, Ca.: Wadsworth Publishing Co., Inc., p. 511).

[12] Ira J. Hutchison, Jr., "Guest Editorial," *Therapeutic Recreation,* 1, no. 2 (1967), 2. Note: The first issues of the *Therapeutic Recreation Journal* were merely entitled *Therapeutic Recreation.*

must have the objective of ameliorating disease or disability with fun being secondary to its purpose.[13]

Extending this notion of the difference between recreation and therapy to settings, he commented:

> We must make a distinction between recreation for the handicapped and therapeutic recreation. A setting where there is recreation for the handicapped must first include a clinical team for its work to be rehabilitative; and its work must first be addressed to treatment rather than to fun for it to be therapeutic.[14]

The issue ends on a somewhat pessimistic note with the final article "Recreation and the Therapeutic Environment." Tracing the emergence of ideas concerning the nature of recreation (therapy versus fun), Miller perceived that this dichotomy had

> . . . led to confusion and to what can probably best be described as inter-therapeutical disputes which no mediator will ever resolve. What has emerged have been two categories of personnel—those who see themselves as therapists and those who see themselves as recreationists. The former concern themselves with illness and employ recreation as treatment in the rehabilitation process, the latter with leisure time and patients' recreative needs.[15]

It is particularly interesting to note the divergent views concerning the nature of recreation held by representatives of the medical profession during the mid-1960s. Probably the most notable physican to support the "recreation for recreation's sake" versus the "therapy" position was Dr. Paul Haun, a British-born psychiatrist. In his classic work *Recreation: A Medical Viewpoint,* he stressed the importance of preserving recreation's "extraclinical" nature while denegrating the position that recreation can be directly equated with treatment. He wrote:

> It is my belief that "recreational therapy" cannot successfully answer rigorous questions . . . that must be put to it if it is to be taken seriously as another form of treatment. If the recreation worker claims access to the sick primarily as a therapist and fails to demonstrate the equivalence, if not the superiority, of his contribution fairly measured against that of other supportive medical disciplines, it would seem unwise for hospital administrators to devote their always limited financial resources to such programs or even the salaries of recreation personnel. It seems both hazardous and unnecessary to me for those interested in recreation to place their figurative eggs in so gossamer a basket as "therapy"; hazardous because I know of no evidence that recreation is an effective treatment instrument and unnecessary since I am persuaded that highly relevant arguments can be advanced for providing recreation services in

[13] Jack M. Goodzeit, "Therapeutic Recreation vs. Recreation for the Handicapped," *Therapeutic Recreation,* 1, no. 2 (1967), 9.

[14] *Ibid.,* p. 31.

[15] Norman P. Miller, "Recreation and the Therapeutic Environment," *Therapeutic Recration,* 1, no. 2 (1967), 34.

terms other than therapy. I am so fully persuaded of the value of recreation that I am alarmed at the possibility of its being unjustly discredited through laying claim to an effectiveness it cannot possess.[16]

Less than one year after this statement appeared in Haun's text, Arthur Stillman, a physician and clinical director of a large state mental hospital, took strong exception to the notion that recreation could (and should) not be perceived as therapy. According to Stillman, a therapy consisted of the following elements:

— A planned conscious intervention
— A body of techniques to produce change
— Techniques based on the patient's or client's needs as realized from understanding the factors that brought the patient or client to his present status
— Techniques intended to alter the patient or client from his initial posture to a predetermined goal
— Techniques that are not passive, accidental or happenstance process, but ones that are known, understood and demonstrable.[17]

In his opinion, recreation, as a therapy, met these criteria. Furthermore, he felt the efficacy of recreation as an intervention was directly dependent upon the skills, abilities, and creativity of the recreation therapist, as in other healing modalities. His forum for these beliefs was also an article in the *Therapeutic Recreation Journal*.

Reacting strongly to the "Is recreation therapy?" debate in 1968, Humphrey suggested that this question be relegated to what he termed the "kindergarten level of our professional development."[18] Citing recent trends such as the initiation of the therapeutic community concept in institutional settings and the comprehensive Mental Health–Mental Retardation Center in the community, he felt that the greatest philosophical challenge facing the field was the abandonment of the strict "medical model" approach to service. Noting that deviating from the medical model "in no way precludes goal oriented approaches related to the disability or symptomatic behavior," it was his opinion that such an orientation could "emphasize the tremendous potential contribution which is lost if our approach does not change to a positive one oriented to residual strengths at the earliest possible moment."[19]

The emphasis placed on goal-oriented approaches and residual strengths of the individual client advocated by Humphrey appears to be evident in the position paper on therapeutic recreation service developed at the Ninth Southern Regional Institute on Therapeutic Recreation at the University of North Carolina in 1969.

[16] Paul Haun, *Recreation: A Medical Viewpoint*, eds. Elliott M. Avedon and Francis B. Arje (New York: Teachers College Press, 1965), p. 60.

[17] Arthur T. Stillman, "In Response To: The Sound of One Hand," *Therapeutic Recreation*, 2, no. 1 (1968), 21.

[18] Fred Humphrey, "Interpreting the Role of Therapeutic Recreation to Other Disciplines," *Therapeutic Recreation Journal*, 2, no. 4 (1968), 33.

[19] *Ibid.*, p. 36.

This document contained an introductory statement concerning the nature of recreation services, several phrases outlining the elements of the therapeutic recreation process and the types of individuals who could benefit from therapeutic recreation, a program method framework for such service, and a listing of essential resources for effective therapeutic reaction practice. The following definition of therapeutic recreation was extended in this paper:

> Therapeutic recreation is a special service within the broad area of recreation services. It is a process which utilizes recreation services for purposive intervention in some physical, emotional, and/or social behavior to bring about a desired change in that behavior and to promote the growth and development of the individual. Therapeutic recreation provides opportunities for participation on one's own volition in activities that bring pleasure or other positive personal rewards.
>
> Therapeutic recreation services are provided by recreational personnel who are qualified by education, training, and experience to provide the individual with opportunities for optimal recreative experiences in relation to the desires of the individual and the total goals of the agency.
>
> The therapeutic recreation specialist is prepared to function as an agent for social, emotional, and physical change and to work effectively with other disciplines also concerned with services to the client.[20]

In a reaction statement drafted in the year following the development of this position, Dr. E.M. Avedon proposed an alternative approach to conceptualizing the term *therapeutic recreation service* and a corresponding rival definition.[21] Based on the assumptions that recreation denoted aspects of a "system" used for a specific purpose, that recreation was not therapy but had therapeutic implications (as advocated by Haun), and that service referred to a system of recreation "packaged and delivered to recipients" he posited that "Therapeutic Recreation Service is a matrix of assistance calculated to contribute to the modification and amelioration of an inhibiting disorder."[22]

To explain each of the major points in this definition, Avedon provided the following conceptual model, which determined that therapeutic recreation service is:

1. A matrix of assistance; i.e.—an aggregate of services formed into a specific system
2. Calculated to contribute; i.e.—consciously selected and designed, based on education and experience
3. To the modification and amelioration of an inhibiting disorder; i.e.—to help an individual who is unable to have adequate recreative experience, to use his abilities so that he may have more adequate experience.[23]

---

[20] "Therapeutic Recreation Position Paper," (Developed at the Ninth Southern Regional Institute on Therapeutic Recreation, University of North Carolina, 1969).

[21] E. M. Avedon, "A Critical Analysis of the National Therapeutic Recreation Society Position Statement."

[22] *Ibid.*, p. 13.

[23] Ibid., p. 14.

Taking a different approach to philosophically defining the field of therapeutic recreation, Ball suggested a model in 1970 which appears to be consistent with, and in some ways reconciles, the previous notions of recreation and therapy. Operating on the fundamental assumptions that the concept of therapeutic recreation could be interpreted as "pleasing refreshment that is remedial," that the recreation experience could be adapted by the use of a modifier, and that recreation is concerned basically with the healthy aspects of a personality, she suggested a continuous range of recreational experiences. The model in Figure 3-1 was proposed to take into account clients' intraindividual differences in skills, knowledges, and attitudes toward leisure.[24]

EXPERIENCE	TYPE OF TIME	MAJOR MOTIVATION
1. Activity for Sake of Activity	Obligated Time	Drive is Outer Directed
2. Recreation Education	Obligated Time	Drive is Outer Directed
3. Therapeutic Recreation	Unobligated Time	Motivation is Inner Directed but Choice of Experiences is Limited
4. Recreation	Unobligated Time	Motivation is Inner Directed

Fig. 3-1   Ball's Service Continuum Model. From Edith L. Ball, "The Meaning of Therapeutic Recreation," *Therapeutic Recreation Journal*, 4, no. 1 (1970), 18. Reprinted by permission of National Therapeutic Recreation Society/National Recreation and Park Association.

In 1971 Shivers, expressing his concepts of therapeutic recreation service and recreation in general, offered a philosophy which was quite consistent with the previously outlined range of recreational experiences. Theorizing that recreation was vital to creating and maintaining a homeostatic balance in the individual, he implicitly supported the "activity-for-activity's sake" and the "recreation" segments of Ball's model. Postulating that the recreationist has the "professional capacity to enter into a therapeutic relationship with a client" and to "provide guidance and counseling to those ill/handicapped persons who require assistance in finding social, physical, or emotional outlets during their leisure", he also appeared to support the therapeutic recreation and recreation education components.[25]

In 1973 Rusalem disturbed whatever calm had been generated by continuum-of-services or range-of-experiences proponents by imploring the field of therapeutic recreation to adopt an alternative to the therapeutic model in therapeutic recreation.[26] In his opinion, the field of therapeutic recreation was still closely aligned philosophically with a treatment model. This paradigm held that:

[24] Edith L. Ball, *"The Meaning of Therpeutic Recreation,"* *Therapeutic Recreation Journal*, 4, no. 1 (1970), 17–18.

[25] Jay S. Shivers, "One Concept of Therapeutic Recreational Service," *Therapeutic Recreation Journal*, 5, no. 2 (1971), 51–53, 93.

[26] Herbert Rusalem, "An Alternative to the Therapeutic Model in Therapeutic Recreation," *Therapeutic Recreation Journal*, 7, no. 1 (1973), 8–15.

— Clients had disabling, disadvantaging conditions which rendered them less effective in everyday living situations and led to frustrations.

— The function of professional workers (including therapeutic recreation personnel) was to recognize and identify pathology.

— Leisure activities and experiences were used to effect desired changes in disabled individuals, therefore activity programs were evaluated and consequently modified as necessary.[27]

According to this author, the basic flaw in this approach was the emphasis placed on "redesigning" the individual rather than dealing with the cause of the pathology, the external environment. In lieu of the treatment orientation, an "ecological" model was proposed which would see the therapeutic recreation specialist as part of a larger social and political movement striving for human rights through consumerism and advocacy. Inherent in this approach is a "shift of professional emphasis from the therapy of people to the therapy of environments," a reduction in the importance of activities which do not relate to the "ecological leisure prescription," and a lack of dependence on other professions.[28]

Interestingly, while Canada lacked a national professional organization such as the NTRS, the first Canadian journal devoted exclusively to leisure and disabled persons *Leisurability,* provided a forum for the philosophical debate concerning therapeutic recreation's service philosophy. Two articles published in the first year of its existence viewed therapeutic recreation as following various categories of service. The first, authored by Martin in 1974 recognized that "the approaches to and the methods of recreation service that are applicable in a given therapeutic setting are intimately associated with the degree of acceptance and recognition of the value of a professional recreation service within the particular medical or rehabilitative environment."[29] Following this assumption, he suggested that our vocational activities could be incorporated within the following orientations:

Fun and Games—in which activity patterns approximate discretionary time outside the therapeutic environment

Personal Adjustment—wherein recreation assists the individual to adjust to an illness or a disability

Therapeutic—wherein recreation is prescribed in addition to medication

Educative—including counseling and referral during and after the therapeutic process

In a similar vein, Jolicoeur, drawing heavily upon traditional views of therapeutic recreation proposed three categories of service in 1975: recreation, education for leisure, and therapeutic recreation.[30] The content of these categories closely resembled the services proposed by Ball and Martin.

[27] *Ibid.,* p. 8.

[28] *Ibid.,* p. 15.

[29] Martin, "Therapeutic Recreation Practice," p. 22.

[30] Pierre W. Jolicoeur, "Recreation for Special Groups," *Leisurability,* 2, no. 1 (1975), 28–34.

Although feeling that the field of therapeutic recreation could potentially demonstrate its remedial or therapeutic potential, Littlefield expressed the sentiment in 1975 that it could only lay claim to the previously described "recreation" or "fun-and-games" service orientation. Echoing Haun's earlier concern over the lack of documentation relating to the efficacy of recreation as a treatment modality, he issued the following statement and challenge to therapeutic recreation specialists:

> Recreation therapy and recreation therapists are by and large nothing more than recreation leaders running recreation programs for developmentally disabled or hindered clients. Do we have concrete statistical evidence or indications of what a leisure activity contains that is inherently therapeutic?[31]

Scarcely two years passed after the challenge before the recurring debate over the therapy question again emerged. This time the issues revolved around the basic terminology used to describe the professional field of therapeutic recreation. The initial impetus for this controversy was a brief article by Witt entitled "Therapeutic Recreation: The Outmoded Label," which appeared in the second quarter, 1977 issue of the *Therapeutic Recreation Journal*. Based on earlier writings such as those of Rusalem, this position statement posited that the term *therapeutic recreation . . . does not adequately describe current philosophy or primary approaches to service. Its continued utilization restricts growth and evolution of needed services due to the tendency to let the label suggest direction instead of the other way around.*[32]

Citing trends such as the service concepts of *enabling, advocacy,* and *leisure education,* Witt suggested that a *therapeutic* orientation could sharply limit service to disabled persons, particularly in community settings. As alternatives to the professional term *therapeutic recreation* he suggested titles from the general leisure service field such as *recreators, leisure facilitators,* or *leisure advocates.*

These recommendations were applauded by certain individuals such as Rowthorn who felt that the term *therapeutic recreation* (like its predecessors *hospital recreation, recreation for the ill and handicapped, recreation therapy* and *recreational therapy*) was a political title adopted to gain respect from the allied health fields.[33] Feeling that the "attribute—therapeutic—is implied in the single term—recreation," she characterized *therapeutic recreation* as a redundant term, and, like Witt, suggested the adoption of *recreation* as a comprehensive and descriptive term for the field.

Witt's position, however, drew swift rebuttal from others including then President of the National Therapeutic Recreation Society, Gary Robb. Reacting to the view that *therapeutic recreation* was outmoded, he made the following points:

[31] Steven R. Littlefield, "So You're a Recreation Therapist," *Therapeutic Recreational Journal,* 9, no. 3 (1975), 107.

[32] Peter A. Witt, "Therapeutic Recreation: The Outmoded Label," *Therapeutic Recreation Journal,* 11, no. 2 (1977), 40.

[33] Anne W. Rowthorn, "An Open Letter to Peter Witt: A Response to His Article, 'Therapeutic Recreation: The Outmoded Label,'" *Therapeutic Recreation Jornal,* 12, no. 1 (1978), 7–9.

— While mainstreaming efforts have been significant, most (80–90%) of therapeutic recreation specialists are employed in institutional settings with moderately to severely handicapped persons.

— By and large, recreators working with disabled persons in the community are not engaged in "therapeutic recreation."

— "Therapy" is still an essential element in most approaches to service within the field. Special skills are therefore required from those providing service.[34]

In summary, he suggested that the term *therapeutic recreation* still remained an appropriate descriptor, yet he appointed a committee to examine the relationship between therapeutic recreation intervention and recreation for special populations. History would reveal that this was the initiation of a systematic quest for a unifying professional philosophy which would encompass the next five years.

Meanwhile, the controversy concerning the notion of therapy in therapeutic recreation service again surfaced in the journal *Leisurability*. Shivers, focusing on the therapeutic relationship he had outlined in previous writings, took a strong stand supporting earlier notions of recreational therapy as prescribed and interventionist.[35] Witt again countered, citing opposing trends in human service with disabled people,[36] and Korn took exception to what he termed "the deification of therapy" in a second rebuttal article.[37] Representative statements from each of these position papers are summarized next.

Why Not Recreational Therapy?!
Jay Shivers

— Therapeutic recreational service is defined as directly interventionist, prescribed, involuntary, very specific in some instances, and rehabilitation oriented.

— The only way to insure client participation, despite lack of choice, is to offer the *appearance* of choice.

— Furthermore, recreationists should know, better than patients, what is beneficial for that patient.

— There is really no reason to believe that forced participation will destroy the value that recreational activity can have for the individual.

— If the activity is not oriented toward rehabilitation or recuperation, it is not therapeutic recreational service.

— Those activities of a recreational nature which are classified as therapies are so designated because they have been applied as specifics in directed treatment programs. Moreover, they furnish results which can be evaluated and measured.

[34] Gary M. Robb, "Letter to the Editor," *Therapeutic Recreation Journal,* 12, no. 1 (1978), 5.

[35] Jay Shivers, "Why Not Recreational Therapy?!" *Leisurability,* 4, no. 4 (1977), 4–9.

[36] Peter A. Witt, "Recreational Therapy: Who Cares?" *Leisurability,* 4, (1977), 13–14.

[37] Max Korn, "The Deification of Therapy," *Leisurability,* 4, no. 4 (1977), 10–12.

The Deification of Therapy
Max Korn

— Thus, the medical model implies that the client is perceived as a "sick patient" who, after being "diagnosed," is provided with some form of "treatment" or "therapy" for his or her "disease" in a "clinic" or "hospital," usually by "doctors" or other "paramedical" or "therapeutic" staff working toward a "cure."

... therapeutic modalities founded on the medical model reinforce the historically prominent role perception of devalued individuals (e.g., handicapped, or elderly) as "sick" persons whether in fact they are sick or not. Similarly, many clients engaged in recreational therapy are not sick, but the demands and expectations we make reinforce their role as "patient" being helped under the "disease model."

... why must we refer to even the most basic recreational activity as therapy?

Recreational Therapy: Who Cares!
Peter A. Witt

— We seem to be moving away from institutionalization, medically dominated practices, notions of prescription, and notions of passive patients.

— *Recreation therapy, therapeutic recreation,* or whatever medically based terminology individuals choose to use fails to recognize the trends within leisure services and human services more generally.

— Legislation, the efforts of advocate associations, and the statements of disabled individuals themselves indicate that we must change our basic orientation to opportunity provision, leisure education efforts, and skill upgrading.

— We should devote our energies to enabling individuals to improve their capacity and appreciation for recreational experiences. This is the heritage of our field.

It is noteworthy that one of our most closely related allied health care professions, *occupational therapy,* was undergoing an identical self-examination at precisely the time these words were being written. It is extremely coincidental that this critique focused upon the same fundamental issues as the therapy debate—identification with the medical model and treatment approaches to rehabilitation. In an article entitled "The Derailment of Occupational Therapy," Shannon described the soul-searching for professional identity which the field of occupational therapy was undergoing. These words, which appeared in the *American Journal of Occupational Therapy* in 1977, could also have been most appropriately applied to the field of therapeutic recreation at that time:

> Occupational Therapy cannot be defined descriptively (What is it) nor is there agreement on a normative definition (What it ought to be). It is not surprising, therefore, that society places little value (political and financial support) on a profession plagued with the problem of role confusion yet faced with the moral imperative of *right conduct* in response to society's increasing demand for accountability.[38]

[38] Phillip D. Shannon, "The Derailment of Occupational Therapy," *American Journal of Occupational Therapy,* 31, no. 4 (1977), 230.

Alleging that occupational therapy had, to its detriment, "walked the primrose path with medicine" in an attempt to define itself philosophically, Shannon extended the following argument. His line of reasoning parallels that of advocates for hospital recreation and of the recreative experience point of view in therapeutic recreation.

> Occupational therapy abandoned its more substantive concern for health in adopting the rationality of the medical model with its focus on pathology. Its systematic approach to wholesome, healthy living as seen in the processing of competency behaviors was replaced with the narrow perspective of the medical model based on the homeostatic principle of symptom reduction. Its epistemological base shifted from the social sciences to the functional requirements of the physical sciences and a focus on the minute and measurable. This attachment to the medical model, an attachment that was less than visionary, signaled the beginning of the derailment process.[39]

To avoid this fate, Shannon urged a return to the traditional view of clients as individuals who occupy roles "that demand a set of skill competencies acquired in play, processed through work, and extended to leisure."[40]

Textbook Efforts

Textbooks in the field of therapeutic recreation provide focal points for the examination of philosophical positions which have been applied to the field at given points in time. The authors of such texts have been able not only to review the various writings of others to date, but also to extend positions which transcend current state-of-the-art thinking. The authors of major texts have, in many cases, been active members of professional organizations in therapeutic recreation. Therefore, they have influenced (and been influenced by) endeavors to conceptualize our vocation. An examination of four major textbooks, published over the past decade at two-year intervals (1972, 1974, 1976, 1978), reveals an interesting evolution in thought concerning the nature of therapeutic recreation.

The earliest of these writings, *Therapeutic Recreation: Its Theory, Philosophy and Practice* by Virginia Frye and Martha Peters (1972), viewed therapeutic recreation as: "A process through which purposeful efforts are directed toward achieving or maximizing desired concomitant effects of a recreative experience."[41]

While this definition does, in fact, suggest a process, as Meyer suggested the term *concomitant* itself does not denote or imply a causal relationship between the recreative experience and "its" effects.[42]

Like those of the previous authors, Avedon's 1974 text *Therapeutic Recreation Service: An Applied Behavioral Approach* recognized therapeutic recreation's general therapeutic effect, but he did not believe it to be a specific therapy per se.

---

[39] *Ibid.*, p. 231.

[40] *Ibid.*, p. 234.

[41] Virginia Frye and Martha Peters, *Therapeutic Recreation: Its Theory, Philosophy and Practice* (Harrisburg, Pa.: Stackpole Books, 1972), p. 44.

[42] Meyer, "Philosophical Alternatives," p. 16.

The following quotes extracted from Chapter 3 of his text are illustrative of this notion:

> Specialists in therapeutic recreation service concern themselves primarily with the human situation rather than limiting concern to activity participation in circumscribed situations. Emphasis is upon the provision of service framed within the context of the field of recreation and modified to function within various social institutions. Because the *results* of service are non specific—theoretically they have a nonspecific effect upon the person rather than a measurable specific effect—they are said to have therapeutic value; however, this effect should not be construed as ''therapy'' per se.[43]
>
> Most personnel in health-related professions are primarily concerned with amelioration or modification of behavior with respect to pathology.
>
> Personnel in therapeutic recreation service are primarily concerned with non-pathological factors, and therefore focus upon enabling an individual to strengthen aspects of personality that are not affected, in order to prevent further limitation or greater functional loss.[44]

O'Morrow's 1976 text *Therapeutic Recreation: A Helping Profession* recognized the importance of the recreative experience concept of therapeutic recreation, yet differed sharply from the preceding texts in two ways. *First,* this author felt that the process of therapeutic recreation could be used to bring about specific desired changes in behavior. *Second,* he outlined the role of therapeutic recreation service in relation to this process. His distinct notions of the therapeutic recreation process and therapeutic recreation service led him to devote separate chapters in his text to these concepts. His definitions of therapeutic recreation as a *process* and a *service* are as follows:

> Because of the therapeutic implications of recreative experiences, therapeutic recreation can certainly be considered a process wherein recreative experiences are used to bring about a change in the behavior of those individuals with special needs and problems. The focus of the process is on the use of recreative experiences to (1) enhance growth and development of the individual and (2) enable the individual to meet his responsibility for fulfilling his own leisure needs.[45]
>
> While recognizing the importance of the concept of therapeutic recreation as a process, therapeutic recreation service may be defined as those professional recreation services that are specifically designed to bring about a change in behavior of a special population member as well as to assist that member to move toward achieving the fullest recreative experience possible.[46]

Although the recognition of therapeutic recreation as both a process and a service was extremely useful in attempting to define this complex field, certain problems arose from this process. Gunn and Peterson, in *Therapeutic Recreation Program Design: Principles and Procedures* (1978), suggested that the therapy-

---

[43] Elliott M. Avedon, *Therapeutic Recreation Service: An Applied Behavioral Science Approach* (Englewood Cliffs, N.J.: Prentice-Hall, Inc., 1974), p. 19.

[44] *Ibid.*, p. 20.

[45] Gerald S. O'Morrow, *Therapeutic Recreation: A Helping Profession* (Englewood Cliffs, N.J.: Prentice-Hall, Inc., Reston Publishing Company, Inc., 1976), p. 121.

[46] *Ibid.*, p. 122.

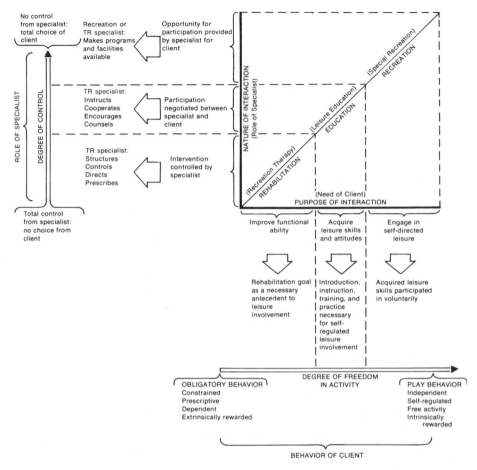

Fig. 3-2 Therapeutic Recreation Service Model. From Scout Lee Gunn and Carol Ann Peterson, *Therapeutic Recreation Program Design: Principles and Procedures*, 1978, p. 15. Reprinted by permission of Prentice-Hall, Inc.

versus-recreation issue, for example, "has resulted from attempts to define therapeutic recreation service as a specific process, with most of the emphasis placed on therapeutic recreation rather than on service."[47] Rather, they suggested that the term *therapeutic recreation* identifies a type of service which uses many processes, stating that

> Rather than being a philosophical statement of one specific process, therapeutic recreation service identifies (1) a group of professionals who possess recreational activity and facilitation skills and who are interested in using those skills to bring about some type of change with (2) special-need populations, such as the mentally retarded, emotionally disturbed, mentally ill and physically handicapped. The specific needs of the consumer determine (a) the type of change, whether in a functional-skill area or a

[47] Scout Lee Gunn and Carol Ann Peterson, *Therapeutic Recreation Program Design: Principles and Procedures* (Englewood Cliffs, N.J.: Prentice-Hall, Inc., 1978), p. 11.

leisure-skill area, and (b) the ways that the therapeutic recreator employs his or her activity and facilitation skills to bring about the change.[48]

Figure 3-2 was then proposed to illustrate the continuum of services inherent in therapeutic recreation.

STUDY GUIDE QUESTIONS

1. Do you agree that the profession of therapeutic recreation has functioned largely at a pre-paradigm stage to date? Do you find this unusual, considering the number of years individuals have been providing "therapeutic recreation" services?

2. If the field has been functioning at a pre-paradigm stage with respect to its values and beliefs concerning an occupational philosophy, have our efforts toward credentialling and the development of standards and research been at a paradigm or postparadigm stage? If so, are there any dangers inherent in this situation?

3. Review the conditions cited by Meyer as being an impetus for the generation of a philosophical position statement. Do you agree that these are major factors necessitating the creation of such a statement? Can you identify any additional factors which would make the development of a statement particularly urgent?

4. Meyer identified *hospital recreation, recreational therapy,* and *recreation for ill and handicapped* as being three major perspectives in the early development of the field. Which viewpoint do you feel is most pervasive in the field today?

5. In our pre-paradigm stage of development, we appear to have drawn heavily upon the opinions of individuals in other disciplines (particularly medicine and the social sciences) to help us define our identity and our reason for being. Do you feel that this was appropriate and desirable? What advantages and disadvantages are associated with this practice?

6. Review some earlier models which have been used to conceptualize therapeutic recreation service such as that of Ball. Do you feel that these models adequately define the field of therapeutic recreation as it exists today? Defend your answer!

7. Do you agree with Rusalem's position that therapeutic recreators are chiefly concerned with "redesigning the individual rather than dealing with the cause of the pathology, the external environment"?

8. In 1975 Littlefield questioned whether "we have concrete statistical evidence or indications of what a leisure activity contains that is inherently therapeutic." Do you feel that this was a valid question at the time? If so, has our body of knowledge advanced adequately to answer this question?

9. In 1977 Witt charged that the term *therapeutic recreation* was unduly restrictive because it could curtail such practices as "enabling," "advocacy," and "leisure education." Do you feel this was (and is) a valid criticism? Are there terms which could more adequately and appropriately be applied to the field?

10. What similarities and parallels do you see between the comments of Shannon relative to the development of occupational therapy and our own professional development? Do you feel all professional disciplines go through a similar process of self-questioning and analysis in their development?

11. Authors of textbooks pertaining to therapeutic recreation over the past decade have passed through stages of emphasizing the "nonspecific" effects of recreation, therapeutic recreation as a process and a service, and therapeutic recreation as a service

[48] *Ibid.,* p. 12.

containing many processes. Which of these positions do you personally identify with? Which position do you feel most adequately represents our profession?

TOWARD A POSTPARADIGM RESOLUTION

In May, 1982, a Philosophical Position Statement was adopted by the NTRS. As indicated by the previous review of literature, this event signaled the culmination of over ten years of effort by the Society to reach a consensus concerning an ideological occupational perspective. The chronological sequence of events leading to the adoption of this position statement is as follows.

While the previously reported definition of therapeutic recreation generated at the 1969 Ninth Southern Regional Institute on Therapeutic Recreation has never been officially accepted, debate over its content has continued. As mentioned, in 1976–77, Mr. Gary Robb, then president of NTRS, appointed a committee headed by Dr. David Compton to study the philosophical issue and make recommendations to the society. Although this committee developed a philosophical position, the document was not officially adopted. During the presidency of Mr. David Park (1979–80), Dr. Lee Meyer was asked to develop a research paper describing the philosophical basis of therapeutic recreation as a field of service. The extensive document which Dr. Meyer authored, entitled "Philosophical Alternatives and the Professionalization of Therapeutic Recreation," identified three alternative philosophical positions which NTRS could choose to adopt as its statement of identity. The Philosophical Issues Task Force of NTRS then reviewed these orientations and extended them to four positions. Position C was eventually chosen as the official statement. A summary of these positions and study guide questions based upon the implications of each of them follow.[49]

Position A
(Recreation)

This position simply states that therapeutic recreation is the provision of recreation services and opportunities to persons with disabling conditions. The main purpose of these services, then, is to provide the opportunity for these individuals to have the most meaningful recreative experience possible. This position holds that these services can be, and are, provided in a variety of settings including hospitals, institutions, and community-based agencies. Regardless of the setting, the primary

[49] These positions are extracted from a survey conducted by the NTRS in the summer of 1981. The study guide questions are paraphrased from the implication sections of this questionnaire. Drs. Carol Peterson, Fred Humphrey, and Jerry Kelley developed clarifications and implications of the positions. The task force which generated the material contained in the survey consisted of Ms. Andi Farbman-Morris, Ms. Viki Annand, Dr. Jerry Kelley, and Mr. David Park.

purpose is still the same, namely, to provide opportunities for this special population of individuals to have a recreative experience.

This position further states that the recreative experiences provided can have therapeutic effects, simply because meaningful recreation experiences, by definition, provide fun, enjoyment, and fulfillment. The provision of these services and opportunities for persons with disabling conditions can become a very important part of, or a supplement to, the therapy or treatment being provided. This position further holds that the opportunity to participate in recreative experiences is a basic human need of all individuals and is necessary for the achievement of growth, development, and balance in one's life. This is equally true for disabled persons and, as such, should be an integral part of all treatment, rehabilitation, education, and other service programs.

According to this position, the uniqueness of therapeutic recreation is the knowledge of the special characteristics of disabled populations and the skill and ability to modify and adapt recreative opportunities and facilities to enable and facilitate participation of disabled persons. This knowledge, skill, and ability, along with the knowledge and skills of a general recreation specialist, comprise the essential body of knowledge of the therapeutic recreation specialization.

STUDY GUIDE QUESTIONS—POSITION A

1. If this position had been adopted, could the name *therapeutic recreation* have been retained to identify the field? What confusion might arise concerning such terms as *special recreation* or *recreation for special populations* if this position had been accepted? Do you feel that this position would be readily embraced by consumer groups of disabled persons?

2. If this position had been embraced, what would have constituted the essential body of knowledge of the therapeutic recreation profession? Would this body of knowledge differ significantly from that of the general recreation field?

3. If this position had been adopted, would it have been compatible with the current movement toward curriculum accreditation promoted by the NRPA? Would this position have compelled our profession to seek sanction from the allied health service field?

4. Which of the following occupational groups would it have been appropriate to affiliate with, if this position had been adopted: (1) the allied health field, (2) the recreation and park field, or (3) a separate, but coequal, field? Defend your choice!

5. In the past, the field of therapeutic recreation has emphasized that recreation is an integral part of treatment to organizations such as the Joint Commission on Accreditation of Hospitals and the Council on Accreditation of Rehabilitation Facilities. If this statement had been adopted, how would it have affected our negotiations with these bodies?

Position B
(Treatment)

This position has as its foundation the idea that therapeutic recreation is the provision of recreation services and opportunities for treatment or therapy (i.e., health restoration, remediation, habilitation, rehabilitation) to those persons who have been determined to be in need of them. More specifically, the latter part of the statement refers to individuals who have a disability or to those persons who are significantly limited in their functional abilities due to illness, disability, maladaptation, or other conditions to the extent of creating a level of dependency. The primary purpose, then, of therapeutic recreation is to utilize the recreation experiences and opportunities to help treat, change, or otherwise ameliorate effects of illness and disability. Stated in another way, the primary purpose is to help the individual to overcome a position of dependence due to illness, disability, or dysfunction. The goal would be to provide services which would contribute to the achievement of optimal functioning and independence.

This position states that therapeutic recreation services would not be restricted or limited to settings which are traditionally viewed as treatment settings, but *could* be provided in a wide variety of settings including hospitals, institutions, schools, and community-based agencies. The service would not be defined by where it is provided, but instead by the nature and purpose of the service. Therefore, if the service were provided as a means of treating, overcoming, or ameliorating the effects of disability or illness, it would be therapeutic recreation. This position holds that the clients of therapeutic recreation are individuals who are experiencing conditions of dependency due to illness or disability, and that the attention of the therapeutic recreator is focused on those who need expert assistance in overcoming that dependence. When those individuals have achieved a certain level with that expert assistance, they are entitled to the same recreation services available to other individuals.

This position further holds that the types of services provided would be diverse and would be related to the identified deficits of the individuals. These services might include prescribed activities, leisure education, leisure counseling, or, in some instances, recreation activities. The uniqueness of therapeutic recreation is found in the skill of the practitioner to use the recreation activity, service, or environment as a technique to facilitate remediation, restoration, and rehabilitation outcomes which promote optimal functioning of the individual. The focus is not on the activity participation per se, but on the behavioral outcomes in relationship to objectively determined needs of the individual. The important distinction is that whatever methodology or technique utilized, the strategy is conceptualized and implemented as a purposeful intervention designed to achieve specific objectives or measurable outcomes. Those outcomes could be either corrective, restorative, rehabilitative, or habilitative, but each is designed to optimize the total functioning of the individual.

STUDY GUIDE QUESTIONS—POSITION B

1. Would the term *therapeutic recreation* still be applicable if this position had been adopted? What differences in connotation would the term have, if retained? If this position had been accepted, would *recreational therapy* have been a more appropriate (and desirable) name for the field?

2. What would be the essential body of knowledge related to this position statement? What skills, abilities, and knowledges would have to be emphasized or developed in our curriculums?

3. Would we be able to maintain our existing accreditation with the general recreation and park field under position B? Do you feel a new and separate accreditation process would have been necessitated if this position had been accepted?

4. Would the adoption of this position have facilitated or hindered current credentialling efforts in the field of therapeutic recreation?

5. Which of the following occupational groups would it have been most appropriate to affiliate with, if this position had been adopted: (1) the allied health field, (2) the recreation and park field, or (3) a separate, but coequal, field? Defend your choice!

6. Therapeutic recreation specialists have described their efforts as being both a treatment, or therapy, modality and a general recreation service. If this position had been adopted, could this practice have continued? How could the distinction between treatment and general recreation be articulated to legislators and rehabilitation agencies?

Position C
(Treatment/Education/Recreation)

This position states that therapeutic recreation is the provision of recreation services and opportunities to assist individuals in establishing and expressing an independent leisure life-style. Accordingly, the primary purpose of therapeutic recreation is to assist the client in eliminating leisure barriers, to develop leisure skills and attitudes, and to optimize leisure functioning. This position states that the uniqueness of therapeutic recreation is that it utilizes three specific types of services as part of a comprehensive approach to enabling leisurability. The three types of services offered are therapy, leisure education, and recreation participation, and the therapeutic recreation specialist is equally prepared to provide all three services. The decision as to where and when each of the services is provided is based on the assessment of client need. Different individuals have a variety of different needs related to leisure utilization. For some clients, improvement of a functional behavior or problem (physical, mental, social, or emotional) is a necessary prerequisite to meaningful leisure experiences. For others, acquiring leisure skills, knowledge, and abilities is a priority need. For others, special recreation participation opportunities are necessary, based on place or residence or because assistance or adapted activities are required. This approach utilizes the need of the client to give direction to program service selection. In some situations, the client may need programs from all three service components. In other situations, the client may need only leisure education, recreation participation opportunities, or both. An example of this might be a physically handicapped child in a community setting. The fact remains, this position is based on a variety of identified client leisure needs rather than on a philosophical preference for one or another type of service.

Another important consideration of this position is the relationship between and among the three service components. Therapy is not an independent entity within the continuum. In other words, the purpose of therapy is not to just improve any functional behaviors or problems. Rather, therapy is viewed as legitimate for the therapeutic recreator when the client has a functional (physical, mental, social, or emotional) limitation that relates to, or inhibits, leisure involvement. This distinction enables the therapeutic recreator to make decisions regarding when therapy is needed and what types of behaviors are appropriate to address within the therapeutic recreation domain of expertise and authority. This approach places therapy within a comprehensive model and ties its functions to eventual leisurability.

Leisure education is also a significant component of this position. These services are basically defined as opportunities to acquire skills, knowledge, and attitudes related to leisure utilization. Many clients in residential treatment and community settings appear to need leisure education services in order to initiate and engage in leisure experiences. For many special populations, it is the absence of leisure learning opportunities and socialization into leisure that blocks or inhibits their leisure experiences. Thus leisure education programs provide the opportunity for leisure behaviors to develop without assuming sickness or disability as the primary barrier.

The last component of this position is recreation participation. Briefly stated, human beings, despite illness or disability and regardless of residence, are entitled to recreative experiences. Most practitioners agree that recreation is a need and a right of clients. Within this position, this need is acknowledged and given an equal amount of emphasis in terms of conceptualization and implementation considerations.

Equally important is the concept of generalizability within this position. The model provides appropriate program direction regardless of type of setting or type of client served. This attribute allows the model to be acceptable throughout the therapeutic recreation profession. A practitioner working in a treatment setting can see the extension of the model into the community environment. Likewise, community therapeutic recreators can view their services within a perspective of previous services received or possible future needs. Thus this position provides a comprehensive approach to service, not just within a given setting, but between and among settings as well.

STUDY GUIDE QUESTIONS—POSITION C

1. This position specifies that all therapeutic recreation specialists will have to be prepared to provide general recreation, leisure education, and therapy services. Those not able to do so are not included in this field. Do you feel this is a desirable situation for our profession? Under this position, are general recreation services termed *therapeutic recreation*?

2. How do the competencies called for under this position differ from those demanded by position A (recreation) and position B (treatment)? Are there competencies consistent with those now outlined under the NTRS guidelines for accreditation?

3. Do you feel that the three major areas of competency called for under this position will be easily accepted by and "sold to" other allied health care professions? Which area(s) of service do you feel would most easily be accepted by health service professions? Which would be the least readily accepted? Defend your choice!

4. Is continued affiliation with the recreation and park field desirable under this position? If so, what measures should our professional organization take to strengthen its role within the general recreation field?

5. Are the concepts and language contained in this position consistent with existing federal legislation relating to recreation and other human services for disabled persons?

Position D
(Treatment and Recreation)

This position states that therapeutic recreation is *both* the provision of recreation services and opportunities for treatment to those persons who have been determined to be in need of it *and* the provision of recreation services and opportunities to persons with disabling conditions. It states that therapeutic recreation is comprised of two distinct specializations that together make up the profession of therapeutic recreation. Under this position, the provision of leisure education services would be subsumed under the treatment or therapy specialization. It also implies that the two specializations have unique purposes and therefore encompass different knowledge, skills, and competencies. The two specializations combined, however, would make up the therapeutic recreation profession.

The primary purpose of the first group would be to treat, change, or otherwise ameliorate effects of illness and disability and to promote optimal healthy functioning. The purpose of the second group would be to provide recreation services and opportunities for persons with disabling conditions. Under this position, the therapeutic recreation field would cover all recreation services for disabled people, and it would divide the roles and functions into the two specializations. The rationales for the roles and functions, and the services to be provided, would be the same as described in the positions outlined earlier. The advantage of this position would be that it would include all persons currently viewed as therapeutic recreators and, at the same time, would delineate differences among the specific roles and functions.

STUDY GUIDE QUESTIONS—POSITION D

1. If this position had been adopted, would it have required giving two separate names to the specializations contained under its "umbrella"? If so, what names would you suggest for the two distinct specializations?

2. What suggestions would you make for delineating the roles and responsibilities of those providing therapeutic recreation and general recreation services under this position?

3. What effects would this position have had upon current and future accreditation efforts within the field of therapeutic recreation? What, if any, specific problems would it have created relative to this process?

4. Reflect upon the previous question with respect to the process of credentialling and the development of standards for practice.

5. With respect to professional affiliation, what type of organizational structure is implied or mandated by this position?

After the drafting of these positions and the implications developed by selected professionals, a questionnaire developed by David Park was sent to the membership of NTRS during the presidency of Carol Peterson. This survey polled the general membership of the society to determine their reactions to the four positions. Although the overall response rate was low, as indicated, an overwhelming proportion of the membership favored the adoption of position C when questioned as to which statement provided best for the development of the field. Table 3-1 indicates by employment setting the specific responses to this inquiry. Following this strong consensus of the membership for position C, the board of NTRS voted to accept it as the current philosophical stance of the society. President Vaughan then charged the Philosophical Statement Committee with generating a written version of the position. The following document is the statement which was adopted in May 1982.

TABLE 3-1   National Therapeutic Recreation Society Membership Survey Response to Philosophical Position Paper

POSITION	COM-MUNITY	CLINICAL REHAB.	PUBLIC SCHOOL	CORREC-TIONS	HIGHER EDUC.	OTHER	TOTAL
A	4 (9.5%)	4 (1.9%)	0	0	4 (8.3%)	1 (2.8%)	13 (3.7%)
B	2 (4.8%)	61 (28.5%)	2 (22.2%)	0	13 (27.1%)	2 (5.6%)	80 (22.9%)
C	31 (73.6%)	125 (58.4%)	6 (66.7%)	0	29 (60.4%)	28 (77.8%)	220 (62.9%)
D	5 (11.9%)	24 (11.2%)	1 (11.1%)	0	2 (4.2%)	5 (13.9%)	37 (10.6%)
TOTALS	42 (12.0%)	214 (61.1%)	9 (2.6%)	0	48 (13.7%)	36 (10.3%)	350 (100%)

SOURCE: *National Therapeutic Recreation Society Philosophical Issues Survey, Summary Report,* 1982, p. 9. Reprinted by permission of National Therapeutic Recreation Society/National Recreation and Park Association.

PHILOSOPHICAL POSITION STATEMENT OF THE NATIONAL THERAPEUTIC RECREATION SOCIETY

Leisure, including recreation and play, are inherent aspects of the human experience. The importance of appropriate leisure involvement has been documented throughout history. More recently, research has addressed the value of leisure involvement in human development, in social and family relationships, and, in general, as an important aspect of the quality of life. Some human beings have disabilities, illnesses, or social conditions which limit their full participation in the normative social structure of society. These individuals with limitations have the same human rights to, and needs for, leisure involvement.

The purpose of therapeutic recreation is to facilitate the development, maintenance, and expression of an appropriate leisure lifestyle for individuals with physical, mental, emotional, or social limitations. Accordingly, this purpose is accomplished through the provision of professional programs and services which assist the client in eliminating barriers to leisure, developing leisure skills and attitudes, and optimizing leisure involvement. Therapeutic recreation professionals use these principles to enhance clients' leisure ability in recognition of the importance and value of leisure in the human experience.

Three specific areas of professional services are employed to provide this comprehensive leisure ability approach toward enabling appropriate leisure lifestyles: therapy, leisure education, and recreation participation. While these three areas of service have unique purposes in relation to client need, they each employ similar delivery processes using assessment or identification of client need, development of a related program strategy, and monitoring and evaluating client outcomes. The decision as to where and when each of the three service areas would be provided is based on the assessment of client needs and the service mandate of the sponsoring agency. The selection of appropriate service areas is contingent on a recognition that different clients have differing needs related to leisure involvement in view of their personal life situation.

The purpose of the *therapy* service area within therapeutic recreation is to improve functional behaviors. Some clients may require treatment or remediation of a functional behavior as a necessary prerequisite to enable their involvement in meaningful leisure experiences. *Therapy*, therefore, is viewed as most appropriate when clients have functional limitations that relate to, or inhibit, their potential leisure involvement. This distinction enables the therapeutic recreator to decide when *therapy* service is appropriate, as well as to identify the types of behaviors that are most appropriate to address within the therapeutic recreation domain of expertise and authority. In settings where a comprehensive treatment team approach is used, *therapy* focuses on team identified treatment goals, as well as addressing unique aspects of leisure related functional behaviors. This approach places therapeutic recreation as an integral and cooperative member of the comprehensive treatment team, while linking its primary focus to eventual leisure ability.

The purpose of the *leisure education* service area is to provide opportunities for the acquisition of skills, knowledge, and attitudes related to leisure involvement. For some clients, acquiring leisure skills, knowledge, and attitudes are priority needs. It appears that the majority of clients in residential, treatment, and community settings need *leisure education* services in order to initiate and engage in leisure experiences. It is the absence of leisure learning opportunities and socialization into leisure that blocks or inhibits these individuals from participation in leisure experiences. Here, *leisure education* services would be employed to provide the client with leisure skills, enhance the client's attitudes concerning the value and importance of leisure, as well as learning about opportunities and resources for leisure involvement. Thus, *leisure education* programs provide the opportunity for the development of leisure behaviors and skills.

The purpose of the *recreation participation* area of therapeutic recreation services is to provide opportunities which allow voluntary client involvement in recreation interests and activities. Human beings, despite disability, illness, or other limiting conditions, and, regardless of place of residence, are entitled to recreation opportunities. The justification for specialized *recreation participation* programs is based on the clients' need for assistance and/or adapted recreation equipment, limitations imposed by restrictive treatment or residential environments, or the absence of appropriate community recreation opportunities. In therapeutic recreation services, the need for *recreation participation* is acknowledged and given appropriate emphasis in recognition of the intent of the leisure ability concept.

These three service areas of therapeutic recreation represent a continuum of care, including *therapy, leisure education,* and the provision of special *recreation participation* opportunities. This comprehensive leisure ability approach uses the need of the client to give direction to program service selection. In some situations, the client may need programs from all three service areas. In other situations, the client may require only one or two of the service areas.

Equally important is the concern of generalizing therapeutic recreation service across diverse service delivery settings. The leisure ability approach of therapeutic recreation provides appropriate program direction regardless of type of setting or type of client served. A professional working in a treatment setting can see the extension of the leisure ability approach toward client needs within the community environment. Likewise, those within the community can view therapeutic recreation services within a perspective of previous services received or possible future needs.

All human beings, including those individuals with disabilities, illnesses or limiting conditions, have a right to, and a need for, leisure involvement as a necessary aspect of the human experience. The purpose of therapeutic recreation services is to facilitate the development, maintenance, and expression of an appropriate leisure lifestyle for individuals with limitations through the provision of *therapy, leisure education,* and *recreation participation* services.

The National Therapeutic Recreation Society is the acknowledged professional organization representing the field of therapeutic recreation. The National Therapeutic Recreation Society exists to foster the development and advancement of this field in order to ensure quality professional services and to protect the rights of consumers of therapeutic recreation services. In order to provide consistent and identifiable services throughout the field, the National Therapeutic Recreation Society endorses the leisure ability philosophy described herein as the official position statement regarding therapeutic recreation.

STUDY GUIDE QUESTIONS[50]

1. Do you agree with the fundamental purpose of therapeutic recreation as outlined in paragraph 2 of the position statement?
2. Do you feel that the three areas of service—therapy, leisure education, and recreation

[50] Some of these questions are based upon "A Reaction to the Philosophical Position Statement of the National Therapeutic Recreation Society" by R.P. Reynolds. This paper was presented at the National Recreation and Park Association Annual Congress in Louisville, Kentucky, October 1982. David Fields, Becky Gaffney, Sue Logan, Andrea Hayward, Joseph Kelly, and James Wheeler assisted in the formulation of these issues.

participation—encompass the roles undertaken by the majority of therapeutic recreation specialists? Do you agree with the definition of purpose of each of these areas? Which area(s) of service do you feel will increase in the future? Which may decrease?

3. The terms *therapy, leisure education,* and *recreation participation* are used to define areas of professional service and to denote specific methods or techniques. Is it desirable to distinguish between processes, techniques, and areas of service in such a mission statement?

4. Do you feel that substantial overlap exists between the areas of service described in the position statement? Is it readily discernible when a client is involved in therapy, leisure education, or recreation participation?

5. Do you agree with the ultimate goals of leisure service to and for our clients as described in the document? Are there current societal trends which may cause these goals to be altered in the future?

6. Could defining three separate areas of service, as the philosophical statement does, result in different ''tracks'' of professional preparation and certification? Would this be desirable?

7. Can graduates from nonaccredited university degree programs reasonably be expected to possess competencies in all the areas of service outlined in the position statement?

8. Is the philosophical statement consistent with the goals and practices of both clinically oriented and community-based therapeutic recreation specialists?

CONCLUSION

As with all professions, therapeutic recreation must face the challenge of continuously examining and, when needed, redefining its occupational philosophy. This process will become increasingly critical as the field matures against the backdrop of a constantly changing society. Practitioners, consumers, and educators share equally the responsibility for this endeavor. Together they can and must shape the ideology which represents the basis for the provision of a most vital area of human service.

Due to the extensive discussion of each of the references provided within this chapter, an annotated bibliography has not been included. The reader is encouraged to consult the original references and the resources listed in the preceding chapter.

CHAPTER FOUR
CREDENTIALLING—
WHICH PATH?

The mark of prestige and status in postindustrial societies that is constituted by having one's occupation termed *professional* has been noted. One hallmark of professionalism is credentialling. Credentialling is the comprehensive process which encompasses the total spectrum of professional and technical verification. According to Carter, "Credentialling is a process whereby the competency level of a professional is ensured as a provider of quality service delivery."[1] From a more narrow perspective, specifically health-related, credentialling encourages and assists professionals through a process of inspection, education, and conciliation to meet and maintain preestablished standards and to maintain or improve the quality of health care.[2]

For over ten years the federal government has been concerned with credentialling in our field. Its initial attention was reflected in 1970 with the passage of the Health Training Improvement Act. Of specific concern within the act appeared to be the long-term workforce demands, those factors associated with the competency of the workforce, and the implications for quality health care.

Generally speaking, the evolution of credentialling was several concurrent

[1] Marcia J. Carter, "State Licensure: Trend or Fad" (Paper presented at the National Therapeutic Recreation Institute, Congress of Parks and Recreation, Louisville, October 24, 1982.)

[2] J. W. Cashman, "Medicare Standards of Service in a New Program—Licensure, Certification, Accreditation," *American Journal of Public Health*, 57, no. 7 (1967), 1107–1108.

efforts which became a coordinated function to better assist professionals in coping with emerging responsibilities, roles, and services. In short, the credentialling picture and the credentialling process are complex.

FORMS OF CREDENTIALLING

There are three basic forms of credentialling. Although all three are closely related, they are by definition and action distinctly different. The forms are (1) accreditation of institutions (for example, health and education) by regional or national agencies or organizations, (2) certification or registration of personnel, and (3) licensure of individual occupations. Accreditation and certification are under the control of private agencies, professional associations, or governmental agencies, whereas licensure is under the control of an agency of government. We will examine here, in brief, each of the forms of credentialling from a general perspective and its development and existence within NRPA–NTRS.

Accreditation

Accreditation is "the process by which an agency or organization evaluates and recognizes an institution as meeting predetermined qualifications or standards."[3] It applies only to institutions and their services or program of study. By means of accreditation, organizations (i.e., Joint Commission on Accreditation of Hospitals), associations or institutions (i.e., North Central Association of Colleges and Secondary Schools, one of six regional accrediting associations), and official state agencies make known to the public those colleges and universities, elementary and secondary schools, hospitals, clinics, and other institutions serving the public which meet required standards of quality determined by the accreditation agency.

Accrediting bodies, for the most part, are classified as voluntary agencies. They are lacking in the essential legal authority to compel, for example, institutions of higher learning or hospitals to become accredited. In other words, colleges and universities and hospitals, at least in theory, are free agents in determining whether or not they will seek accreditation. Be that as it may, a vast majority of educational institutions and hospitals feel a strong compulsion to submit themselves to an evaluation both from within and from without by their peers to become accredited. So strong is this compulsion for some that accreditation is regarded as a matter of life and death. Denial of accreditation will sometimes arouse deep resentments and criticisms in both the institutions and the community.

Accreditation is an American phenomenon. Technical excellence of American hospitals is in part measured by the Joint Commission on Accreditation of Hospitals (sponsored by the American Hospital Association, the American College

[3] U.S. Department of Health, Education and Welfare, *Health Resource Statistics 1976–1977*, DHEW Publication No. (PHS) 79-1509 (Washington, D.C.: U.S. Government Printing Office, 1977), p. 6.

of Physicians, the American College of Surgeons, and the American Medical Association). The commission is also involved in the accreditation of psychiatric facilities, long-term care facilities, and other facilities which will be discussed in the next chapter. The standards for accreditation are exacting and have provided by and large a valuable resource for continued upgrading of technical components of hospital services.

Accreditation of educational institutions, programs, or both in other countries is a form of review and regulation under control of governmental agencies. Accreditation in the United States has evolved as a from of voluntary self-evaluation under the auspices of nongovernmental organizations or agencies. Historically, it started in the formulation and adoption of the Constitution of the United States, which took care to provide for separation of church and state and made certain that legal control over education was a power of the state.[4] Later, during the late nineteenth century, there was a rapid proliferation of small public and private institutions alongside well-established institutions. The states were only partially able to provide the necessary controls to bring a semblance of order to these institutions. It was in this climate that a practice known as accreditation was devised.[5] Responsibility for the accreditation function was first exercised by regional associations which were originally established to improve relations between secondary schools and higher institutions and to improve college admission standards and requirements. Later the associations adopted the practice of accrediting general institutional programs. It was not until this century that professional associations began establishing procedures for accrediting professional schools and programs of study.[6] These associations are recognized by the National Commission on Accreditation which was established in 1949 to coordinate those professional organizations involved in professional accreditation activities.

Specifically related to allied health education, the accreditation of such programs is through the AMA Committee on Allied Health Education and Accreditation. The committee and twenty-nine collaborating organizations are the consortium that accredits education programs for allied health organizations. As of 1977, twenty-three allied health occupations were accredited through this committee.[7]

There are two types of accreditation in the educational arena, institutional and specialized. Institutional accreditation means that the total institution has met the standards established by the accrediting agency (i.e., North Central Association of Colleges and Secondary Schools). Specialized or program accreditation means that a part or parts of an educational institution have met certain criteria, relating usually to a single profession (i.e., parks and recreation program of study accredited by the

[4] John McCormally, "The Root of Opposition to Federal Support," *Educational Digest*, 23, no. 4 (1961), 32–33.

[5] William K. Selden, *Accreditation: A Struggle over Standards in Higher Education* (New York: Harper & Row, Publishers, Inc., 1960), pp. 7–81.

[6] National Commission on Accreditation, *Accreditation in Teacher Education (Washington, D.C., 1965), pp. 20–21.*

[7] DHEW, *Health Resource Statistics*, p. 484.

NRPA Council on Accreditation). Specialized accrediting developed as the result of the desire of professional groups to regulate the quality of the educational preparation for their professions. Usually an institution of higher education will possess institutional and several specialized accreditation programs, (i.e., teacher education, psychology, social work, business).

Very generally stated, the purposes of accreditation are fivefold.

1. To offer guidance to the public in the selection of an institution lay people may wish to patronize
2. To encourage institutions to improve their programs by providing standards on criteria established by competent bodies
3. To facilitate the transfer of students from one institution to another
4. To inform those who employ graduates of an institution or who examine its graduates for admission to professional practice, about the quality of training which the graduates received
5. To raise the standards of education for the practice of a profession.[8]

NTRS–NRPA and Accreditation.   The accreditation movement within the park and recreation field to 1977 has been well documented by Dr. Ira Shapiro. In brief, the American Recreation Society (one of the societies which merged to form the NRPA) initiated a committee in 1959 to study approaches to accreditation. By the early 1960s, the Federation of National Professional Organizations for Recreation, a consortium of recreation organizations, established the National Committee on Accreditation. In 1965 the committee published a draft of its standards and evaluative criteria which was later revised after pilot studies at several colleges and universities. Between 1966 and 1974 several informal and formal requests for recognition were made to the National Commission on Accreditation by the Committee on Accreditation. Unfortunately, the commission rejected the applications. In 1974 the NRPA established the present Council on Accreditation with approval by the NRPA Board of Trustees in 1975.[9] Since the mid-1970s, revisions have been made in the accreditation standards including the addition of therapeutic recreation accreditation standards in 1976. Also, the original accreditation process involved both undergraduate and graduate (masters) programs, but as of 1981 only the undergraduate program is considered for accreditation.

The general purposes of accreditation were stated previously. The following are the specific purposes of accreditation, as determined by the NRPA Council on Accreditation:

1. To serve the public by promoting and maintaining standards of professional preparation in recreation, park resources, and leisure services.

[8] National Commission on Accreditation, *Accreditation in Teacher Education*, pp. 12-13; Lloyd E. Blanch, ed., *Accreditation in Higher Education* (Washington, D.C.: U.S. Government Printing Office, 1959).

[9] Ira G. Shapiro, "The Path to Accreditation," *Parks and Recreation*, 12, no. 1 (1977), 29–31, 68.

2. To assist the academic unit and the administration of the institution in establishing and attaining appropriate goals and programs for recreation, park resources, and leisure services professional preparation.
3. To insure continual self-study for the purposes of development and improvement of professional preparation programs.[10]

At this juncture the reader may question the attention paid to the broad field of parks and recreation instead of to therapeutic recreation. The rationale is rather simple. No parks and recreation program of study can be solely accredited in therapeutic recreation unless the program has first met those accreditation standards associated with the basic foundation and orientation in professional preparation for recreation, leisure services, and resources. In other words, the total recreation, leisure services, and resources program is evaluated by degree level for accreditation, not a specific area of specialization such as therapeutic recreation. The therapeutic recreation specialization is evaluated according to therapeutic recreation accreditation standards after the general program meets the initial accreditation standards. If the general program meets accreditation standards, the program will be so accredited. Likewise, if the therapeutic recreation option or specialization meets the standards, it will be included within the total program of study.

Certification and Registration

Recognition of the competence of individual practitioners may be accomplished by membership in the professional association, by certification, or by registration. Certification is a voluntary and national process "by which a governmental or nongovernmental agency grants recognition to an individual who has met certain predetermined qualifications set by a credentialling agency or association."[11] Certification is often considered a personal credentialling alternative to either licensure or registration. Further, certificiation may be looked upon as a base for state licensing standards.

Registration, on the other hand, is "the process by which qualified individuals are listed on an official roster maintained by a governmental or nongovernmental agency."[12] A registry may be the product of a national-level certification program sponsored by a professional association, a state-level licensure program approved by state government, or both.

Historically, the development of certification was the result of members of the same occupation banding together for comradeship. Accompanying this association was an interest in advancing the knowledge or in perfecting the skills of the occupation by sharing experiences and counsel. Although most of the early professional

[10] Council on Accreditation, *"Standards and Evaluative Criteria for Recreation, Park Resources and Leisure Services Baccalaureate Curricula* (Alexandria, Va.: National Recreation and Park Association, 1981, Rev.), p. 1.

[11] U.S. Department of Health, Education and Welfare, *Credentialling Health Manpower*, DHEW Publication No. (OS) 77-50057 (Washington, D.C.: U.S. Government Printing Office, 1977), p. 4.

[12] DHEW, *Health Resource Statistics*, p. 6.

groups or societies were local, they eventually met in state and, later, national conferences to discuss mutual interests and concerns. Often they published outstanding professional findings, along with proceedings of their annual meetings.

An additional motive for association was a desire to gain status for the entire membership. As a result, associations began to sponsor and urge the adoption of certification plans which would not only protect their status but also indicate to the public their concern for the public's needs. Thereafter followed the establishment of a register of "qualified" practitioners. Once certification was achieved, the next logical step was licensure, although a number of other historical factors entered into this procedure.

Some professions have established certification boards, specialty boards, or registries for the purpose of distinguishing quality. Qualifications for certification or registration may include graduation from an accredited program of study, acceptable performance on a qualifying examination, or completion of a given amount of work experience. In some instances, persons who meet certain requirements of education, experience, and competency and who pass an examination given by the certification or specialty board can use specific professional titles.

It is not unusual to find confusion existing among accreditation, certification, and licensure regarding the concept of competency. Theoretically, licensure is supposed to assure minimal competence, whereas accreditation and certification are designed to promote high standards of education and practice. In reality, certification is often used in place of licensure and only assures minimal competence. However, according to Benjamin Shimberg at the Educational Testing Service in Princeton, New Jersey, the "purpose of certification is to enable the public in general and employers in particular to identify those practitioners who have met a standard that is usually set well above the minimum level required for licensure."[13] One is inclined to assume that reference in the previous statement is being made to educational qualifications because the National Commission for Health Certifying Agencies makes a similar reference but definitely alludes to educational qualifications.[14]

In December, 1977, sixty-five professional health associations formed the National Commission for Health Certifying Agencies as the result of an acknowledged need to develop and encourage high standards of professional conduct and service among health-certifying agencies. The commission has developed nationwide standards for the certifying agencies which attest to the competence of the individuals who participate in the health care delivery system.[15]

[13] Benjamin Shimberg, "Testing for Licensure and Certification," *American Psychologist*, 36, no. 10 (1981), 1139.

[14] National Commission for Health Certifying Agencies, "Background on Issues," in *Perspectives on Health Occupational Credentialling*, DHHS Publication No. (HRA) 80-39 (Washington, D.C.: U.S. Government Printing Office, 1980), p. 10.

[15] National Commission for Health Certifying Agencies, "Bylaws and Criteria for Approval of Certifying Agencies," December 1978 (personal copy). See also, National Commission for Health Certifying Agencies, "The Development of Commission Standards," in *Perspectives on Health Occupational Credentialling*, DHHS Publication No. (HRA) 80-39 (Washington, D.C.: U.S. Government Printing Office, 1980), pp. 95–103.

NTRS–NRPA and Certification and Registration.   The roots of the therapeutic recreation certification and registration movement are found in the National Voluntary Registration of Hospital Recreation plan established in 1956 by the Council for the Advancement of Hospital Recreation. An excellent description of this movement is provided by Dr. Marcia Jean Carter in a 1981 article "Registration of Therapeutic Recreators: Standards from 1956 to Present."[16] Since 1956 the plan has undergone several revisions designed to upgrade and recognize appropriate training and educational qualifications. In fact, it appears that NTRS has completed a circle in its certification plans. Originally there was a two-level plan, which went to a six-level plan during the 1970s, and has now returned to a two-level plan. Of special note was the extensive research associated with the present plan, which began in 1980, to bring the plan more in line with existing allied health programs and the revised therapeutic recreation competencies established by the Council on Accreditation. These efforts resulted in the implementation of a two-level certification plan—Professional (Therapeutic Recreation Specialist) and Paraprofessional (Therapeutic Recreation Assistant) in 1981.

Occurring simultaneously with the proposed revision of the certification plan was a move to reorganize the NTRS Registration Board, so as to address in a more specific and comprehensive fashion the credentialling needs of therapeutic recreators. This concern resulted in the establishment of the National Council for Therapeutic Recreation Certification (NCTRC) in 1981. The council is a policy-making body financially independent of NTRS. Its present board arrangement consists of nine members, with representation from the professional and para-professional levels of certified members, consumers, supervisors or employers, and one appointment from both the NRPA Board of Trustees and NTRS. A Certification Review Board, a standing committee of the council, reviews applications three times yearly. The purposes of the Council are:

1.   To establish national evaluative standards for the certification and recertification of individuals who attest to the competencies of the therapeutic recreation profession.
2.   To grant recognition to individuals who voluntarily apply and meet the established standards.
3.   To monitor the adherence to the standards by the certified therapeutic recreation personnel.[17]

In addition to these purposes, the council promotes the delivery of quality therapeutic recreation services, distributes a registry, and communicates with other credentialling professional groups.[18] In sum, the establishment of the council and of the two-level certification plan brings the therapeutic recreation credentialling movement into closer alignment with other recognized credentialling systems and

---

[16] Marcia Jean Carter, "Registration of Therapeutic Recreators: Standards from 1956 to Present," *Therapeutic Recreation Journal*, 15, no. 2 (1981), 17–22.

[17] National Council for Therapeutic Recreation Certification, "Fact Sheet" (Alexandria, Va., n.d.).

[18] *Ibid.*

aids in the overall credibility and recognition not only of NTRS, but also of therapeutic recreators as professionals.[19]

Licensure

By definition licensure is "the process by which an agency of government grants permission to persons meeting predetermined qualifications to engage in a given occupation and use a particular title."[20] A license to practice within a state, issued by a state agency, is a means of identifying individuals within given professions or occupations who have attained the minimal degree of competency necessary to ensure that the public health, safety, and welfare of the citizens within that state will be reasonably well protected. Licensure is a government responsibility whose function is to protect society from malpractice by incompetent individuals. Some of the professions and occupations usually licensed are within the health care areas, and some are not. As of 1977, more than thirty occupations in the health field were licensed in one or more states,[21] although Carter estimated that forty-five different occupations were licensed as of 1981.[22]

Licensing is viewed by government as a regulatory device. Licensing to regulate the right to practice a profession or trade has long been accepted as a proper exercise of the police power of the states. Modern regulatory processes are an outgrowth of practices that date far back in history. Many of the system's organizational features, its basic concept of protection, and its status in law were to a large degree well defined long before there was a New World. There is considerable evidence that the modern occupational associations in some of their aspects are analogous to the medieval guilds of merchants, craftsmen, and the professions.

By the end of the sixteenth century, however, the medieval concept of the guild as a self-regulatory system of industrial control had for all practical purposes broken down. Although features of the guild system (departmentalization of labor into master, journeyman and apprentice; legal regulations for apprentices; and authority of the state to regulate prices) came to colonial America with skilled artisans and men of professional backgrounds, the guild concept never took firm root. Although the economic revolution in the early nineteenth century encouraged the development of some examination and licensing of occupations, it was not until after the Civil War that standards of training and competence were established within occupations. This was achieved primarily through the efforts of local, state, and national associations or societies which adopted and, to an increasing extent,

---

[19] The National Council for Therapeutic Recreation Certification Standards can be found in Appendix A. The National Council for Therapeutic Recreation Certification (NCTRC) and its certification should not be confused with the National Certification Board (NCB) and the Model Certification Plan for Recreation, Park Resources, and Leisure Service Personnel, which was also approved in 1981. The NCTRC and its plan are for therapeutic recreation personnel only whereas the NCB and its plan are directed toward other park and recreation personnel who provide leisure services.

[20] DHEW, *Health Resource Statistics*, p. 7.

[21] *Ibid.*

[22] Carter, "State Licensure."

enforced codes of ethics and standards of competence. Accompanying this activity, the states reversed their pre–Civil War position and assumed the responsibility of regulating the professions as a means toward greater protection of the public from incompetency, fraud, and quackery. Nor were the professions alone affected by new trends. By the opening of the twentieth century there was a rapid increase in the number of regulatory statutes enacted by both the federal and state governments to protect the nation's resources and labor and the public's health, welfare, and morals.[23]

State government understandably became more complex as it legislated in an expanding area of public service. Services which customarily had been local responsibilities—education, health, and welfare—now gradually became the responsibility of state government. It was in such a pattern of economic and governmental development that our present occupational licensing system appeared.[24]

If one were to review historically the trends in occupational organization relative to licensing, the following would appear: (1) State agencies have replaced private associations as the chief instrument for regulating admission to and practice in various professions and trades, (2) licensing has increasingly become a centralized function, (3) in each occupation there is a natural trend from optional certification to compulsory licensing, (4) the number of licensed occupations is increasing, and (5) there is continual demand for raising and tightening of qualifications for issuance of licenses.

There are two basic kinds of licensing laws for individuals, mandatory laws (sometimes referred to as *compulsory acts*) and permissive laws (sometimes referred to as *voluntary acts*). Mandatory laws forbid any person from performing the activities and assuming the responsibilities of a particular licensed profession or occupation unless legally licensed or functioning within the proper scope of another licensed profession or occupation for which he or she has been granted a license. In essence, a mandatory act is the legal right to practice. Permissive laws do not forbid unlicensed persons from engaging in the activities and assuming the responsibilities of the particular licensed profession or occupation, but they do forbid unlicensed persons from using the designation authorized by law for licensed individuals or from indicating to the public that they have been awarded licenses.[25]

A licensing law for a professional, usually called a *practice act,* has four basic elements: (1) definition of practice; (2) provision establishing a board of examiners, usually consisting exclusively of others in the profession, to implement and administer the law; (3) enumeration of criteria and qualifications for licensure and procedures to be followed in granting and renewing licenses to qualified applicants; (4) description of conduct in violation of the law and of conduct that establishes a

[23] The Council of State Governments, *Occupational Licensing Legislation in the States* (Chicago, 1952), pp. 11–27.

[24] *Ibid.*

[25] U.S. Department of Health, Education and Welfare, *Development in Health Manpower Licensure: A Follow-Up to the 1971 Report on Licensure and Related Health Personnel Credentialling*, DHEW Publication No. (HRA) 74-3101 (Washington, D.C.: U.S. Government Printing Office, 1971), p. 21.

basis for suspension or revocation of a person's license. Under a typical licensing statute, certain educational and training requirements must be satisfied. More than likely, the applicant will be expected to successfully complete an examination and possess satisfactory personal qualities. The function of the board of examiners usually consists of, but is not limited to, the following: determining eligibility of applicants, setting standards of ethical conduct, disciplining unethical and perhaps incompetent practitioners, and assessing the qualifications of applicants who possess out-of-state licenses.

The elements described here can be found in most professional practice acts. However, state laws governing the various professions are not identical; they vary somewhat from state to state. This variation is a direct result of our federal system. Each state is free to decide which professions and occupations to license and whether a particular licensing law should be mandatory or permissive. Individual states may also define each licensed profession or occupation and establish the qualifications (i.e., certification by one's own professional organization or graduation from an approved or accredited program of study before taking the examination) and the manner of selection of board members. In short, states are able to determine all aspects of the licensing plan, subject only to constitutional limitations.

Professional-practice acts contain the definition of the specific professions' practice, but they are not always cast in identical language. What usually occurs is that the national association of the profession develops a "Model Practice Act," which is then shared with respective state associations. Thus, in some states, there is little or no modification of the Model Practice Act; in other states the language of the definition is considerably different. For the most part, the definition is conceptual in approach, with a listing of a few techniques and procedures.

NTRS–NRPA and Licensure.   Although a number of states have licensure plans relative to parks and recreation personnel in general, only two states at present have therapeutic recreation licensure laws—Utah (1975 and amended in 1981) and Georgia (1981). During the past decade, more than a dozen states have considered professional-practice legislation, but only Utah and Georgia have enacted such.

In Georgia, both kinds of licensure laws exist for therapeutic recreators; "mandatory licensure for therapeutic recreation professionals in a medically based agency or institution and permissive licensure for therapeutic recreation professionals in a municipal, county, or other nonmedically based agency or setting."[26] Their professional-practice statement follows.

"Practice of Therapeutic Recreation" means, but is not limited to, the following:
(1) Assessment of leisure functions; determining an individual's present level of recreative and leisure behavior and performance by using standardized procedures which include history taking, observation, staff, client, and family interviews, test of

[26] Board of Recreation Examiners, *Law for the Georgia Board of Recreation Examiners* (Atlanta, 1981), p. 3.

leisure interests, motor and perceptual skills, social skills, and learning skills; and activity analysis for the purpose of preparing an individually prescribed leisure plan which will be goal oriented and stated in behavioral terms and which will provide a schedule of service and evaluation, and

(2) Therapeutic recreation services, which is a process that uses recreation services for purposive intervention in some physical, emotional, or social behavior to bring about a desired change in that behavior and to promote the growth and development of that individual.[27]

The purposes and definitions of the Recreational Therapy Practice Act, which is mandatory licensure in Utah, read as follows:

Purposes of Act.

The purposes of this act are to safeguard life and health, to promote emotional, social, physical and intellectual growth through the prescription and application of therapeutic recreation activities, to protect the public interest and welfare, to ensure high quality service, and to protect both the individual who receives such services and the qualified persons rendering it in good faith, by licensing and identifying to the people of this state those individuals practicing recreational therapy within the State of Utah who meet the qualifications set forth in this act.

Definitions.

"Recreational Therapist" means any person licensed to perform recreational therapy under the provisions of this act including: therapeutic recreation technicians, therapeutic recreation workers, and master therapeutic recreation specialists.

"Practice of professional therapeutic recreation" means the performance for compensation or personal profit of any act in the initiation, prescription, direction, supervision, performance, or participation in any sport, game or other recreational or leisure activity while representing the same to be a treatment with the purpose to improve, maintain, prevent or retard the development of emotional, social, intellectual, or physical pathology in others; in the supervision or teaching of other persons to perform such acts; or in the performance of any service requiring substantial specialized judgement and skill in the use of recreation for treatment of others based on knowledge of principles of biological, physical, social, psychological, and recreational sciences.[28]

In sum, licensure attempts to regulate for the benefit of the people as a whole. It is in this social environment that groups seek legislation to license occupations in order to raise standards of practice, eliminate fraud and incompetence, and, thereby, protect public health and welfare. But this same goal—improving the social environment—has also brought concern over potential monopoly, restriction in consumer choice, and added barriers to the right of individuals to select their own vocations. These factors and others in association with credentialling will be discussed shortly.

---

[27] *Ibid.*, p. 1.

[28] Division of Registration, *State of Utah Recreational Therapy Practice Act* (Salt Lake City, 1981), p. 1.

THERAPEUTIC RECREATION
CREDENTIALLING: PROS
AND CONS

Most, if not all, therapeutic recreation educators and practitioners support the concept and importance of credentialling. It is one of the major vehicles for professional status, and it certainly is the chief avenue for acceptance of therapeutic recreation practitioners within health care settings, especially those which are medically oriented. Yet there are pitfalls and problems associated with credentialling; more so with certification and licensure than with accreditation. Our intent here is to consider for your future discussion both the pros and cons of credentialling.

Accreditation

Almost every profession has adopted accreditation as a means of suggesting how its practitioners should be prepared. Unfortunately, like any form of regulation which involves controls and restraints, accreditation has never been completely accepted as necessary or desirable by all park and recreation educators, including therapeutic recreation educators. As one university president commented to one of the authors recently, "Accreditation is self-serving."

The truth is that our accreditation movement has been forced upon us by a variety of internal factors, even though we recognize that the major objective of accreditation is to raise by external sources the standards of education for the practice of our profession. As a result, some therapeutic recreation educators have taken a laissez faire approach to the development of therapeutic recreation course content or programs of study which do respond to public and health service needs regardless of setting. In other instances, departments have indicated to potential students that they have a therapeutic recreation option when in fact they have none. Thus the "competitor," if you like, and the student need to be protected. External forces are many, but probably the most important one is the fact that the vast majority of allied health personnel are graduates of accredited educational programs in their fields. Therapeutic recreation practitioners in the health setting must interact with personnel from these other disciplines. Graduation from an institute offering an accredited therapeutic recreation option attests to a minimum of academic quality and provides recognition, respectability, and prestige.

In considering the pros and cons of accreditation, it seems appropriate to identify some influences of accreditation relative to therapeutic recreation. There is no question that, as a result of the accreditation movement, there is more balance and less diversity. Therapeutic recreation courses; their content and sequencing, fieldwork standards, and experiences; and the program of study in general have been strengthened, whether the overall department program has been accredited or not. Further, accreditation has tended to improve the quality of therapeutic recreation faculty, research efforts, and finances. On the other hand, one criticism of therapeutic recreation accreditation frequently heard, if not in relation to park and recreation curricula as a whole, is the human factor which makes it impossible to have a uniform interpretation and application of therapeutic recreation standards. Specifically, criteria for evaluation are not applied evenly. Other arguments frequently heard against therapeutic recreation accreditation include, but are not limited to, the following: (1) Accreditation emphasizes minimal or acceptable quality rather than high quality; (2) accreditation standards are universal and do not consider local or regional standards or concerns; (3) accreditation standards lack consensus on what professional preparation should include, and, until such consensus can be reached, it is presumptuous to establish national standards; (4) accreditation criteria promote uniformity of standards and practices and discourage innovation and experimentation; (5) accreditation perpetuates self-preservation rather than public good; and (6) successful compliance by the student with therapeutic recreation accreditation standards does not necessarily mean successful professional performance.

This last point has a number of supporters. In fact, a number of investigators have questioned the relationship between professional educational standards and job performance. In those studies relating to health care, researchers found that health care employers tend to demand too much education for the job rather than considering the performance of the individual on the job. Hoyt upheld this notion after his review of studies relating to college success and postcollege accomplishments found that there was no more than a very modest correlation between college success and adult success, "no matter how you defined it."[29] Berg also reinforced this point in an elaborate study of education and job performance in a number of vocations including paramedical work, medicine, and administration by those who hire health personnel. He found that there was a tendency for persons to be in jobs that utilize less education and less professional techniques than they had obtained. Berg further suggested that more emphasis be placed on the task to be performed and the work environment. He stated that the "critical determinants of performance are not increased educational achievement but other personality characteristics and environmental conditions."[30] Berg's study makes one consider the proposition that under certain conditions too much education can cause or create difficulties.

The arguments in favor of therapeutic recreation accreditation are impressive, and they are as follows: (1) Accreditation improves the quality of professional practice, (2) accreditation assists in the successful building of a public image of therapeutic recreation as a profession, (3) accreditation provides reliable information to NCTRC and licensure boards for certification and licensure purposes, (4) accreditation assists in neutralizing political and group pressures from internal and external sources, (5) accreditation helps to overcome diversity in therapeutic recreation courses and curricula in some programs of study in relation to other health professions, (6) accreditation reflects the scope of therapeutic recreation, (7)

[29] Donald P. Hoyt, *The Relationship between College Grades and Adult Achievement: A Review of the Literature* (Iowa City, Iowa: American College Testing Program, 1965).

[30] Ivar Berg, *Education and Jobs: The Great Training Robbery* (New York: Praeger Publishers 1970), p. 73.

accreditation facilitates communication with other professional accrediting agencies, and (8) accceditation discourages governmental involvement in control of curricula.

It may be concluded that the two sets of arguments appear to offer no specific consensus on whether there should or should not be accreditation. Such arguments, however, do not nullify or even reduce the need for establishing accreditation and applying standards and requirements in the education of potential therapeutic recreation practitioners. Quite to the contrary, accreditation is worth the effort, time, expense, and problems because a profession that fails to judge itself and its processes will surely soon lose its right to respect from those it serves. Any sort of accreditation must take into account a concern for the public. But at the same time, as Frank Dickey, a former director of the National Commission on Accrediting, states, "Voluntary, nongovernmental accreditation is the single most important indication of quality."[31]

Certification and Registration and Licensure

Because certification and registration and licensure are closely related and in some instances overlap, we will consider the pros and cons of these forms of credentialling together. It needs to be noted initially, however, that licensure draws considerably more criticism than certification and registration. In fact, there is little criticism of certification and registration independent of licensure. Perhaps this is the result of a complex society and the extraordinary increase in state legislation requiring governmental examination and licensure in order to practice the professions. It is a difficult process for legislators and administrators to forge conflicting group demands into responsible public policies.

We will begin our discussion by listing several positive and negative aspects of licensure which have implications regarding therapeutic recreation practice. Following this will be a more in-depth discussion of some related factors relative to the health workforce and therapeutic recreation in particular. We will conclude with comments about the future of certification and licensure for therapeutic recreators.

Beneficial consequences of licensure may be summarized as follows:

First, in modern urban society, government agencies are responsible for insuring adequate knowlege and competence among those ministering to the public and its health and well-being. This can only be accomplished by defining the conditions of admission to, and retention in, the specific occupations involved in providing services.

Second, the intense specialization in all fields that is characteristic of our complex society often means that the public may fail to distinguish between compe-

---

[31] Frank Dickey, "The Continuing Need for Non-Governmental Accreditation" (Paper delivered at the National Conference on Accreditation of Public Post-Secondary Occupational Education, Atlanta, November 12, 1971).

tent and incompetent practitioners. State licensing therefore performs a vital function in protecting the people from fraud and poor service.

Third, licensing only competent and well-trained personnel protects the health of people.

Fourth, the boards of examiners provide the citizen who has limited time and money with a simple and inexpensive administrative avenue for redress against malpractice.

Fifth, through penalties imposed in various statutes, such as revocation of a person's license, the board can force licensed practitioners to be accountable to high standards.

Sixth, licensing boards, composed of experts, are able to keep pace with advances in the field and see that the standards of service available to the citizen are in reality put into effect.

Despite these potential benefits, the following criticisms are raised:

First, licensing may limit the number of entrants to an occupation by establishing unduly restrictive experiential and educational requirements. This may tend to create an artificial scarcity of personnel.

Second, by creating monopoly conditions through the erection of barriers to admission for licensing, licensure may raise the price a person pays for a service and restrain competition to a degree detrimental to society as a whole.

Third, the licensing board may incorporate the ethics, standards, and particular interests of the profession into administrative regulations and thus give the status of public law to essentially private rules.

Fourth, by defining the limits of a particular profession to include only certain practices and to exclude others, the board may inhibit the development of new techniques and skills necessary to improve services for people.

Fifth, the board may take arbitrary and unreasonable action in revoking the rights of persons to practice the occupation of their choice.

Sixth, professional associations are inclined to resist the participation on boards of consumers, who are seen as lacking sufficient experience and technical qualifications to make policy determinations affecting practice in demanding and sophisticated health fields.

According to some, credentialling of the health workforce tends to represent a gyroscopic instrument, because it provides balance without forward progress. The intent of licensing, as indicated earlier, is to protect the public from incompetent practitioners as well as to upgrade the particular profession or occupation. Until recently, the credentialling function was thought to be of concern only to professional organizations and individuals. Now that health has become a national priority, Americans are witnessing a shift in attitudes concerning public interests and accountability. Can therapeutic recreation in its present stage of development as a profession be accountable to the public for its services regardless of setting? In other words, does therapeutic recreation rank high enough to inspire true public confidence in what we say we do? According to Goode, laymen usually cannot evaluate professional services adequately, especially the services of a new profession.[32]

The following statement appears to describe very succinctly the present adequacy or inadequacy of the licensure process:

> If an occupation validates its right to call itself a profession, it becomes a monopoly in the public interest. The members of the occupation get the right to call others incompetents or quacks, and this enables the occupation to eliminate competition from outsiders and to validate its claim to be serving society in an honorable way . . . Further, since the work of a profession involves an essential service which no one else can perform, no one else can claim the right to tell the members of the profession how to do it or even how it should be evaluated. Consequently, professionals attain great autonomy and power. Still another advantage is that one can control entry, decide what the qualifications of people who seek entry shall be, organize their training, and thus decide who one's colleagues are going to be. One gets to control the process of one's services by the control of competition and influence on state and federal lawmakers, through professional association and other pressure groups. One gets to control the behavior of the members of the occupation and hence is able to enforce standards and maintain whatever values the occupation thinks are desirable.[33]

Licensing laws are receiving much criticism, as we have alluded to, because in many circles citizens believe laws have contributed to the inherent inefficiency of the health care system. It is charged that licensing limits the number of practitioners, allows the particular profession to have control over the educational curriculum, and allows further professional control by placement of its own members on the state licensing boards and on accreditation committees. Licensing, then, does not necessarily mean that the profession's standards and requirements have been elevated or approved as being a valuable element for society; it only means that the licensed individual has met standards set by his or her profession. The argument that is voiced by the professionals and the professional associations in setting and maintaining all of the controls is that members of a profession are the most qualified to judge performance and to establish educational standards.[34]

There are other factors in the credentialling process that beg consideration. At a time when innovations are needed in the delivery of services, the licensure system has an inhibiting effect. According to Hershey:

> The major effect of our mandatory licensing system for professional and occupational specialists in the health field is to establish a rigid categorization of personnel that tends to interfere with the organization of services by health institutions to meet the demand of patient service.[35]

[32] William J. Goode, "Encroachment, Charlatanism, and the Emerging Professions: Psychology, Sociology amd Medicine," *American Sociological Review*, 25, no. 12 (1960), 902.

[33] Edward Gross, "When Occupations Meet: Professions in Trouble," *Hospital Administration*, 12, no. 3 (1967), 40–41.

[34] Mark R. Arnold, "An Assault on Professionalism," *National Observer*, April 13, 1970, p.m.

[35] Nathan Hershey, "The Inhibiting Effect upon Noncertification on the Prevailing Licensure System" (Paper delivered to the New York Academy of Science, New York City, March 28, 1964).

Another factor is that, as new professions or occupations enter the health arena, such as therapeutic recreation, they frequently cross the lines of old disciplines. Licensure laws have been inept in delineating the latitude of functions for particular occupations. Therefore it is difficult to define those duties that rightfully should be the sole responsibility of a particular profession and those that can be shared with other professions. For example, how does therapeutic recreation fare with occupational therapy?

Other impediments in the licensure system concern geographic and career mobility. With respect to geographic mobility, recognition of licensure from state to state is achieved in either of two ways: by endorsement or by reciprocity. Theoretically the two differ, but practically the two terms are used interchangeably. They both involve equivalence of licensure requirements. The practice act establishes the qualifications for licensure. The fact that these criteria differ from state to state has been pointed out. Thus persons licensed to practice in one state may be barred from practicing in another unless they obtain a second license. This can become a serious problem when a new service system is developed, because it precludes the possibility of transferring licensed health workers throughout an organized health system.

What are the issues inherent in licensure that affect career mobility? Licensure practices are criticized on the grounds that they "lock in" individuals to certain positions and exclude others. The professions are criticized for controlling who enters their ranks on the basis of licensure and certification procedures. Some feel that practitioners skills and competence in job performance should be the criteria for upward mobility. Several states have enacted career mobility legislation so as to allow recognition of limited education or experience to facilitate upward mobility.

To offset some of the problems associated with licensure, a number of proposals by individuals and national health organizations have been offered. *Institutional licensure* is one such proposal by an individual which has received support in some circles as an alternative to individual licensure. Although not as strong a movement today as it was in the early 1970s, it is still being discussed. Under institutional licensure, a single license would be issued to employing institutions, replacing the licensure of individual practitioners. Individuals, except physicians, would be hired or promoted on the basis of skill, education, and training rather than on the basis of licensure.[36] Another proposal is that of the American Hospital Association. They propose, within a plan called *AMERIPLAN*, a national licensure system as a basic guarantee of qualifications in lieu of individual licensure.[37]

As noted, the state government is responsible for licensing; however, the federal government from time to time has also been concerned. In fact, PL 91-519, which was enacted on November 2, 1970, contained an amendment to the Public Health Service Act which instructed the Secretary of HEW to:

. . . prepare and submit to the Congress, prior to July 1, 1971, a report identifying the major problems assocated with licensure, certification, and other qualifications for practice or employment of health personnel together with summaries of the activities of Federal agencies, professional organizations, or other instrumentalities directed toward the alleviation of such problems and towards maximizing the proper and efficient utilization of health personnel in meeting the health needs of the Nation.[38]

[36] 3/M, "An Alternative to Mandatory Licensure of Health Professionals," *Hospital Progress*, 50 (1969), 73–79.

[37] American Hosptial Association, *AMERIPLAN—A Proposal for the Delivery and Financing of Health Services in the United States* (Chicago, 1970).

[38] U.S. Department of Health, Education and Welfare, *Report on Licensure and Related Health Personnel Credentialling*, DHEW Publication No. (HSM) 72-11 (Washington, D.C.: U.S. Government Printing Office, 1971), p. 71.

The Committee on Licensure ended its report with the following recommendations:

1. All states are urged to observe a two year moratorium on the enactment of legislation that would establish new categories of health personnel with statutorily-defined scopes of functions . . . It would be unwise to develop new statutes that define functions narrowly and that establish rigid requirements for education and training . . .
2. All States are urged to take action that will expand the functional scopes of their health practice acts and that will extend broader delegational authority—both of which will facilitate the assignments of additional tasks to qualified health personnel . . .
3. All States are encouraged to adopt and utilize, fully, national examination for those categories of health personnel for which such examinations have been prepared . . .
4. The Department (HEW) encourages the development of meaningful equivalency and proficiency examinations in appropriate categories of health personnel for entry into educational programs and occupational positions . . . Educational institutions, accrediting agencies, and certifying bodies are asked to continue to formulate programs that accept alternatives to formal education for entry into career fields . . .
5. State licensing boards are urged to take—with the active support of the professional associations—new steps that will strengthen the boards and that will allow them to play an active role in maintaining high-quality health service . . .
6. The professional organizations and States are urged to incorporate a specific requirement for the assurance of a continued level of practitioners' competence as one condition in the recredentialling process . . .
7. The concept of extending institutional licensure . . . has important potential as a supplement or alternative to existing forms of individual licensure. Demonstration projects should be initiated as soon as practicable . . . [39]

Also of interest is that, in 1977, the Department of Health and Human Services (formerly HEW) requested state legislative bodies to provide documentation for five criteria to use in determining the appropriateness of licensure for health personnel. The questions asked were:

1. In what way will the unregulated practice clearly endanger the health, safety, and welfare of the public and is the potential for harm easily recognizable and not remote or dependent on tenuous argument?
2. How will the public benefit by an assurance of initial and continuing professional competence?
3. Can the public be effectively protected by means other than licensure?
4. Why is licensure the most appropriate form of regulation?
5. How will the newly licensed category impact upon the statutory and administrative authority and scopes of practice of previously licensed categories in the State?[40]

Before proceeding, it is important to draw to the reader's attention the concern of NTRS for those other than therapeutic recreators who enter the field and for the need for continuing education, both of which items were a part of the recommenda-

[39] *Ibid.*, pp. 73–77.
[40] Carter, "State Licensure."

tions made by the Committee on Licensure.

Historically, the NTRS has always provided opportunities for those without a baccalaureate degree in either recreation or therapeutic recreation to enter the career field of therapeutic recreation. A combination of criteria has been used including experience, completion of the NTRS 750 Hour Training Program, and various degree programs.

It has become apparent in our dynamic society that the more professionalized occupations become, the more a lifelong process of education is required. Therapeutic recreation educators and practitioners have offered and participated in continuing-education programs in a variety of ways to upgrade skills and retain competence. Since 1977 the NTRS has had a Continuing Professional Development Review Board whose purpose it is to review applications submitted by sponsors of continuing professional therapeutic recreation training programs and to study the issue of continuing competence of therapeutic recreation personnel. In almost all of the medical and allied health professions, one must be prepared to learn new techniques in order to keep occupational skills current. The growth during the late 1960s and the 1970s in America of the continuing-education movement and its specialized institutions was a response to this need. A variety of methods were being used—academic studies, in-service education, workshops, extension studies, institutes, seminars, lectures, conferences, and home study programs.

Today there exists considerable controversy about continuing education. The question of mandatory versus voluntary continuing education is being debated in every state among examining boards and within professional organizations. In fact, mandatory continuing education is at a standstill. It is for this reason that the NCTRC certification plans do not at present recognize continuing education units, even though they approve of continuing education in principle. The major criticisms of continuing education are many and varied depending upon whom you are discussing the matter with and what books or reports you have recently read. Record keeping and transfer of evidence of continuing education is one reason. Research is also lacking as to the value of continuing education in association with the competency of the practitioner. Evaluation of the experience does not support the time and money required, and "forced feeding" of the practitioner may not change a person's mind-set regarding new techniques and services. Finally, instructors may have no clear objectives in mind relative to the content of the learning opportunities to be provided. What criteria would be established, and by whom, for deciding that continuing education properly relates to job performance and meets either the therapeutic recreation licensure or certification requirement? It is not enough to determine that continuing education is a "good thing." Rather, does it do what it purports to do—insure continued competency in practice?

It is well for us now to summarize our discussion about credentialling and pose a few questions. Many forces have contributed to the complex problems of regulation of health personnel. The philosophy of accountability and the changing concept of accountability are directly challenging the professional and occupational power structure. Issues of accountability pose very serious questions: Where should the authority for accreditation and credentialling really reside? Who should resolve these issues—a governmental agency, the dominant profession's association, the public, or the educational institutions responsible for the various educational programs?

This issue gives you the opportunity to debate with our therapeutic recreation practitioners what credentialling path therapeutic recreation should follow. Before you make up your mind, allow the authors to add some additional comments. According to the approved NTRS Philosophical Position Statement, the implications of credentialling are as follows:

> Current action and movement toward an independent certification body and toward national examination would be consistent with this position. Efforts would have to span the scope of the three services and develop and maintain liaisons and contacts with both the allied health field and the recreation field.[41]

Dr. Carter raised a number of important issues and questions concerned with therapeutic recreation credentialling during the 1982 NTRS Institute in Louisville. Some of the issues voiced relate to items discussed above—geographic and career mobility, variance among states regarding the organization and operation of state boards and agencies, and differences in the Practice Act from state to state. Another concern centers around the issue of control and authority. Dr. Carter asked the question of where to locate power for the administration of a therapeutic recreation credentialling program—In the professional organization or in professional practice legislation? In recent years, she continued, courts appear to be functioning as certification agents, proclaiming that to license unqualified professionals is to deny the consumer the protection of the law.[42]

Licensing boards possess a large array of power. The manner in which they exercise this influence affects the economy and the public at large. Through the examining power and the power to establish, within limits, qualifications for applicants, boards may determine how many persons shall be permitted to practice. In fact, such power could have a direct impact on the quality, availability, and cost of service to the consumer. By defining who may practice and how they function, laws affect the cost of health care because more types of personnel must be employed. And, if adequate numbers of such individuals are not available, the services may not be provided or may be extremely costly.

In a more positive vein, as indicated earlier, certification in many instances acts as a base for state licensure standards. Licensing legislation usually makes special provision for utilizing such expert knowledge in formulating standards of training and admission requirements and in determining compliance. Thus the professional associaton concerned is invited to participate in determining standards of admission and conditions of continuance in practice. However, some states have

---

[41] David C. Park, *Philosophical Alternatives Monograph* (Arlington, Va.: National Recreation and Park Association, n.d.), p. 20.

[42] Carter, "State Licensure."

developed bipartisan regulatory boards, while others, in relation to the specific occupation, have excluded or prohibited the appointment of representatives of the occupational group, and they use an advisory council of professionals to advise them. In this regard, Dr. Carter posed the question: "Is therapeutic recreation ready for such a partnership?"[43]

Before reacting to the response of Dr. Carter relative to the credentialling issue, you may wish to respond to some other questions concerning credentialling which she has posed, specifically:

1. Can we easily define our scope of practice?
2. What is meant by the phrase "quality therapeutic recreation service"?
3. What are the specialty areas and unique techniques employed in therapeutic recreation?
4. Can therapeutic recreation document financial accountability?
5. Does a core curriculum in therapeutic recreation exist?
6. Can we adequately delineate the functions performed by entry level therapeutic recreators?
7. Do we know how frequently our professionals need to renew their competence?[44]

Dr. Carter concluded her presentation as follows:

Increased public demands for the assurance of practitioner competence as well as practitioners' interest in professional recognition have contributed to the growth and concern for an appropriate credentialling program for therapeutic recreators. A credentialling trend exists. Licensure for therapeutic recreators is a premature priority. Therapeutic recreators lack the solid theoretical and practical base and the political astuteness to develop and maintain or justify the existence of state licensure. A more appropriate posture for the present is to coordinate licensure and certification efforts of NCTRC and state licensure bodies.[45]

SUMMARY

There has been an extraordinary increase, over the last two decades, in state legislation requiring governmental examination and licensure in order to practice one's profession. One professional group after another has sought legislative and administrative support for enactment and enforcment of legislation to establish educational and experiential qualifications, to require passage of an examination, and to provide for issuance of a state license—all as prior conditions for entrance into the occupation. This raises the general question as to the degree to which professional groups integrate their interests and activities with those of society. Some basic questions are as follows: Under what circumstances are governments becoming

[43] *Ibid.*
[44] *Ibid.*
[45] *Ibid.*

more dependent upon professional contributions and cooperation? Conversely, to what extent and under what circumstances are professional groups, like therapeutic recreation, becoming more dependent upon government sanctions and protection? What are the effects of governmental sanctions and protection of older professions in relationship to the emerging professions like therapeutic recreation, whrein there is some overlapping and there are possibly some competing areas? Under what conditions might therapeutic recreation licensing, as an example, establish professional monopolies that lead to social rigidity and that do not reflect the needs of society?

In conclusion, Wilensky, in an historical study of the process of professionalization in eighteen occupations, found that where the area of competence is not clearly exclusive, legal protection of the title (certification or registration) is the aim; where definition of the area of competence is clearer, a licensure act (Practice Act) is established. Further, licensure laws usually come toward the end of the professionalization process; therefore, occupational groups "cannot claim this as a unique feature of their development."[46] Still further, he inferred that turning toward legal protection, regardless of form, is usually the result of internal debates among occupational members hoping to enhance status; or it may be forced upon them, resulting from public demand for protection.[47]

Whether proceeding toward licensure or certification, responsiblity for assuring service quality through self-regulation has been a definitional characteristic of groups which seek the designation of *profession*. Professional associations create codes of ethics and standards for training, to guarantee the technical competence of their members. Among health professionals, all manner of societies attest to a certain practitioner's achievement of a superior skill in a specialized area. These certifications and recertifications are the most widespread response of various professions to the need for some type of minimal quality control and public accountability.

STUDY GUIDE QUESTIONS

1. Discuss the NTRS's concern for the provision of adequate numbers of qualified therapeutic recreation personnel and its related activities for the past five years.
2. What is the relationship of NCTRC to government?
3. Consider the two therapeutic recreation practice acts in this chapter and respond to the following: (1) What are their positive points? (2) What are their weaknesses?
4. Prepare a Therapeutic Recreation Practice Act.
5. Decide what are the two outstanding credentialling problems facing NCTRC.
6. Review the historical development of the NCTRC certification and registration plan. Outline and discuss the rationale for the various certification and registration plans that have been in existence from 1956 to the present.
7. Develop a 2,000-word paper addressing which credentialling path you would take.

---

[46] Harold L. Wilensky, "The Professionalization of Everyone?" *American Journal of Sociology,* 120, no. 2 (1964), 145.

[47] *Ibid.*

8. Review a barber or beauty operator licensure act and compare it to an allied health occupation or therapeutic recreation licensure act.

9. List other advantages or disadvantages of accreditation; likewise, of certification and licensure.

10. From a therapeutic recreation perspective, respond to those questions found on pages 82 and 83.

11. What is your response to Dr. Carter's summary of certification versus licensure found on page 82.

ANNOTATED BIBLIOGRAPHY

BERG, IVAR, *Education and Jobs: The Great Training Robbery*. New York: Praeger Publishers, 1970. Looks at the relationship of education to employment through a review of early and new studies from a sociological perspecitve.

BULLOCK, CHARLES C., and MARCIA JEAN CARTER, "Status Report: Continuing Professional Development Program for Therapeutic Recreators," *Therapeutic Recreation Journal*, 15, no. 2 (1981), 46–49. Focuses on the efforts of the NTRS Continuing Professional Development Program to maintain quality within continuing education programs.

CARTER, MARCIA JEAN, "Registration of Therapeutic Recreators: Standards from 1956 to Present," *Therapeutic Recreation Journal*, 15, no. 2 (1981), 17–22. An historical review of the NTRS registration program from 1956 to 1981.

HENDERSON, KARLA A., "Continuing Education Needs of Therapeutic Recreation Professionals," *Therapeutic Recreation Journal*, 15, no. 1 (1981), 4–10. Explores the continuing education needs of therapeutic recreation specialists in Wisconsin and offers recommendations to be considered by specialists and institutions in providing continuing-education opportunities.

HENKEL, DONALD, "Certification/Registration: A Necessity, "*Parks and Recreation*, 10, no. 2 (1975), 25, 37–39. A response to David R. Yale's article "Certification/Registration: A Mistake." Reviews efforts toward certification and registration, their importance to the field, and eventual association with educational accreditation.

HOULE, CYRIL O., *Continuing Learning in the Professions*. San Francisco: Jossey-Bass, Inc., Publishers, 1980. Points out the need for professionals to continue expanding their knowledge, based on newer concepts and ideas.

MCCARBERT, PEGGY, "The Efficacy of Continuing Education," pp. 89–99, in *To Assure Continuing Competence*. Report of the National Commission for Health Certifying Agencies, DHHS Publication No. (HRA) 81–5. Washington, D.C.: U.S. Government Printing Office, April 1981. Reviews the various problems associated with continuing education and the need for additional research before issues in the area can be resolved.

O'MORROW, GERALD S., "Therapeutic Recreation: Its Problems and Future," *Therapeutic Recreation Journal*, 15, no. 2 (1981), 31–38. Overviews the history and purpose of accreditation, especially NTRS accreditation, curriculum, and potential future curricula.

SHAPIRO, IRA G., "The Path to Accreditation," *Parks and Recreation*, 12, no. 1 (1977), 29–31, 68. An excellent historical article on the NRPA accreditation movement to 1976.

U.S. DEPARTMENT OF HEALTH AND HUMAN SERVICES, *Perspectives on Health Occupational Credentialling*. Report of the National Commission for Health Certifying Agencies, DHHS Publication No. (HRA) 80–39. Washington, D.C.: U.S. Government Printing

Office, April 1980. Reports on the commission's efforts to assure the public that professionals certified in commission-sanctioned programs are acting within demonstrated ranges of competence. Also reports on a research program designed to provide insight into, and comprehensive perspectives on, health occupation certification.

YALE, DAVID R., "Certification/Registration: A Mistake," *Parks and Recreation*, 10, no. 2 (1975), 24, 36–37. A negative reaction to certification and registration programs as proposed by NRPA. Hints that those without degrees and experience and minorities will not qualify. Further, those with creative ability from other fields will not be able to transfer ability to parks and recreation because they cannot qualify for certification and registration.

BIBLIOGRAPHY

BERNSTEIN, ALAN H., "Licensing of Health Care Personnel, *"Hospitals*, 45 (1971), 128–31.

CURRAN, W.J., "New Paramedical Personnel: To License or Not to License," *New England Journal of Medicine*, 282 (1970), 1085–91.

DELANEY, PATRICIA A., "Presenting Our Professionals, *"Parks and Recreation*, 11, no. 8 (1976), 27–44.

———, "Registration/Certification, *"Parks and Recreation*, 11, no. 7 (1976), 78–79.

DUBIN, S.S., "Obsolescence or Lifelong Education: A Choice for the Professional," *American Psychology*, 27 (1972), 486–92.

FREIDSON, ELIOT, *Professional Dominance: The Social Structure of Medical Care*. New York: Atherton Press, Inc., 1970.

HALVERSHAM, KIP J., "Career Development: Continuing Education Needs," *Leisure Today* (April 1979), 26–27.

HUTCHINSON, IRA J., *Registration and Certification Work Program on Building Professionalism for the NRPA National Council*. Arlington, Va.: National Recreation and Park Association, 1973.

LAWRENCE, PATRICIA, "Certification: The Time Is Now," *Therapeutic Recreation Journal*, 11, no. 3 (1977), 103–4.

MATTRAN, K.J., "Mandatory Continuing Education Increases Professional Competence," in *Examining Controversies in Adult Education*, ed. K.J. Mattran. San Francisco: Jossey-Bass, Inc., Publishers, 1981.

NATIONAL COMMISSION ON ACCREDITING, *Accreditation: Federalization or Nationalization*. Washington, D.C., 1972.

NEVINS, JOHN F., *A Study of the Organization and Operation of Voluntary Accrediting Agencies*. Washington, D.C.: National Commission on Accrediting, 1959.

NEWMEYER, ELLYN, and CAROL PETERSON, "Therapeutic Recreation and the Accreditation Issue," in *Expanding Horizons in Therapeutic Recreation VI*, eds. David J. Szymanski and Gerald L. Hitzhusen, Columbia, Mo: Department of Recreation and Park Administration, 1979, 261–65.

PERRY, J. WARREN, "Career Mobility in Allied Health Education," *Journal of the American Medical Association*, 210 (October 6, 1969), 107–11.

POTTINGER, PAUL S., "Taking Licensure: Competencies for Complacency," *Pro Forum*, 2, no. 2 (1979), 5–7.

RAY, ROBERT O., "Toward Continuing Education: A Preliminary Inquiry into the Professional Development of Therapeutic Recreation Specialists," in *Expanding Horizons in Therapeutic Recreation VII*, ed. Gerald L. Hitzhusen. Columbia, Mo.: Department of Recreation and Park Administration, University of Missouri, 1980.

SELDON, WILLIAM K. and HARRY V. PORTER, *Accreditation: Its Purpose and Uses*. Washington, D.C.: The Council on Postsecondary Accreditation, 1977.

SHARPLES, JOSEPH, "Registration/Certification," *Parks and Recreation,*9, no. 8 (1974), 26–27, 46–47.

SHIMBERG, BENJAMIN, "Testing for Licensure and Certification," *American Psychologist,* 36, no. 10 (1981), 1138–46.

STEINLOFF, R., and B. BLATOWSKI, "Continuing Education Opportunities," *Parks and Recreation,* 11, no. 7 (1976), 67–68.

SZYMANSKI, DAVID J., "Statement of Therapeutic Recreation Credentialling," in *Expanding Horizons in Therapeutic Recreation VI,* eds. David J. Szymanski and Gerald L. Hitzhusen. Columbia, Mo.: Department of Recreation and Park Administration, 1979, 257–60.

U.S. DEPARTMENT OF HEALTH AND HUMAN SERVICES, *To Assure Continuing Competence.* Report of The National Commission for Health Certifying Agencies, DHHS Publication No. (HRA) 81–85. Washington, D.C.: U.S. Government Printing Office, April 1981.

WEISS, CAROL, JUDITH BIEBER, CAROLYN PETERSON, and LINDA WOLD, "Danger: Therapeutic Recreation at Work," *Therapetuic Recreation Journal,* 17, no. 1 (1983), 12–17.

WHITMAN, JEFF, "Mandatory Continuing Education: A Look Before Leaping," *Leisure Commentary and Practice,* 1, no. 5 (1982), 2–3.

WITT, PETER A., "Professionalism/Certification/Accreditation," *Leisure Commentary and Practice,* 1, no. 2 (1982), 1–2.

CHAPTER FIVE
DEVELOPMENT AND IMPLEMENTATION OF PROFESSIONAL STANDARDS

Standards of practice for therapeutic recreation programs and personnel within health care and municipal park and recreation settings have for some time been a subject of interest and concern to therapeutic recreation practitioners and educators and to those concerned with the professionalization of therapeutic recreation. The purpose of standards is to provide or outline a minimal norm of acceptable functioning, activity, and practice. Standards are associated with such terms as *quality of service, quality assurance, assessment, evaluation, accountability, audit*, and *regulations*, to name a few. Standards are also associated with facilities, supplies and equipment, and personal qualifications. Standards have been established by government at all three levels, by various national voluntary regulatory agencies, and by professional organizations and occupational groups. As yardsticks, standards divide matters into two classes—satisfactory or unsatisfactory.

It is the purpose of this chapter to consider those events and factors which have led to the development and implementation of standards in general and of current therapeutic recreation service or program standards in particular. This will include a discussion of the consumer movement in human service and of the role of government in shaping human-service policy, including the various factors which influence the direction of health and human service legislation and which eventually lead to the setting of standards. Thereafter, the discussion turns to the measures undertaken by organizations (governmental and non-governmental) to assure quality service, including therapeutic recreation service, and the problems inherent in attempting to measure the effectiveness of standards with reference to therapeutic recreation standards. An additional theme focuses on the consideration of personal ethics as a standard of conduct that guides individuals in providing a service ideal.

HISTORICAL NOTES

Interest in standards of service, especially those relating to health and human services, is a relatively recent development. Although laws and regulations to improve services date back many decades, widespread concern about the development of adequate standards on the part of health and human-service administrators, professionals, congressmen, business and community leaders, and consumers can be considered essentially a post–World War II phenomenon.

There are numerous reasons for this recent surge of interest, and they include pressures from within the health and human-service field, as well as forces at play on the greater social scene. Forces within the health and human-service field stem from the professions and their members' quest to improve internal quality control. As a result, professionals have moved from narrow inquiries about the success or failure of a given service to an individual to a broader concern about the efficacy of services with larger population groups.

The most significant factor of the recent interest in standards, however, is that it is no longer professionals alone who are asking what hitherto had been academic questions about quality of service. Equal, if not greater, interest in quality service and standards is being displayed by consumers and legislators. It is from these quarters that some of the most pertinent and difficult questions are being posed.

In the health arena for example, consumer concern has been building to a rapid crescendo in recent years. There is discontent with availability of care when needed, dissatisfaction with the quality of care when rendered, and universal criticism of its costliness. Today, quality health care is an expected, essential, and important societal imperative in our culture. Further, medical care is considered to be effective only if it covers the entire range of services, preventive and rehabilitative as well as curative. Accordingly, the American people are becoming increasingly vocal about and dependent upon the need for more and better quality-based health services. In addition, they expect government, at a minimum, to protect them from the unnecessary risks attendant on incompetence, inefficiency, or venality. Although no hard evidence exists of the extent to which people are suffering because of deficiencies in the delivery system, there is ample evidence that many services are ineffective.[1]

Traditionally, consumers have had little voice in shaping health policy and little power to direct and redirect the health system. However, this situation has been changing rapidly. The American people are increasingly adamant about the need for more, better, and quality-based health services. Consumers today are

---

[1] Leon Eisenberg, "The Search for Care," in *Doing Better and Feeling Worse*, ed. John H. Knowles (New York: W.W. Norton & Co., Inc., 1977), pp. 235–446.

involved not only in such things as outreach services, but also in shaping health policies and procedures at many levels. Regarding the latter, for example, it has been suggested by consumers that if professionals are not able to fully enforce standards, *they* will determine program effectiveness and set priorities. Although this option has certain genuine merits, it has an equal number of drawbacks, since the abandonment of professional responsibility for standards of service can ultimately be profoundly harmful.

Paralleling the consumer's concern and action has been the involvement of the federal government in assisting the consumer. In the past the free-enterprise system promoted the notion that the delivery of quality health and human services should be managed by the private sector and that government intervention was inappropriate. However, during the past two or more decades it became apparent that the needs and interests of certain populations and groups of people were not being met. Thus congressional attention more and more began to focus on reminding individuals of their right to service and on making services more economical, comprehensive, satisfying, and accessible. As a result, a plethora of new federal programs came forth designed to encourage modifications and reforms of our traditional American private institutions. In addition, during this period, there was an exponential growth of federal funding and participation in social action programs.

Associated with this expanded role in funding and providing services, the federal government took an increasing responsibility for quality control of services directly and indirectly through inspection, regulations, and development of standards for service. Today the hand of the government appears everywhere in the health care and human-service system. Government funds, government regulations and control, and government programs are all having a growing impact on the system. Federal and state governments are searching out ways to gain control of the health care industry, according to many. Regulatory agencies inaugurated to control costs, extend and improve delivery of care, and promote appropriate utilization of health care resources abound. Governmental influences, felt most sharply with the advent of the Professional Standards Review Organization (PSRO) legislation, are but a "sign of the times" postulated James Igelhart in the *National Journal Report*.[2] In an astute analysis of creeping "regulationism" made as far back as 1973, Igelhart commented:

> This trend will accelerate dramatically in the near future. It began with regulation of prices charged by health institutions. But now it is being extended to the basic workings of the medical profession, to address the nature and quality of health services.[3]

This trend is not entirely negative, because those in need of care are beginning to receive such and the quality of service is improving. Although government regulation is increasing, we have nothing resembling the centralized government control that exists in such countries as England and Sweden.

[2] James K. Igelhart, "Health Report/Executive–Congressional Coalition Seeks Tighter Regulations for Medical-Services Industry," *National Journal Report* (November 10, 1973), pp. 1684–92.

[3] *Ibid.*, p. 1688.

ROLE OF GOVERNMENT

The legal basis for governmental health and human-service activities is found in the Constitution under such clauses as "promote the general welfare." The United States is a federation of states in which broad powers are specifically delegated to the federal government, and all powers not so delegated are reserved for the states. Within the framework of the federal Constitution, state legislatures formulate and operate under their own constitutions. Over the years, the activity of the federal goverment in the health and human-service field has met the test of legitimacy many times in the Supreme Court and has had public support.

Without question, the role of government in health and human services, but especially in health care, has grown enormously since those early days in which the Public Health Service, originating in the marine hospitals, took on the control of entrance to ports in response to such epidemics as yellow fever. Today some sixteen different agencies and departments of the federal government are engaged in health programs alone, with the largest agency being the Department of Health and Human Services. According to some, health service is now big business, the fastest growing industry in the country, employing a labor force of nearly 6.7 million people as of 1981.[4]

When health service is viewed within the complexity of today's bureaucracy, the origins of today's health and human-service programs seem obscure. Perhaps the single greatest impetus to the role of government in human services was the passage of the Social Security Act in 1935. Following the Great Depression, the act was a response to the needs of the vulnerable, in other words, the retired worker, the unemployed, the very young and the aged, and the disabled. The annual amendments to the Social Security Act make it a significant piece of continuing human-service legislation, a lesson in the history of health and human service and of changing federal-state relations.

With the establishment of the Social Security Act and subsequent health and human-service legislation, the federal government started to create an integrated federal-state health and human-service system in which the lower echelons of government were strengthened to become effective instruments of public policy. After authority is delegated to an agency, rules, regulations, standards, and guidelines are explicated; these are essential to implement the various statutes. In time, state and local health departments gradually became organized and strengthened. Grants-in-aid to states are based upon complex formulas of population, income, and the like to match federal with state monies. Grants-in-aid are accompanied by control mechanisms and accountability, uniform records and required service reports, federal audits, statewide plans, and the requirement of a state personnel system. Federal and state consultants have become involved with compliance to standards and regulations.[5]

---

[4] Janet H. Shirreffs, *Community Health: Contemporary Perspectives* (Englewood Cliffs, N.J.: Prentice-Hall, Inc., 1982), p. 241.

[5] John J. Honlon, *Principles of Public Health Administration*, 5th ed. (St. Louis: The C. V. Mosby Company, 1969), pp. 48–68.

With each succeeding piece of health legislation, the administration of health programs and services has grown more complex. In April 1953, for example, the Department of Health, Education and Welfare (HEW) was created, and its head was given a cabinet position. Because of increasing concerns about health and human services in general, HEW was separated into two cabinet level agencies in October, 1979—the Department of Education and the Department of Health and Human Services (DHHS).

By its mode of operation, the federal government has greatly influenced the private, or voluntary, sector. Over the years, the government, in response to specific problems, has extended its involvement to include hospital construction, biomedical research, manpower training, education and rehabilitation of the disabled, Medicare and Medicaid, regional medical programs, comprehensive health planning, and health maintenance organizations.

In addition to federal legislation of health and human-service programs, emphasis has also been placed upon accountability in terms of performance outcomes, particularly in relation to health care reimbursable expenses. For example, the Social Security Amendments of 1972 provided for the establishment of professional standards review organizations. These organizations, composed of physicians, use a "peer review" technique at the local level to assure that medical services paid for by Medicare, Medicaid, and other health programs are medically necessary, meet professionally recognized standards, and are provided for in the most appropriate settings.

Influences on Human-Service Legislation

Reference has been made to the marked expansion in the volume and variety of federal human-service legislation generated by the United States government. Since national health and human-service affairs often have a decided political coloration, it is well to note in brief the influences and climate within which health and human-service legislation arises to enhance the quality of life.

Public policy making is fraught with difficulty. The long-range results are often far afield from the original expectations. This, of course, has been conspicuous in such fields as defense, foreign affairs, and economics. Serious attempts to formulate a national health policy for the delivery of health services or human services in general are relatively new; likewise, in improving the quality of such services. Foreseeing the ultimate result of any policy decision is therefore quite difficult.

Health and human-service goals for the nation, as an example, are contained in the political platform upon which the president is elected. The philosophy and objectives of the candidate's political party are important clues to the kinds of legislation and human-service programs which will be proposed during the coming administration. For instance, should the federal government's budget for health programs be large or small? Should the federal budget be balanced, or should deficit spending be accepted? What is the relationship of the voluntary and private sectors of health care to the public sector?

As the reader well knows, today the relationship between the president and the Congress greatly affects the kind of health and human-service legislation enacted by Congress. The president has the advantage of setting national health goals with budget plans and can indicate which human-service legislation proposed by Congress he will authorize and finally implement. As we are also aware, the president can use the threat of a veto and can appeal to the people on national human-service issues through our public media.

In addition to the president's recommending human-service legislation, congressional members friendly to the administration and to the intent of the proposed program may introduce such. Often, and particularly when the majority political party of the Congress is not the same as the political party of the president, human-service legislation originates in the Congress itself. The details of this legislation and supportive information are supplied and developed by the executive branch, the personal staffs of the Congress members involved, and the staffs of standing or special congressional committees, normally with the assistance of strongly interested outside organizations and lobbies.

In every age, individuals in power have played key roles in bringing public awareness to health and human-service issues facing the nation. Catalysts have emerged and through personal magnetism have aroused the public interest in health and human services. Fortunately, health, as an example, has had advocates and catalysts on the national scene, but there has not always been wide representation of all health disciplines in the determination of national health concerns. The profession of medicine has traditionally had strong legislative advocates, whereas the fields of nursing and social work (and more recently therapeutic recreation) have only begun to have strong and organized professional advocates of their causes and concerns. In the past few years various citizen groups associated with health and human-service matters have also been involved in the pursuit of their causes.

Nothing holds more fascination in national and state political arenas than new and strong health and human-service advocates emerging and exercising leadership in such affairs. Ideas seldom grow in isolation, but rather from the ground swell of activity and experiences of human-service leaders. Some of these individuals are quite adept at capturing public attention through the press, popular literature, and other technologic media and bringing the issues sharply into focus with the pervasive feeling that something must be done and soon. Emerging health and human service advocates must be able to capture the tide of public opinion regarding health and human-service matters through good timing and maintaining a stand on an issue with a constituency. The professional's participation in political activities is an essential extension of public health and human-service policies which foster access to health care and upgrade the quality of human service.

Monetary assistance formerly channeled through federal agencies for categorical programs is now being provided through block grants at the state and local levels. The process broadens the political arena and heightens political action in regional, state, and local government areas through consumer input. Traditionally, the health and human service professional preferred to be insulated against such politics in the laboratory, hospital, or agency. Politics is often regarded as an unwholesome activity, tangential to the real interest of education or service. On the other hand, the professional diligently attends meetings dealing with sources of grant funds he or she seeks to receive to further a particular goal. To express the values one develops regarding one's profession, it is appropriate to influence the decision-making process about the direction of health care and human services and the allocation of the nation's resources. Relative to therapeutic recreation, the funding associated with Sections 311 and 316 of the amendments to the Rehabilita-tion Act of 1978 and therapeutic recreation services as discussed in Chapter 2 are excellent examples of the type of input by professionals that is needed to continue to support therapeutic recreation as a health and human service. Active participation by health workers at all levels of public decision making in health affairs is vital to the future of health and human services.

Dozens of federal laws are passed annually, many with far reaching con-sequences for the health and human service of individuals and groups in this coun-try. On the other hand, even though bills often die in committees, do not pass both houses, or are threatened with presidential veto, the idea often does not die. The public hearings, the debates, and the popular press may sensitize the public. Time between congressional sessions is also used to shape new and better approaches, including compromises reached by the various interest groups.

ASSURING QUALITY
SERVICE

The fact that quality care and service has emerged as an important issue with the rapid growth of health and human services in recent years has been noted. The assuring of quality care and service is found in those standards developed by regulatory bodies or agencies. These regulatory bodies consist of governmental agencies at the national, state, or local level; voluntary agencies such as the Joint Commission on Accreditation of Hospitals; and professional organizations such as the NTRS. The means used in the development and establishment of standards by government are the regulations which follow specific legislation. Voluntary and professional organizations respectively initiate standards or quality-control pro-grams based upon consensually acceptable criteria for optimum quality.

Quality assurance is a pervasive issue in health care. No one can insure absolutely that the four determinants of quality used in the *Forward Plan*—effec-tiveness, safety, cost, and patient satisfaction—will be present to an appropriate degree in every health intervention.[6] Nevertheless, it is the shared responsibility of health professionals and government to provide a reasonable basis for confidence that action will be taken both to assess whether services meet professional recog-nized standards and to correct any deficiencies that may be found. Thus quality assurance is not a guarantee of performance, much less of satisfactory results, but a process that leads to improved health care quality.

[6] U.S. Department of Health, Education and Welfare, *Forward Plan for Health: Fiscal Year 1977–1981*. DHEW Publication No. (HSM) 77-49 (Washington, D.C.: U.S. Government Printing Office, n.d.), p. 14.

The forthcoming sections consider the development of standards by various regulatory bodies or agencies. The discussion starts with a brief overview of the development of regulations by government and the nature of recent governmental health and human-service legislation which has had an effect on the establishment of therapeutic recreation programs and standards of service. Thereafter, attention is given to the various voluntary regulatory agencies which establish standards and impact on therapeutic recreation service. The discussion concludes with an examination of standards developed by professional organizations, focusing on NTRS.

Government Legislation and Regulation

The twentieth century has been marked by an expansion in the volume and variety of federal health and human-service legislation generated by the United States government. Weintraub and his colleagues identified 195 federal laws specific to the handicapped enacted between 1827 and the passage of PL 94-142 in 1975. Of these laws, 61 were passed between March 1970 and the end of 1975.[7] In 1974, 36 federal bills which directly or indirectly affected the handicapped and gifted were signed into law.[8]

Legislation is essential to assure that the rights of individuals will be protected, that services will be provided, and that a basis for quality control will be assured. Implementation of laws governing health and human services is dependent on clear regulations, responsive public and professional advocacy groups, and significant consequences for failure to comply. These conditions have not always existed in the past, but they do appear to exist today. As a result of financing many health and human-service programs in recent years, the government has been able to exercise some control over those providing services, by initiating regulations concerned with the quality of service. One is nevertheless cautious about suggesting a strong role for government in initiating more regulations; in fact, early reference in this chapter implied a "creeping regulationism" on the part of government.[9] A 1982 report of the National Commission for Health Certifying Agencies hints that, as the federal strategy changes to one of retrenchment, the diminished federal presence in the health care system could weaken efforts to assure the quality, availability, and affordability of care. Deregulation can be taken as a symbol of less government interest in these goals.[10]

A regulation is born following the enactment of a law. Congress ordinarily leaves the determination of regulations to the administrative agency charged with implementing the law. A regulation issued in accordance with prescribed processes

[7] F. J. Weintraub and others, eds., *Public Policy and the Education of Exceptional Children* (Reston, Va.: The Council for Exceptional Children, 1976), pp. 103–11.

[8] M. L. LaVor, "Federal Legislation for Exceptional Persons: A History," in *Public Policy and the Education of Exceptional Children*, eds. F.J. Weintraub and others (Reston, Va.: The Council for Exceptional Children, 1976), p. 96.

[9] Igelhart, "Health Report."

[10] National Commission for Health Certifying Agencies, *Federal Regulations of Health Occupations* (Washington, D.C., February 1982), p. 1.

thus has the force of law. After preparing a proposed regulatory approach or specific regulation, an office circulates it to other offices in the same agency. Once approved by directors of the office, division, and bureau responsible for its content, it is forwarded to the secretary of the department. Thereafter it is open to discussion by agencies both inside and outside the department. Additional regulations may be added. The next step is publication of the proposed regulation in the *Federal Register*, at which time the public has sixty days to submit comments, and public hearings may be conducted. After consideration of public comments, there is a redraft and recirculation through the various offices, and eventually the draft is given to the department administrator or secretary for final approval. The finished regulation must be published in the *Federal Register* at least thirty days before its effective date.

One should not confuse regulations with what is referred to as *guidelines*. Because of difficulties created by regulatory requirements, agencies sometimes establish guidelines rather than full-blown regulations. Guidelines do not have the force of law. An agency can also issue guidelines even if it lacks regulatory authority or cannot persuade the administration to approve proposed regulations. There are also times when an agency, rather than acting on its own initiative, receives legislative, executive, or judicial directions to issue regulations. The voices of states, consumers, professional groups, and the press also stimulate new or revised federal regulations.

Following are four important federal legislative acts that have come about as responses to national health and human-service needs and that have, in turn, affected the health and lives of millions of Americans. The enactment of federal laws such as those summarized has impact on the state and local agencies which must often manage the ensuing programs. In the process of establishing these laws, associated regulations were developed.

PL 90-480. In 1968, Congress passed the Architectural Barriers Act, which required that all buildings and facilities constructed in whole or in part with federal funds or leased by the federal government must meet the requirements of the American National Standards Institute (ANSI), *Specifications for Making Buildings and Facilities Accessible to, and Usable by, the Physically Handicapped.*[11] These guidelines are a voluntary standard that gives specifications for making features of the environment accessible. The standards detail how to make a toilet stall usable, how wide a walk must be, at what height a telephone should be for a person in a wheelchair, the type of sign that a blind person can read, and the like. They do not say where and how many of each of these to include. They are intended for use as a reference in regulations and laws and as a guidebook. Only when they become adopted do they become mandatory. All states today have legislation governing

---

[11] American National Standards Institute, *Specifications for Making Buildings and Facilities Accessible to, and Usable by, the Physically Handicapped* (New York, 1961); A project to adapt and extend these standards was completed in 1977, at Syracuse University School of Architecture, but the new ANSI standards have yet to be released.

facilities with state funds, and most states possess matching legislation for buildings renovated with state funds. Increasing numbers of local jurisdictions are requiring accessibility through ordinances, building codes, and similar regulations.

PL 92-603. A major mechanism for assessing and assuring the quality of care for the individual patient is the Professional Standards Review Organization, (PSRO), enacted into law in the 1972 Amendments to the Social Security Act. This body has four components: National Professional Review Council, Statewide Professional Standards Council, Regional Professional Standards Review Organization, and Advisory Council. The legislation applies only to government-sponsored programs—Medicare, Medicaid, and Maternal and Child Health Care. In reality, it is a tool for the control of both cost of health care and quality of care only in institutions (hospitals, nursing homes, etc.).

PSROs are nonprofit associations of physicians, primarily at the regional or local level, specifically concerned with determining whether hospitalization is medically necessary, is of appropriate duration, and meets recognized professional standards of quality. PSROs must also determine whether patient care could have been given as effectively or more economically in other types of facilities or on an outpatient basis.[12] Disagreement on any of these matters can be appealed to the statewide council.

The underlying basis of PSRO activity is peer review, in which physicians play the central role, although many functions are actually delegated to qualified nonphysican assistants (ward-experienced RNs, principally, but also health record analysts and others). Peer review relies not, as in the past, on the individual criteria of the reviewer, but on professionally developed norms, standards, and criteria for care, diagnosis, and treatment. The law stipulates that national norms may be adapted to the practices of local PSRO areas.[13]

PL 93-112. A milestone was reached regarding human-service legislation with the passage of the Rehabilitation Act in 1973. Although this act contained several important parts or features that impact on recreation services, of special note for the reader is Section 504, often compared with Title VI of the Civil Rights Act of 1964, and at times referred to as the handicapped Bill of Rights. One sentence within this section which is mandated and which has far-reaching implications for recreation services reads as follows: "No otherwise qualified handicapped individual in the United States shall, solely by reason of his handicap, be excluded from participation in, be denied the benefits of, or be subjected to discrimination under any program or activity receiving federal financial assistance."[14]

---

[12] U.S. Department of Health, Education and Welfare, *Social Security Amendments of 1972* (Washington, D.C.: U.S. Government Printing Office, 1972), p. 102. William Jessee and others, "PSRO: An Educational Force for Improving Quality of Care," *New England Journal of Medicine*, March 27, 1975, p. 670.

[13] U.S. Department of Health, Education and Welfare, *PSRO Factbook.* DHEW Publication No. (RSA) 77-12 (Washington, D.C.: U.S. Government Printing Office, 1977), p. 21.

[14] U.S. Department of Health, Education and Welfare, "Rehabilitation Act: (Washington, *Federal Register*, Part IV, 42 August 23, 1973), 163.

While recipients of federal funds are required to have each of their programs or activities accessible to and usable by handicapped individuals (Subpart C: Program Accessibility), the subpart does not require every existing facility or parts of existing facilities be accessible. Further, PL 90-480 refers to physical accessibility, while Section 504 of PL 93-112 refers to program accessibility. Thus a recreation program may require a combination of both provisions.

PL 94-142.   Perhaps the most important single piece of legislation currently affecting handicapped children is the *Education for All Handicapped Children Act* enacted in 1975 by Congress, which became effective in 1978. This law, which amended PL 90-380 and greatly expands educational opportunities for handicapped children, was designed to insure a free and appropriate public education for all special children between the ages of three and twenty-one. Children may be served in schools, institutions, or their own homes. The law provides a formula by which the federal government makes a commitment to pay an increasing percentage of the cost associated with special-education services necessary for handicapped children. Through this legislation, the federal government has attempted to assure that the rights of special children are protected, by helping subsidize the cost of services involved in special educational programs of various types. Further, the law attempts "to assure that the rights of the handicapped and their parents and guardians are protected."

Major emphasis within the act is on the word *appropriate,* and specific guidelines are given for what is considered appropriate education. The key to the definition of *appropriate* is the requirement of an individual education plan (IEP) for each child which includes an overall assessment of present level of educational performance, the establishment of specific educational goals, a statement of services to be provided to reach those stated goals, and at least an annual evaluation.

Recreation professionals feel the law has monumental importance to the field of parks, recreation, and leisure services. Although recreation service is considered a related or supportive service, it is the first time recreation has been included in educational legislation. This law begins to promote leisure and recreation as a very significant aspect of the total education of handicapped persons. In fact, the term *recreation* in this act incorporates the assessment of leisure function, therapeutic recreation services, recreation programs in schools and community agencies, and leisure education. According to Coyne,

> . . . recreation is authorized when assessment determines that leisure services are required to assist the child. After this need is determined, a statement of the specific recreation services to be provided to the child along with related goals, instructional objectives, evaluative procedures, and timelines must be included in the child's IEP.[15]

A case in point concerns a family in Massachusetts who refused to sign their daughter's IEP in the academic years of 1979–80 and 1980–81 because it did not

[15]Phyllis A. Coyne, "The Status of Recreation as a Related Service in PL 94–142," *Therapeutic Recreation Journal*, 15, no. 3 (1981), 5.

include recreation services. After some twenty-four hours of testimony (from Dr. Gerald Fain, Boston University; two therapeutic recreation practitioners; and the parents of the child involved) and over 100 pages of documents supporting the child's need for leisure services as well as the qualifications of and the validity of the therapeutic recreation profession to meet these needs, the hearing officer decided in favor of the child and parents.[16]

Voluntary Regulatory Bodies

A major voluntary regulatory body is the Joint Commission on Accreditation of Hospitals (JCAH). The JCAH is a private, not-for-profit corporation that is provider sponsored and provider oriented. It was organized in 1951 as an outgrowth of an accreditation program started and sponsored by the American College of Surgeons in 1918. The JCAH has a quasi-governmental role in that it was named in the Medicare Act passed by Congress in 1965 as a bench mark for eligibility of hospitals to participate in the Medicare program. Schlicke has asserted that JCAH accreditation has become "the most powerful standard setter and police agent for the medical profession, completely superseding the token requirements of legal licensing agencies."[17] Moreover, as Grosby commented, "JCAH has been the model for most efforts to improve services through accreditation programs and their associated quality assurance activities."[18]

In addition to accrediting general medical and surgical hospitals, the JCAH is also responsible for the accreditation and quality of care in a number of other health care facilities. In 1966 JCAH assumed responsibility for accreditation of extended-care facilities, nursing care facilities, and resident care facilities. As a consequence, nursing facilities are subject to many of the same service standards and procedures as are hospitals. An accreditation program was begun in 1972 by the Accreditation Council for Facilities for the Mentally Retarded (ACR), which had been established three years earlier by the JCAH. In 1979, however, as a result of internal differences, there was an incorporation of a new independent council outside of JCAH. Today JCAH limits its accreditation through the Accreditation Council for Services for Mentally Retarded and Other Developmentally Disabled (AC/MR–DD) to those developmental disability programs that are operated by hospitals and psychiatric facilities. In mid-1972 accreditation also became possible for public and private psychiatric hospitals, psychiatric outpatient clinics, psychiatric partial hospitalization facilities, psychiatric facilities serving children, and community mental health centers. Later, alcoholism and drug abuse facilities were added to the accreditation process. The program is conducted by the Accreditation Council for Psychiatric Facilities for the JCAH.[19]

[16] "Decision," Massachusetts Department of Education, Division of Special Education. Bureau of Special Education Appeals #3231, n.d. (personal copy).

[17] Cited in Kenneth G. Grosby, "Accreditation and Associated Quality Assurance Efforts," *Professional Psychology*, 13, no. 1 (1982), 132.

[18] *Ibid.*

[19] As a result of deregulation, it is anticipated that, by 1986, psychiatric units of general hospitals will be accredited by the JCAH *Accreditation Manual for Hospitals*, not by the JCAH *Consolidated Standards for Children, Adolescents, and Adult Psychiatric, Alcoholism, and Drug Abuse Facilities.*.

The mission of the JCAH is to determine how health services shall be provided so as to assure the best possible quality of care.[20] Hospitals are surveyed by a team of physicians, hospital administrators, and quite possibly other health personnel, who review the patients' charts, the quality of care in the hospital, and the hospital's facilities. While there are critics, including physicians, health personnel, and consumers, most agree that the various voluntary accreditation programs have had a major influence on improving the quality of care in the United States.

There is one other voluntary quality control on health care facilities from external sources that needs to be mentioned—the Commission on Accreditation of Rehabilitation Facilities (CARF). This nonprofit, private, national organization was formed in 1966, and it is concerned with establishing and maintaining standards of quality associated with facilities providing services to individuals with disabilities. The structure of the commission includes representatives from such organizations as the American Hospital Association; Goodwill Industries of America, Inc.; National Association of Jewish Vocational Services; National Easter Seal Society; United Cerebral Palsy Association, Inc.; National Association of Rehabilitation Facilities; and the National Rehabilitation Association. The standards relate to inpatient or outpatient organizations, to basic program services (i.e., assessment and evaluation; program management, treatment, and training; referral, discharge, and follow-up) and to individual programs or services (i.e., spinal cord injury, chronic-pain management, outpatient medical rehabilitation, infant and early childhood development, vocational evaluation, work adjustment, psychosocial programs).[21] Therapeutic recreation by title is a recognized service within the standards.[22]

Although various public and private health insurance programs are not regulatory agencies, they are concerned about the quality and the variations in service. Public programs (Medicare and Medicaid) do indicate a level of service for reimbursement purposes and, in so doing, address occupational (personnel) standards. Because the federal reimbursement programs provide hospitals and nursing facilities, as an example, with large shares of their revenues, these occupational standards have great influence over facility-based professions.

Private programs such as Blue Cross plans are a principal source of insurance reimbursement for hospital expenses. There are eighty Blue Cross voluntary, nonprofit prepayment plans in the United States and Puerto Rico. All plans are separately incorporated, locally administered units loosely linked by the Blue Cross Association. Local power resides in the separate plans, and this accounts for the wide variation in benefits, a fact often dependent on local history and custom. Most Blue Cross plans offer service benefits, and payment is made directly to the hospital or other provider.[23] In addition, Blue Cross, like other insurance companies, also processes claims and reimbursements for Medicare, Medicaid, and other public-

[20] Joint Commission on Accreditation of Hospitals, *Accreditation Manual for Hospitals* (Chicago, Il.: the Commission, 1976), p. 3.

[21] Commission on Accreditation of Rehabilitation Facilities, *Standards Manual for Rehabilitation Facilities* (Tucson, Ariz., 1980), pp. v–viii.

[22] *Ibid.*, pp. 40–47, 74.

[23] U.S. Bureau of the Census, *Statistical Abstract of the United States 1975* (Washington, D.C.: U.S. Government Printing Office, 1976), p. 484.

health programs.[24] In some plans, therapeutic recreation is a reimbursable expenditure.

In 1974 more than seven hundred companies in this country were writing health insurance policies. There is enormous variability in coverage offered—even greater than is true of Blue Cross—although in most communities there exist commercial health policies paralleling Blue Cross offerings in coverage as well as in cost. According to some sources, commercial companies have not succeeded better than the "Blues" in controlling either the cost of care or its quality.[25]

Medicare, a health insurance program for the aged, was created by Title 18 of the Social Security Act of 1965 and went into effect July 1, 1966. The act contains two parts; Part A provides insurance for hospital care (i.e., inpatient), posthospital extended care (i.e., skilled nursing facility), and home health benefits and is financed entirely by Social Security taxes levied on the working population and their employers. Part B, which is voluntary, provides medical insurance that covers not only care by physicians but also hospital outpatient services, physical therapy, diagnostic x-rays, and so forth. Those who elect Part B must pay a monthly premium.

Medicaid was created by the same 1965 Social Security Act (Title 19) that brought Medicare into existence. Medicaid is used to help pay the health care costs of the poor and the medically indigent of all ages. Unlike Medicare, Medicaid is not a federal program. Each state has its own Medicaid program and determines its own eligibility requirements and its own Medicaid benefits. Each state finances a percentage of its own Medicaid program, while the remaining financial support comes from the federal government.

As a result of skyrocketing hospital costs, Congress approved in 1983 a Medicare prospective-pricing plan for most inpatient services as part of the Social Security Amendments of 1983. Prospective pricing is a concept based on the grouping of direct patient cost data as determined by the diagnosis, treatment, and age of a patient. This concept is referred to as diagnosis-related group (DRG) and is a financial attempt to stabilize the Medicare program while at the same time allowing hospitals to benefit financially from improvements in management.

Under this plan the hospital is paid a preestablished rate of payment based on the discharge diagnosis, the age, the treatment procedures, and the discharge status of the patient. Itemized bills for services are no longer used. All costs for nonphysician services are included in one payment. It is anticipated that this prospective-payment procedure will encourage hospitals to contain costs by reducing the length of stay, by reducing the number of diagnostic tests, and by finding other ways to produce services for less money.

The DRG pricing system, which began in October, 1983, will be phased in over a four-year period. It applies to all hospitals except children's—psychiatric, rehabilitation, long-term, and rural hospitals with fewer than fifty beds. Although a

[24] U.S. Committee on Ways and Means, *National Health Insurance Resource Book* (Washington, D.C.: U.S. Government Printing Office, 1974), p. 209

[25] *Ibid.*

large percentage of employed therapeutic recreation specialists are found in the exempted hospitals, such hospitals are likely to be added at a later date if costs are actually reduced.

Critics of the new system fear emphasis on cost control without adequate quality control. Further, according to some therapeutic recreation practitioners, the advent of DRG billing may threaten the very existence of therapeutic recreation programs.

Professional Organizations

Professional associations play an important role in the health and human-service affairs of the nation. Further, associatons are frequently forces for change in the health field. According to a report by the National Commission for Health Certifying Agencies, "the strongest outside influence on federal regulations comes from professional associations."[26] Professional organizations, especially large ones, maintain and fund government liaison committees to monitor the course of regulations and legislation. These committees further advise government agencies about the state of the art in a profession and about perceived regulatory gaps and inconsistencies. The Health Care Financing Administration (HCFA), an agency within DHHS for example, is particularly solicitous of professional input. A case in point was the proposed regulations for hospitals participating in Medicare and Medicaid; specifically, staff requirements relative to therapeutic activities in psychiatric hospitals in March 1983. The proposed regulations recommended that hospitals select "qualified therapists and support personnel" rather than specifically mentioning "occupational, recreational, and physical therapy."[27] According to Farbman, the response from NTRS membership to HCFA was excellent,[28] and this reaction, along with resistance from the other professional organizations, caused the proposed new regulation to be put on hold.

NTRS Standards   The first major effort to develop therapeutic recreation standards is credited to Dr. Doris Berryman in 1971, who sought to define such standards relative to residential institutions in association with a grant funded by the Children's Bureau, HEW.[29] According to Van Andel, who chaired the NTRS Professional Standards Committee for many years, Berryman's results served as a major reference in the development of standards through the 1970s. Also in 1971, the NTRS Board of Directors adopted the "National Therapeutic Recreation Society Standards for Psychiatric Facilities."[30] These standards, along with others recommended by representatives of other professional organizations, provided the

---

[26] National Commission for Health Certifying Agencies, *Federal Regulations, p. 40.*

[27] Andi Farbman, "Legislative Alert," Washington, D.C.:The George Washington University, Department of Human Kinetics and Leisure Studies, February 17, 1983, personal copy.

[28] Andi Farbman, "Legislative Update," *NTRS Newsletter,* 8, no. 3 (Spring 1983), 4.

[29] Doris L. Berryman, *Recommended Standards with Evaluative Criteria for Recreation Services in Residential Institutions* (New York: New York University, School of Education, 1971).

[30] Glen E. Van Andel, "Professional Standards: Improving the Quality of Services," *Therapeutic Recreation Journal,* 15, no. 2 (1981), 24.

basic content for the JCAH, *Accreditation Manual for Psychiatric Facilities*.[31] Simultaneous with these efforts was the development and publication of *Standards for Residential Facilities for the Mentally Retarded,* by the JCAH's Accreditation Council for Facilities for the Mentally Retarded, which included recreation service standards.[32] A similar endeavor was the development of therapeutic recreation standards by the National Accreditation Council for Agencies Serving the Blind and Visually Handicapped.[33]

By the late 1970s, a document containing general standards had been developed for use in nine major settings (Drug Abuse Centers, Alcohol Rehabilitation Facilities, General Medical Hospitals, Pediatrics, Child/Adolescent and Adult Psychiatric Centers, Physical Medicine/Rehabilitation, Developmental Disorders Centers, Mental Retardation Facilities, and Skilled and Intermediate Care Facilities).[34] At the same time, as a result of an expansion of community programs for special populations, there developed a need for program standards in association with community facilities. In 1978, the NTRS Board of Directors approved community therapeutic recreation standards.[35] Since 1979, three documents have been published: *Guidelines for Community-Based Recreation Programs for Special Populations, Standards of Practice for Therapeutic Recreation Service*, and *Guidelines for Administration of Therapeutic Recreation Service in Clinical and Residential Facilities*[36]. To further assist therapeutic recreation educators and practitioners with therapeutic recreation standards, the Department of Leisure Studies, University of Illinois, in cooperation with NTRS, published *Quality Assurance: Concerns for Therapeutic Recreation.*[37]

MEASURING QUALITY ASSURANCE

As we have noted, increasing attention is being paid to improving and appraising the quality of health of individuals and human services in general. According to Van Andel, ''The primary purpose of professional standards is to upgrade and improve

---

[31] Jerry D. Kelley and B. L. Smith, "Standards for Therapeutic Recreation in Psychiatric Facilities," *Therapeutic Recreation Journal*, 6, no. 2 (1972), 53.

[32] Cited in National Therapeutic Recreation Society, *NTRS 1972 Yearbook* (Arlington, Va.: National Recreation and Park Association, 1972), pp. 100–108.

[33] National Accreditation Council for Agencies Serving the Blind and Visually Handicapped, "Social Work and Leisure and Recreation Services," *Accreditation Manual* (New York, 1973), Section D-5.

[34] Judith Goldstein and Glen E. Van Andel, *NTRS Guidelines for Therapeutic Recreation Service in Clinical and Residential Facilities*, n.d. (personal copy); and Van Andel, "Professional Standards," p. 25.

[35] Van Andel, *Ibid.*

[36]Jacquelyn Vaughan and Robert Winslow, eds. *Guidelines for Community-Based Recreation Programs for Special Populations* (Alexandria, Va.: National Recreation and Park Association, 1979); *Standards of Practice for Therapeutic Recreation Service* (Alexandria, Va., National Recreation and Park Association, 1980). National Therapeutic Recreation Society Standards Committee, *Guidelines for Administration of Therapeutic Recreation Service in Clinical and Residential Facilities* (Alexandria, Va.: National Recreation and Park Association, 1982).

[37] Nancy Navar and Julie Dunn, eds., *Quality Assurance: Concerns for Therapeutic Recreation* (Urbana-Champaign, Ill.: University of Illinois, Department of Leisure Studies, 1981).

the quality of the professional service being provided.''[38] In addition, Van Andel stated that standards relative to therapeutic recreation can be used:

> . . . to identify and define basic components needed to provide quality programs, . . . to evaluate the degree of change and/or improvement in service delivery, . . . to achieve compliance with current accreditation standards (JCAH and other accreditation review organizations), *and* . . . to help therapeutic recreation personnel document legitimate problems or limitations in therapeutic recreation service which may help justify program or personnel changes at their agencies.[39]

In summary, applying professionally determined standards and criteria assures quality in service provision.

To achieve such quality assurance implies that quality can be measured. According to many, however, quality, as a concept, is a remarkably difficult term or notion to define. The heart of the quality issue, as pointed out by McDermott, lies in widespread misconceptions about objectives and methods. He continued by saying that such basic issues as what is worthwhile measuring to assess quality, the state of the methodology, and the societal gains from alternative efforts at assuring quality have not been adequately probed or even clarified.[40]

Quality has several meanings, each of which tends to shade into the others. One is that the quality of something is identical with its nature. Another is *rank order* or *degree of excellence*. The adjectival form, *qualitative*, is the antonym of *quantitative:* whatever quality is, therefore, it cannot be quantitated. There is also a somewhat elusive connotation of wholeness in its meaning, wholeness in the sense of being greater than the sum of the parts; if one removes a component of quality, the quality itself is lost. From all this, one might reasonably conclude that quality cannot be quantitated or fragmented, but it can provide a basis for a rank order. In other words, quality can be measured, though without any degree of precision.

On the other hand, perhaps the definition of quality may be at such a fundamental level that the criteria of quality are nothing more than value judgments that are applied to several aspects, properties, ingredients, or dimensions of a process called human services. As such, the definition of quality may be almost anything anyone wishes it to be. It is to be hoped that in this vein it would be a reflection of values and goals current in the health and human-service system and in the larger society of which it is a part.

Few empirical studies delve into what the relevant dimensions and values are at any given time in a given setting. One study the authors stumbled across found that twenty-four ''administrative officials'' gave eighty criteria for evaluating *patient care.* They concluded that patient care, like morale, cannot be considered as a unitary concept and ''. . . it seems likely that there will never be a single com-

---

[38] Van Andel, "Professional Standards," p. 26.

[39] *Ibid.*

[40] Cited in Eli Ginzberg, "Health Services, Power Centers, and Decision-Making Mechanisms," in *Doing Better and Feeling Worse*, ed. John H. Knowles (New York: W.W. Norton & Co., Inc., 1977), p. 207.

prehensive criterion by which to measure the quality of care.''[41] Thus one is left with the fact that whichever of a multitude of possible dimensions and criteria are selected to define quality, they will, of course, have profound influence on the approaches and methods employed in the assessment of service.

The need to find methods stems from the impetus to determine accountability and be definitely assured of quality service. Concerning the quality of service, it is widely believed and accepted that the level of health and human service in a given community will improve if the shortcomings of the service can be identified, measured, and reported back to those providing it. Thereafter, these findings can become the basis for corrective training of professionals and for improvement of curricula for students, for example, in therapeutic recreation. Relative to accountability are a number of issues, such as the need for methods of evaluating returns of public investment in health and human services, professional and legislative standards, possible certification and recertification of personnel, demonstrated ability to contribute to the solution of problems, and some basis for comparative studies of the effectiveness of the health and human service delivered, again, as an example, by therapeutic recreation specialists.

With respect to therapeutic recreation, it is not so much a question of developing and implementing standards along with having the standards accepted by administrators and accrediting bodies, but more whether the standard assures quality. Quality-assurance activities are concerned with the expectation that, as examples, health status will be improved or patient satisfaction will be enhanced. Therapeutic recreation is not alone in attempting to assure quality, but, being the ''new kid on the block'' so to speak, we are open to more challenges than other professional organizations. As Navar and Dunn have pointed out, ''an accurate 'state of the art' description of therapeutic recreation quality assurance involvement is still unknown.''[42]

Unfortunately, the development of standards of therapeutic recreation as opposed to other professional association standards is at a somewhat primitive level, especially those relating to community settings. Further, our standards are extremely broad and have had to interface with specific facility standards of accrediting bodies. Understandably, the several sets of standards procedures which exist can produce considerable confusion and frustration for those attempting to implement their own standards and at the same time comply with organization standards. Such confusion has been described as significantly hampering implementation of quality assurance efforts.[43]

Our intent here is not to critically review and evaluate what guidelines NTRS has developed or what kinds of standards need to be developed, but rather, to consider approaches to quality-assurance procedures that will improve our standards. In so doing we need to recognize that the initial purpose of an evaluation of a

[41] M. W. Klein and others, "Problems of Measuring Patient Care in the Out-Patient Department," *Journal of Health and Human Behavior*, 2, no. 4 (1961), 138–44.

[42] Navar and Dunn, *Quality Assurance*, p. 2.

[43] Kenneth P. Drude and Ronald A. Nelson, "Quality Assurance: A Challenge for Community Mental Health Centers," *Professional Psychology*, 13, no. 1 (1982), 85–90.

health, and in some instances, a human-service facility or agency is regulatory. Such an appraisal is designed to match a facility against specific standards that determine its acceptability for the purpose of the regulatory or accrediting agency. It is intended to correct abuses and raise the general level of service to an acceptable minimum, as has been noted. The second purpose of appraisals is closely related, if not superimposed upon the first—that of serving as a stimulus for the improvement of quality. The standards may be minimum or optimum levels. The third purpose is to study the effects of specific programs or procedures on the quality of service. We may refer to this purpose as *program evaluation*. Certain procedures, such as leisure education in preparation of the individual for leisure involvement, are believed to improve functioning for daily living.[44] It is essential that the effectiveness of a procedure on the consumer be examined.

In our approach to standards and quality assurance we must also keep in mind that agency service is multidimensional. It is a service provided by a group of professional, technical, and other workers. In health care settings such a group is usually coordinated by a physician. The quality of service received by the consumer is affected by the adequacy of the agency facilities and their maintenance, by the administration and organization of the agency, by the competence of the personnel, and by the interpersonal relations among staff as well as between staff and consumer.

In considering any measurement of standards, one is confronted with how the specific standards were established. It appears that our standards are based on both *empirical* and *normative* sources.[45] *Empirical standards* are derived from actual practice. They enjoy a certain degree of credibility and acceptance because they rest on demonstrably attainable levels. Their major shortcoming, however, is that service may appear to be adequate in comparison to that in other settings and yet fall short of what is attainable through the full application of current therapeutic recreation knowledge and practice.

Normative standards, on the other hand, are derived from knowledge and practice of what is already known. In other words, they are drawn from standard textbooks or publications, from highly qualified practitioners who serve as judges within the professional group, or from others outside the profession after consultation with those inside the profession. Normative standards have the advantage of being able to be set high, to represent the "best" in service, or to be calibrated at a more modest level signifying "acceptable" or "adequate." In any event, their distinctive characteristic is that they stem from a body of legitimate knowledge and values rather than from specific examples of actual practice. As such, they depend for their validity on the extent of agreement concerning facts and values within the profession or, at least, among its leadership.

This brief commentary on the development of our standards focused on the kinds of evidence pertaining to the validity of our standards that is needed to assure the appropriateness of the services to be delivered and the quality of these services.

[44] Navar and Dunn, *Quality Assurance*, p. 150.

[45] Van Andel, "Professional Standards," p. 24.

Clearly, more empirical research is needed to support the standards we have developed. Empirical studies of the therapeutic recreation process and continuum would contribute greatly to the identification of dimensions to be incorporated into standards. In reality, we are implying a hypothesis that, given certain criteria—professional training, certification, organizational structure, supplies and equipment, facilities, and the like—the desirable quality of standards is achieved. This hypothesis should be recognized and tested explicitly so that valid criteria can be used in a more formal fashion and to better purpose.

Quality, though intangible to a great degree, is not an abstraction. Nor is the judgment of quality capricious or a purely personal whim. While agreement cannot be expected to be complete, there are numerous ways to measure quality. One such way to evaluate program or procedures on the quality of service is by considering quality from three perspectives: *outcome*, *process*, and *structure*.[46]

Outcome is a frequently used indicator of the quality of service. The validity of outcome as a dimension of quality is seldom questioned. Moreover, outcomes tend to be fairly concrete and, as such, seemingly amenable to more precise measurements. However, a number of considerations limit the use of outcomes as measures of the quality of service. The first is time. In some instances it may take a prolonged period of time before relevant outcomes are manifest. Thus results are not available for appraisal when they are needed. Although some outcomes are generally unmistakable, other outcomes are not so clearly evident. These could include consumer attitude and satisfaction, social restoration, and physical disability and rehabilitation.[47] Finally, although outcomes might indicate good or bad service in the aggregate, they do not give insight into the nature and location of the strengths or deficiencies to which the outcomes may be attributed.

Another approach is to examine the *process* of service itself rather than its outcomes. The concern here is not in achieving results as such, but in whether what is now known to be "good" or "best" service has been applied. Judgments are based on considerations such as the appropriateness, completeness, and redundancy of information obtained through technical competence in the performance of diagnostic and assessment data; the acceptability of service to the recipient; the statement of goals and objectives in writing; the following of documentation procedures; and so on. This approach requires that a great deal of attention be given to specifying the relevant dimensions, values, and standards to be considered. However, it does draw attention to whether therapeutic recreation is properly practiced.

The last approach, *structure*, is concerned with the adequacy of facilities and equipment, the qualifications of personnel, the administrative organization and operations of programs within the service, and the like. The assumption is made that, given the proper facility, personnel, supplies and equipment, good service will follow. Although this approach offers the advantage of dealing, at least in part, with

---

[46] Herbert C. Schulberg, "Quality-of-Care Standards and Professional Norms," *American Journal of Psychiatry*, 133, no. 7 (1976), 1047–51.

[47] Herman R. Kelman and Allen Willner, "Problems in Measurement and Evaluation of Rehabilitation," *Archives of Physical Medicine and Rehabilitation*, 43, no. 2 (1962), 172-81.

fairly concrete and accessible information, the relationship between structure and process or structure and outcome is not well known.[48]

The methods used to evaluate quality, based on standards, can easily be lacking in rigor and precision. However, these methods have been adequate for the administrative and social-policy purposes that have brought them into being. This is not to say that a great deal does not remain to be accomplished in therapeutic recreation in developing the precision necessary for our purposes. A great deal of effort has gone into the development of standards which are presumed to lend stability and uniformity to our service, and yet this effort has not always been empirically demonstrated. However, empirical research to support standards so as to assure quality service is not enough. Taking a page from psychology, Claiborn reminds his fellow psychologists that

> If the profession is to make a significant effort to ensure quality of service and to enforce standards of quality, it must have a strong commitment of the membership and a willingness to act (*reference here is to their Code of Ethics*). The system must be prepared to withstand challenges from those who are judged by it. Members of the profession must be willing to judge their peers (*reference here is to their State licensing–certification boards*). Perhaps most important, the basis for judging competence should be rooted in a well-based knowledge of what constitutes quality care.[49]

Although the suggestions above can be applied to recommended standards for community-based recreation programs for special populations, the effects, directly or indirectly, of federal efforts to regulate recreation service are difficult to describe because they vary so greatly from one locality to another, depending on tradition and the response of the community. Although in theory the consumer has benefited from federal legislation that affects recreation services, limited information is available in the literature to determine whether such a theory is correct. The only in-depth study reported is Coyne's study of recreation services and PL 94-142.[50] In this specific instance, the law appears to have had limited positive effect, except in isolated situations, in educating handicapped children through recreative experiences. In fact, one of Coyne's recommendations was "to formulate and implement a systematic plan of action based on the specific power structure of the state and local education agencies."[51]

In sum, the emerging profession of therapeutic recreation, relating specifically to health and human-service therapeutic recreation standards, appears to be in a state of active frustration. It is frustrated by the inability to develop faster professionally, by changing public expectations, by increasing (if not decreasing in the future) government regulations, and by the dilemmas inherent in its existing form of organization. Each year it seems to become more difficult for the field of therapeutic

---

[48] Jack Zusman, "Mental Health Service Quality Control," *Archives of General Psychiatry*, 13, no. 11 (1972), 497–506.

[49] William L. Claiborn, "The Problem of Professional Incompetence," *Professional Psychology*, 13, no. 1 (1982), 156.

[50] Coyne, "The Status of Recreation," pp. 4–15.

[51] *Ibid.*, p. 14.

recreation to maintain a traditional organizational structure in face of the onslaught of new internal developments, new regulations, and changing public demands. As consumers become yet more sophisticated in their demands, the need for greater quality assurance will increase. Therapeutic recreation has shown extraordinary adaptive capacities, but to continue to do so will require further research into standards of practice so as to ensure quality assurance. The practical task of establishing reliability and validity in our standards is formidable, but it must be done.

CODE OF ETHICS

While a professional ideal and recommended personal behavior, a commonly held goal, and agreed-upon ways of achieving it, are seen by many scholars to be the very heart of the idea, *profession*, the code of ethics is the glue that holds a profession together. A profession is concerned with both its service ideal and the quality of its professional activities. The existence of a code of ethics commits the practitioner to a high level of skill in practice as well as the enforcement of standards of practice to meet the professional ideal.

It is reasonable to expect that practitioners should seek to govern and regulate entry into their profession, monitor the practice and performance of those who are admitted, and establish procedures for the dismissal or expulsion of persons who do not meet or adhere to the practices and standards of the profession. Without the latter, there can be no code of ethics because there can be no standard of practice.

Generally speaking, codes of ethics serve a variety of purposes. They provide one basis for developing preservice curricula for the particular professional group. They help to orient new practitioners to their professional responsibilities, rights, and privileges. They recommend behaviors which are deemed most likely to result in achievement of the ideal toward which the profession is focused and which will preserve and enhance the profession for continued usefulness. They furnish the guide for distinguishing scrupulous and unscrupulous conduct. They serve as a basis for regulating the relationship of the practitioner to the consumer of the professional service, to the profession itself, to society, and to co-workers within and outside the profession. They provide the profession with a basis for excluding or reprimanding the unscrupulous or the incompetent practitioner and for defending the member who is unjustly accused of wrongdoing. They serve as a guide to the public for understanding the characteristics of professional conduct. Finally, they give the general public some sense of assurance that reliance on members of the profession is not misplaced.

A code of ethics is usually the last attribute to be developed in the process of professionalization.[52] However, the rationale for its being the last attribute developed is not clear. Some sociologists and scholars observing professional characteristics indicate that it is the nature of the process. Others suggest that the

---

[52] Harold L. Wilensky, "The Professionalization of Everyone?" *American Journal of Sociology*, 70, no. 2 (1964), 145.

profession is still technical in nature or that its members are yet to become united toward a common mission or goal. Still others say that its students are unaware that the so-called emerging profession serves a social purpose.[53]

Codes of ethics are not new. They can be traced back to ancient times. A study of the Old Testament reveals a system of laws and codes under which the Hebrew people lived. The Oath of the Hindu Physicians probably dates to 1500 B.C., and it emphasizes the ethics of the physician's conduct toward his patients. Hippocrates, known as the Father of Medicine and as the ideal physician, was born in Cos in 460 B.C. He rejected many then-current beliefs regarding medicine. To him, medicine was a science, not a mystery. To Hippocrates, medicine was the study of human beings through observation, examination, recording and analysis of findings, and application of the wisdom of the clinician. He placed emphasis on the environment and its components in order of their importance—weather, water, soil—and on the habits of people such as eating, drinking, and exercise. His respect for the personal rights of individual patients, the esteem in which he held members of the profession, and the ethical standards he established and inspired were quite remarkable. These standards have endured through the centuries.[54] Today the American Medical Association code, adopted in 1847 and revised four times, consists of ten sections treating such subjects as consultations and precedence, scientific competence, professional courtesy, cooperation with nonphysician health personnel, solicitation of patients, fees, conditions of practice, and confidentiality.[55]

Because the NTRS is, by design, a branch of the NRPA, its "Statement of Professional Ethics" is found within the *Suggested Principles of the Code of Ethics of the Recreation and Park Profession*, which was adopted in 1977, following a series of code of ethics committee actions beginning in 1973. Growth and change in the therapeutic recreation movement and shortcomings in the old code made it desirable to develop this new code of ethics. It reads as follows:

NATIONAL THERAPEUTIC RECREATION SOCIETY STATEMENT OF PROFESSIONAL ETHICS

Introduction

The National Therapeutic Recreation Society (NTRS), a branch of the National Recreation and Park Association (NRPA), is a professional organization committed to the provision of recreation services for all persons regardless of age, race, sex, national origins, religious beliefs, or physical, social or mental abilitites. NTRS maintains open membership to all persons employed in an occupation which provides recreation services for special populations (e.g. mentally ill, retarded, physically handicapped, aged, correctionally incarcerated, socially disadvantaged, etc.), and who subscribe to

[53] *Ibid.*, p. 146.

[54] Harry E. Sirgrist, *History of Medicine* (New York: Oxford University Press, Inc., 1951). William E. Peterson, *Hippocratic Wisdom* (Springfield, Ill.: Charles C. Thomas, Publisher, 1946).

[55] American Medical Association, *Ethical Principles of the American Medical Association* (Chicgo, Ill., 1955).

the professional standards and ethical practices endorsed by the governing board of the society.

The National Therapeutic Recreation Society affirms its commitment to the goals of the park and recreation movement as represented by the Constitution of the National Recreation and Park Association and acknowledges its a priori adherence to standards and principles embodied in the related health disciplines from which it draws much of its heritage of concern and standards of practice.

In this spirit, the therapeutic recreation professional subscribes not only to the ethical code adopted by NRPA, but equally subscribes to those general principles of ethical conduct endorsed by all health related disciplines.

The Statement

I. The therapeutic recreation professional believes in the value and importance of special recreation services for persons who are limited in their opportunities because of physical, social or mental disabilities. He/she is committed to the continuous task of learning and self-improvement to increase his/her competency and effectiveness as a professional.

II. Above all else, the therapeutic recreation professional is guided by the accepted responsibility of encouraging and providing quality service to the client/consumer. He/she demonstrates respect for the dignity of the client/consumer as an individual human being. He/she makes an honest effort to meet the habilitative, rehabilitative and leisure needs of the client/consumer and takes care that the client/consumer is not exploited or otherwise abused. This includes but is not limited to the guarantee of basic human rights under law.

III. The therapeutic recreation professional engages only in those activities which bring credit to himself/herself and to the profession. He/she shows respect for fellow colleagues in word and deed. When he/she becomes aware of unethical conduct by a colleague or fellow professional, appropriate and prescribed professional channels will be followed in reporting said conduct.

IV. The therapeutic recreation professional observes the principle of confidentiality in all written and verbal communications concerning clients/consumers, fellow colleagues and/or matters of professional privilege.

V. The therapeutic recreation professional serves as an advocate for therapeutic recreation by interpreting the purposes and values of the profession to client/consumers, other professionals, and the community at large. He/she accepts responsiblity for improving communications and cooperative effort among the many professional fields serving special populations. He/she encourages and participates in demonstration and investigative projects aimed at upgrading professional services and communicates the results of his/her efforts.

VI. The therapeutic recreation professional obligates himself/herself to providing consultation service to consumers, other professionals, community agencies and institutions. Fees for services, where appropriate, are made known to client/consumers prior to entering into any contractual relationships.[56]

Concepts of Ethics

In any discussion of a code of ethics, one is influenced by values or ideals held by the individual, the society, and the profession. Codes of ethics flow from values or ideals. They are, in fact, values in action. Values are formulations of preferred behavior held by individuals or groups. They imply a usual preference for certain

[56] National Recreation and Park Association, "National Therapeutic Recreation Society Statement of Professional Ethics," in *Suggested Principles of the Code of Ethics of the Recreation and Park Profession* (Washington, D.C., 1976), Section III.

means, ends, and conditions of life, often being accompanied by strong feelings. Although behavior may not always be consistent with values held, possession of values results in a strain toward consistent choice of certain types of behavior whenever alternatives are offered. The meaning attached to values is of such an impelling emotional quality that some individuals will make personal sacrifices and work hard to maintain them, while groups will mobilize around the values they hold to exert approval and disapproval in the forms of rewards and penalties (sanctions).

Terms used to express values are varied, and no two experts agree on them. A value can usually be defined only in other value terms equally prone to varied meaning, carrying their own loads of overtones and nuances. Two sources are used in the search for understanding of the term *value*. The literature of value clarification sees values as (1) guides to behavior, (2) growing out of personal experiences, (3) modified as experiences accumulate, and (4) evolving in nature.[57] This literature provides additional understanding about the nature of values by noting that the conditions in which values operate often have conflicting demands; that is, several values or end states are functioning. One example of this in therapeutic recreation may be found when working with a recently physically disabled woman. In such a case, the specialist is confronted with values of physical safety and self-determination. The disabled woman wants to participate in an activity, but it is not safe for her to do so in her present condition. Which value should take precedence? A value judgement is called for.

Milton Rokeach defined *value* as ''an enduring belief that a specific mode or end state of existence is personally or socially preferable to an opposite or converse mode or end of existence.''[58] He went on to state that values, rather than standing alone, exist in systems; that is, individual values are organized in such a manner that they have a relative importance to other values. He construed values as being relatively enduring, as beliefs upon which persons act by preference, and as modes of conduct or end states of existence. Value beliefs are conceptions of what is desirable; there is an emotion or feeling aspect to them; and they lead to action.

Perhaps another way of thinking about values is to think of what the individual or group would like to see happen; what their conception of an ideal world may be; what they would preserve from the present and what they would change if given the power to do so; what they take for granted as proper or to be expected; how they think society *should* be organized, what individuals *should* be like, what kinds of personality and conduct they wish could be developed in all people. Given a conception of what should be, groups and individuals tend to choose means and modes of life which help achieve the things they conceive of as ideal, and a system of preferences emerges.

On the other hand, the field, or discipline, of ethics concerns itself with the fulfillment of the human personality and the ideal of human action, expressed in terms such as *good* and *bad*, *right* and *wrong*, *better* and *worse*. It seeks to determine criteria by which to formulate ultimate social goals or ideals, to choose

[57] Lewis Raths, Merrill Harmin, and Sidney R. Simon, *Values and Teaching* (Columbus, Ohio: Charles E. Merrill Publishing Company, 1966).

[58] Milton Rokeach, *The Nature of Human Values* (New York: The Free Press, 1973), p. 5.

between conflicting or competing values, and to determine which should have priority. The result of such consideration may be gathered together as a body of principles referred to as *the ethics* or *ethic* (of a group, profession, etc.). Even more specifically, they may be reduced to detailed prescriptions such as *codes*.

"Ethical" behavior is behavior selected according to some common understanding as to what has been formally or informally adjudged "ideal" or "good," following approved principles or priorities by which selection among different "good" behavior is made. *Ethics* thus refers both to the process by which ideals are established and to the product of the process.

The terms *ethics* and *ethical* may have more definite connotations than *value*, but they are also hard to define and elastic in application to specific situations. General usage indicates that ethics may be thought of both as a discipline and a code, and this causes problems in working out the interrelation of professional values and ethics. Although there are many philosophic positions on this distinction, it appears that in relation to cohesive groups, like professions, there are interacting influences between values and ethics. Ethics may be thought of as a philosophic discipline which determines what is right and wrong and helps develop principles by which values, "what is preferred or best," are selected. These accepted values, in turn, influence what a group may codify as indisputably its ethical norms for right and wrong conduct.

Associated with the place of values and ethics in any profession is the service idea. Any profession stands for something which it deems highly essential to the common good of society, and which its practitioners firmly believe they have a unique part in providing as a service to the rest of society. However partial the actual fulfillment of this ideal, the ideal is there as a central, indispensable theme in all professional activity. Medicine visualizes a state of increasing longevity and optimum health; law upholds the idea of universal order and justice; education idealizes general possession of knowledge and intelligent use of humanity's accumulated experience; library science hopes for preservation of and easy accessibility to humanity's collected learning and creative thought; and therapeutic recreation wants "an appropriate leisure lifestyle for individuals with physical, mental, emotional, or social limitations."[59] These ideals or values are not unique to the profession concerned. In fact, most members in society probably would affirm their desirability in varying degree. However, while many other people may contribute to its realization, working toward the ideal is regarded as the special province of the profession. The enlargement and continuous redefinition of the meaning of the ideal and of means for its attainment are accepted as the paramount responsiblity of every member of the profession. For the professional person, the professional ideal assumes priority among many generally accepted goals for humanity.

Each profession also has idealistic words to describe what it does in its attempt to attain the ideal state to which it ascribes. This parlance often takes on a mystical or symbolic meaning. Traditionally, the clergyman *saves*, the nurse *comforts*, the physician *heals*, and the engineer *builds*. The therapeutic recreator has always *helped*, and more recently *enables* and *facilitates*.

[59] National Therapeutic Recreation Society, "Philosophical Position Statement," adopted May 1982.

The place of values and ethics in any profession, therefore, is in the personal behavior associated with the professional or service ideal. The existence of a recognized code of ethics commits the members of the profession to social values above what might be considered selfish ones of income, power, and prestige. Further, the code recommends behavior which is deemed most likely to result in achievement of the ideal toward which the profession is focused, and which will preserve and enhance the profession for continued usefulness. Still further, the code creates a sensitivity to ethical standards and is concerned with the professional's relationship to the consumer and other professionals.

Ethics in Curricula

Analysts of professional concepts observe that in the process of communicating to new recruits the professional ideal, the approved and expected behavior patterns are an inescapable core which must be deliberately learned through imitation and personal strivings to meet professional expectations. Every professional person must sense what the profession is trying to do, and, within tacitly understood or prescribed limits of variation, act as other members of the profession and the general public anticipate.

As we have noted, a profession has a service ideal, and for therapeutic recreation, like any other occupation or professional group, that ideal is to give service in as effective a fashion as possible. Effectiveness is the product of adequate knowledge and skills and appropriate recognition and use of values and ethics. The practitioner must adhere to an identifiable body of values and display attitudes which stem from these values and which determine the relationship of the person to colleagues, recipients of service, and the community. Given the fact that values and ethical behavior norms are accepted by most professions as prominent distinguishing features which must be transmitted to inductees, why has this aspect of professional preparation frequently been entirely omitted from our therapeutic recreation programs of study? A review of our accreditation standards noted that in only the most recent revised issue of the standards has ethics as a competency appeared.[60] In fact, according to Fain, "At present there is little evidence of investment by recreation and leisure professionals toward the study or promotion of ethical practice." Further, there is no reason to suspect that issues of moral or ethical substance will be vigorously pursued by the recreation and leisure professions in the near future."[61] These views and comments appear to be in agreement with the Meyer investigation reported earlier concerning therapeutic recreation and its professionalization. He reported that in the development of action (statements) needed to be taken to eventually affect the professionalization of therapeutic recreation, a code of ethics was ranked by the thirty-six panel members as fourteen within seventeen major categories. In fact, no therapeutic recreation practitioner or therapeutic recreation

[60] National Council on Accreditation, *Standards and Evaluative Criteria for Recreation, Park Resources and Leisure Services Baccalaureate Curricula* (Alexandria, Va.: National Recreation and Park Association, October 1981, Rev.).

[61] Gerald S. Fain, "Toward a Philosophy of Moral Judgment and Ethical Practices in Leisure Counseling," in *Leisure Counseling: Concepts and Applications*, ed. E. Thomas Dowd (Springfield, Ill.: Charles C. Thomas, Publisher, in press).

educator, when compared to general recreation practitioners and general recreation educators, indicated any action regarding the category.[62] Further, in the final analysis, relative to priorities for professional action, a code of ethics was not even found among the desired action of both groups. In other words, not one panel member ranked a code of ethics as one of the top five priorities in action need for professionalization.[63] Like other professions, therapeutic recreation needs to take pains to develop in its potential members the kinds of attitudes which reflect the values and ethics of its emerging professional status and are considered to be desirable traits of therapeutic recreators. In this regard, Sylvester, in exploring confidentiality in therapeutic recreation practice, found that "some practitioners were partially informed, misguided, or simply ignorant concerning matters of confidentiality.[64]

It is of vital importance that the process of training a professional entail more than transmitting technical skills. It is, in the strictest sense, a process of adult socialization when the values of the professional community are made a part of the person. Professionalization, for the individual recruit, means involvement with a community way of life and "provides life goals, determines behavior and shapes personality."[65] To put it more succinctly, becoming a professional implies incorporating important features into one's identity. As such, the professional, like anyone else, can be expected to seek experiences that will reinforce and confirm it.

Society depends upon this in the face of its inability to judge or evaluate the competence and reliability of what "it is buying."[66] In addition to whatever formal mechanisms a profession may set up to maintain professional standards, the most important mechanism is the professional's own inner controls through the practitioner's sense of personal identity. In the face of this intimate connection between one's profession and one's self, we could expect that any conditions that make demands incidental to or in conflict with a professional's sense of what is important to his or her identity would fail to gain the practitioner's full commitment and possibly lead the person to actively oppose them.

Some of the reasons for not including such matter in the curriculum, in the opinion of the authors, are:

1. There is no clearly defined, explicit demand for a therapeutic recreation service ideal or for values and ethical personal behavior from agencies employing therapeutic recreation students. Further, we do not yet know what values and ethical norms are of practical use.

    Our programs of study must follow practice, and therapeutic recreation has not identified its professional ideal with sufficient clarity to incorporate such content within its program. There is much to back this opinion. Job descriptions, civil service

---

[62] Lee E. Meyer, "An Analysis of Views of Recreation Professionals Toward Therapeutic Recreation and Its Professionalization" (unpublished Doctoral dissertation, University of North Carolina at Chapel Hill, 1978). pp. 101–2.

[63] *Ibid.*, p. 266.

[64] Charles D. Sylvester, "Exploring Confidentiality in Therapeutic Recreation Practice: An Ethical Responsibility in Need of Response," *Therapeutic Recreation Journal*, 16, no. 3 (1982), 33.

[65] Ernest Greenwood, "Attributes of a Profession," *Social Work*, 2, no. 7 (1957),45-55 206.

[66] William J. Goode, "Community within a Community: The Professions," *American Sociological Review*, 22, no. 7 (1957), 194–200.

examinations and specifications in requests for therapeutic recreators seldom list philosophical and ethical principles as such. Just why agencies have so far largely ignored this aspect of professional competence for job performance can only be speculated upon. Job specification statements seem to lean on formal definitions in terms of years of experience, needed self-knowledge, emotional development, and so on. Competence in the area of ethical perception is hard to define and measure. Further, there may also be a tendency to regard value formation and ethical behavior as an inseparable aspect of an employee's internal personality, overlooking elements of professional identification. Still further, because the student is a graduate of an appropriate training program, familiarity with professional values and ethics is assumed.

2. Therapeutic recreation values are not in any way distinctive from those any conscientious person in our North American culture would hold. Although employers want their staff members to be value conscious and ethical on the job, this is largely provided for by the process of growing up in a democratic society such as that to which professional entrants have long been exposed.

    It appears to be true that many of the values which therapeutic recreation affirms had their origins in Judeo-Christian religious beliefs and Anglo-American political and legal philosophies. However, these permeating value traditions take on a variety of forms, and each member of society makes his or her particular interpretation of them and ranks them in importance, guided by personal experiences. The student therapeutic recreator must learn the therapeutic recreation interpretation of value and ethical principles and their application to specific human situations.

3. Values and ethical norms will be learned regardless of any specific planning, because they are an integral, inseparable part of therapeutic recreation. Values and ethics belong to that part of human experience which is a by-product of living. Satisfactory professional value orientation and knowledge of professionally approved and disapproved behavior are a certain by-product of exposure to therapeutic recreation activity and theoretical formulation.

    It is difficult to assume that the therapeutic recreation educational process is pervaded with content involving value judgments and ethical considerations. Depending on the particular faculty member to whom the student is exposed, the priority value judgment and interest of internship supervisors, and the student's own inclination in suggested or optional assignments, the individual student might personally be exposed to therapeutic recreation decisions and points of view. Trusting to "exposure" involves a danger of fragmentation.

4. Values and ethical decisions are wholly a matter of individual choice on the part of each therapeutic recreator and each agency. Each therapeutic recreator must select from a myriad of value systems that which is congenial and meaningful; schools have an obligation not to teach in such a highly personal area. Each agency will ultimately judge whether each therapeutic recreator's approach meets the ethical norms of that particular agency.

    This point of view might be regarded as a laissez-faire handling of the philosophic components of therapeutic recreation, especially in light of faculty who lack knowledge about teaching values and ethics and have no deep concerns about the ethical sights of therapeutic recreators. On the other hand, however, most educators do not take responsibility, in the opinion of the authors, for exposing the student to "desirable" ways of thinking or for commending attitudes which at least conform to some therapeutic recreation demands.

In conclusion, it is of vital importance that the process of training a professional entail more than transmitting skills. It is, in the strictest sense, a process of adult socialization, where the values of the professional community are made a part of the person. Professionalization for the individual recruit means involvement with a community way of life that "provides life goals, determines behavior and shapes personality."[67] To put it more succinctly, becoming a professional implies incorporating important features into one's personal identity. As such, the professional therapeutic recreator can be expected to seek experiences that will be compatible with his or her sense of identity and that will reinforce and confirm it.

STUDY GUIDE QUESTIONS

1. What are some of the problems which have been identified in relation to health and human-service care in the United States?

2. Speculate into the future and describe what you believe therapeutic recreation service in the United States will be like in the year 2020.

3. Describe various health and human-service legislation that has been enacted over the years and discuss its effect upon therapeutic recreation service.

4. Explain the purpose of PSROs and their effect upon therapeutic recreation service.

5. How can therapeutic recreation service be improved regarding quality in both health care and community-based settings?

6. What effect might the prospective-pricing plan have upon the provisions of therapeutic recreation service? Develop strategies to include therapeutic recreation service within the prospective-pricing plan.

7. Does your program of preparation in therapeutic recreation meet NRPA/NTRS accreditation standards? If so, how could these standards be improved? If not, why not?

8. Where in your program of therapeutic recreation education are the following items discussed, if at all?
   a. Civil rights
   b. Therapeutic recreation salaries
   c. Violation of professional ethics
   d. Social-class differences
   e. Standards of personnel practice
   f. Principles of *prevention* versus *cure*

9. Prepare a list of words encountered in therapeutic recreation literature which express or convey value and ethical meaning.

10. Should the teaching of values or ethics be formal and specific or should such be learned as they occur pervasively in the curriculum? Should the emphasis be on proximate and instrumental values, or on abstract and ultimate ones? Or should students be left entirely free to make their own values choices, on the assumption that such individual liberty is consistent with academic freedom. Should the student be "indoctrinated" with the value system of professional therapeutic recreation?

ANNOTATED BIBLIOGRAPHY

AMERICAN NURSES' ASSOCIATION, "Code for Nurses with Interpretive Statements," Pamphlet. Kansas City, Mo.: The Association, 1976. Concerned with nurses' conduct and relationships for ethical practice, including responsibilities to the profession, to other members of the health team, and to the patient.

[67] Ernest Greenwood, "Attributes of a Profession," p. 54.

AMERICAN PSYCHOLOGICAL ASSOCIATION, *Ethical Standards for Psychologists.* Washington, D.C., 1977. Considers the principles or standards which guide the psychologist and the profession, with an interpretation of each.

COMMISSION ON ACCREDITATION OF REHABILITATION FACILITIES, *Standards Manual for Rehabilitation Facilities.* Tuscon, Ariz., 1980. Sets forth standards relative to inpatient and outpatient provision of services to meet needs of disabled people.

COYNE, PHYLLIS A., "The Status of Recreation as a Related Service in PL 94-142," *Therapeutic Recreation Journal,* 15, no. 3 (1981), 4–15. Reports on a national survey to determine the extent of involvement of therapeutic recreation in state and local education agencies.

HALEY, MICHAEL J., "What Is a DRG?" *Topics in Health Care Finance,* 6, no. 4 (1980), 55–61. Discusses the purpose of impact on patient care, and suggested alternatives to prospective rate setting with case examples from New Jersey and Georgia involving prospective price plans.

JOINT COMMISSION ON ACCREDITATION OF HOSPITALS, *Accreditation Manual for Long Term Care Facilities.* Chicago, Ill., 1980. Sets forth standards presumed necessary for achievement of quality care in long-term care facilities such as nursing homes.

JOINT COMMISSION ON ACCREDITATION OF HOSPITALS, *Consolidated Standards for Children, Adolescents, and Adult Psychiatric, Alcoholism, and Drug Abuse Facilities.* Chicago, Ill., 1981. Presents standards presumed necessary for achievement of quality care in psychiatric facilities and in rehabilitation facilities for alcoholism and drug abuse.

MILLER, DULCY B., "Suggested Methodologies for Auditing Programs in Long Term Care Facilities," *Therapeutic Recreation Journal,* 9, no. 3 (1975), 99–105. Denotes various approaches to evaluating therapeutic recreation programs in nursing homes, focusing on use of volunteers, administrative staff, facility staff, families to audit activity programs.

NATIONAL THERAPEUTIC RECREATION SOCIETY, *Standards of Practice for Therapeutic Recreation Service.* Alexandria, Va.: National Recreation and Park Association, 1980. Offers general standards for therapeutic recreation service in both clinical and community-based settings.

NATIONAL THERAPEUTIC RECREATION SOCIETY STANDARDS COMMITTEE, *Guidelines for Administration of Therapeutic Recreation Service in Clinical and Residential Facilities.* Alexandria, Va.: National Recreation and Park Association, 1982. Focusing on guidelines for evaluating therapeutic recreation service within various clinical and residential settings, this is a resource for developing standards for meeting various accreditation bodies' specifications such as the Joint Commission on Accreditation of Hospitals and Commission on Accreditation of Rehabilitation Facilities.

NAVAR, NANCY, and JULIE DUNN, EDS., *Quality Assurance: Concerns for Therapeutic Recreation.* Urban-Champaign, Ill.: University of Illinois, Department of Leisure Studies, 1981. Primarily offers guidelines in the development of therapeutic recreation standards in association with JCAH, *Consolidated Standards Manual for Child, Adolescent, and Adult Psychiatric Association and Drug Abuse Facilities,* but includes sufficient information for use in hospitals and long-term care facilities.

SECHREST, LEE, and PAUL E. HOFFMAN, "The Philosophical Underpinnings of Peer Review," *Professional Psychology,* 13, no. 1 (1982), 14–18. From a psychology profession perspective, sets forth the philosophical basis for peer review and tries to show how that philosophy is being used to develop a coherent point of view reflecting a responsible maturing profession.

SYLVESTER, CHARLES D., "Exploring Confidentiality in Therapeutic Recreation Practice: An Ethical Responsibility in Need of Response," *Therapeutic Recreation Journal,* 16, no. 3 (1982), 25–33. An exploratory study (N = 131) to determine whether therapeutic recreation practitioners differ in their judgments of confidential incidents according to various variables.

"THE UPHEAVAL IN HEALTH CARE," *Business Weekly* (Cover Story), July 25, 1983, pp.

44–56. Reflects the concerns of doctors and hospitals about diagnosis-related groups (DRGs).

VAN ANDEL, GLEN E., "Professional Standards: Improving the Quality of Services," *Therapeutic Recreation Journal,* 15, no. 2 (1981), 25–30. Surveys the development of therapeutic recreation standards, including their purpose and implications for their future.

VAUGHAN, JACQUELYN, and ROBERT WINSLOW, eds., *Guidelines for Community-Based Recreation Programs for Special Populations.* Alexandria, Va.: National Recreation and Park Association, 1979. Offers guidelines for program standards based on a 1979 survey of community-based special recreation programs (N = 113), notes the five most common problems encountered in community special recreation programming, and suggests resolutions.

WEST, RAY E., ed., *Issues and Guidelines for Establishing Third-Party Reimbursement for Therapeutic Recreation.* Alexandria, Va.: National Recreation and Park Association, 1981. A well-developed delineation of the problems and impact of third-party payment issues for therapeutic recreation in clinical settings, which offers guidelines for practitioners in developing third-party reimbursement.

BIBLIOGRAPHY

AMERICAN HOSPITAL ASSOCIATION, "Medicare Prospective Pricing: Legislative Summary and Management Implication," Special Report 3. Chicago, Ill.: The American Hospital Association, Office of Public Policy Analysis, April 1983.

AMERICAN NATIONAL STANDARDS INSTITUTE, *Standards Specifications for Making Buildings and Facilities Accessible to and Usable by the Physically Handicapped.* New York, 1980.

BERRYMAN, DORIS L., *Recommended Standards with Evaluative Criteria for Recreation Services in Residential Institutions.* New York: New York University School of Education, 1971.

DECKER, BARRY, and PAUL BONNER, eds., *PSRO: Organization for Regional Peer Review.* Cambridge, Mass.: Arthur D. Little Publishers, 1973.

DONABEDIAN, AVEDIS, "Advantages and Limitations of Explicit Criteria for Assessing the Quality of Health Care," *Health and Society,* 59, no. 3 (1981), 99–106.

DRUDE, KENNETH P., and RONALD A. NELSON, "Quality Assurance: A Challenge for Community Mental Health Centers," *Professional Psychology,* 13, no. 1 (1082), 85–90.

HAYS, JACK R., "Three Methods of Peer Review in a State Mental Hospital System," *Psychological Reports,* 41 (1977), 519–25.

INGBER, FERN KAUFMAN, "Issues and Guidelines for Establishing Third Party Reimbursement for Therapeutic Recreation." (Unpublished master's thesis, George Washington University, 1978).

JOINT COMMISSION ON ACCREDITATION OF HOSPITALS, *Accreditation Manual for Hospitals.* Chicago, Ill., 1980.

JOINT COMMISSION ON ACCREDITATION OF HOSPITALS, *Standards for Services for Developmentally Disabled Individuals.* Chicago, Ill., 1980.

KELLEY, JERRY D., and B.L. SMITH, "Standards for Therapeutic Recreation in Psychiatric Facilities," *Therapeutic Recreation Journal,* 6, no. 2 (1972), 52–61.

MEREDITH, JACK, "Program Evaluation Techniques in the Health Services," *American Journal of Public Health,* 66, no. 13 (1976), 1069–73.

NATIONAL COMMISSION FOR HEALTH CERTIFYING AGENCIES, *Federal Regulation of Health Occupation.* Washington, D.C., February 1982.

SELDEN, WILLIAM K., *Certification in Allied Health Profession,* Conference Proceedings. Washington, D.C.: U.S. Government Printing Office, 1971.

U.S. DEPARTMENT OF HEALTH, EDUCATION AND WELFARE, *Activities Coordinator's Guide: Long Term Care Information Series 3.* Washington, D.C.: U.S. Government Printing Office, 1978.

U.S. DEPARTMENT OF HEALTH, EDUCATION AND WELFARE, "Medical Assistance Program Intermediate Care Facilities," *Federal Register,* Part III, 39, no. 12, January 17, 1974, 2254–57.

U.S. DEPARTMENT OF HEALTH, EDUCATION AND WELFARE, "Skilled Nursing Facilities Standards for Certification and Participation in Medicare and Medicaid Programs," Washington, D.C.: *Federal Register,* Part III, 39, no. 12, January 17, 1974, 2238–54.

VAN DER SMISSEN, BETTY, *Evaluation of Community Recreation: A Guide to Evaluation with Standards and Evaluative Criteria.* New York: National Recreation Association, 1965.

YOUNG, HURL H., "A Brief History of Quality Assurance and Peer Review," *Professional Psychology,* 13, no. 1 (1982), 9–13.

CHAPTER SIX
THE DILEMMA
OF PROFESSIONAL
PREPARATION

A profession consists of individuals who possess both general and specialized knowledge and skills obtained through education, which allows them to provide specialized services to a public which recognizes and accepts their services. A professional is one who possesses competence in some area shared only by the other members of the same profession. A professional person's services are sought because that person has a competency, a mastery of knowledge and skill, which the recipient of the service does not have. It is this unique competence which determines the relations of professional communities to the larger society. The lack of such competence is a major obstacle to such recognition.

Although enhancement of the social good and promotion of professional self-interest are characteristics of organized professions, these two goals are not always necessarily compatible. One of the crucial points at which consideration of public responsibility and professional self-interest may come into conflict is in the determination of educational standards. The dynamics of the concern of the professions with educational standards are by no means uncomplicated. On the one hand, we see clearly the genuine desire to protect the interests of the society as a whole and of the user of service, specifically by an ever-increasing level of competence. On the other hand, we cannot, in good conscience, avert our eyes and fail to notice another tendency at work, a tendency that seems to be most heavily weighted in the direction of professional self-aggrandizement.

In a mood of pseudoprofundity, but with serious intent, the authors have attempted to express this tendency in the form of a law (with apologies to Professor Parkinson). This law is named the *law of professional velocity:*

> The internal dynamics of the process of professionalization result in an upward and onward motion of the profession which is expressed in a continuous pressure toward extending the educational requirement for desired professional statuses irrespective of the absence of public clamor for such professional velocity.

These remarks are not intended to be an iconoclastic assault on, or a churlish depreciation of, the importance and integrity of professions in general and therapeutic recreation in particular. The concern for putting the professions within a realistic perspective is precisely the conviction that they do play an extremely significant part in contemporary society and that they also attempt to be responsive to the public interest. It is relatively harmless to overlook semantic overidealization of things of little moment, but it can be extremely serious when matters of real importance are involved. It is in this sense that our belief in the need for a look at therapeutic recreation education can be traced to a passionate conviction about the vitality of therapeutic recreation and its potential contribution.

PROFESSIONAL EDUCATION

The function of a profession in society and the demand implicit in its practice determine the objectives of education for that profession. The responsibilities which its practitioners assume designate the content of knowledge and skill to be attained. In this respect, however, one is reminded by Ralph W. Tyler, an early pioneer in the development of professional social behavioral curricula, that in curriculum planning one must guard against confusion of professional and nonprofessional tasks that may clutter up the curriculum with activity courses that can be learned on the job. He emphasized that it is the nature of a profession to base its techniques upon principles rather than rule-of-thumb procedures or simple routine skills. A characteristic of professional education is, in fact, that it teaches a body of principles and concepts for differential use.[1]

The profession also determines the character of the educational experience which students must have to become the kind of person required both to provide competent service and to contribute to the ongoing development of the profession. Thus professional education trains for professional self-dependence. The educational system is not designed to train a few to lead, many to follow, and others permanently to serve under the guidance of more competent members. There will emerge, to be sure, those who will represent the profession, and speak and act for it as a whole. There will be those who will play an identifiable part in determining the profession's growth and in fashioning the shape of things to come by representing it in its intramural and extramural affairs, by administering its programs, by formally

[1] Ralph W. Tyler, "Educational Problems in Other Professions," in *The Role of the Professional School*, ed. Bernard R. Berelson (Chicago: American Library Association, pp. 22–28.

teaching its future members, and by engaging in and directing its research. Be what it may, the basic aim of education from a professional perspective is the same for all students, each one of whom is a therapeutic recreation specialist or a professional person in the making. The contributions of specialists are made in the future. The educational process is aimed at developing leaders for tomorrow's practice, through producing practitioners of high caliber to provide and sustain that leadership. The members of our emerging profession, like members of other professions at all operating levels, are charged with the responsibility of advancing learning and conveying such learning to colleagues and students.

The significant role of professional programs of study is supported by the fact that they are the only current gateway to a profession. The performance of professional preparation is therefore a signal service to both the profession and the public. Professional programs of study collect from a wide variety of sources a wealth of facts, ideas, principles, and technical procedures appropriate to the field. These are systematically organized with a view to their application to professional service and to their mastery by students. Educational programs unite in a curriculum a group of subjects which are intended to develop the intellectual comprehension, the practical skills, and the professional attitudes a student of the profession must possess.

As a framework for further discussion, McGlothlin has said that professional education must help the student to achieve five sets of attributes. They are as follows:

1. Competence to practice his profession, with sufficient knowledge and skill to satisfy its requirements.
2. Social understanding, with sufficient breadth to place his practice in the context of the society which supports it.
3. Personality characteristics which make possible effective practice.
4. Zest for continued study which will steadily increase knowledge and skill needed by practice.
5. Competence in conducting or interpreting research so that he can add to human knowledge either through discovery or application of new facts.[2]

The first attribute postulates that in a profession there is a recognized body of knowledge and skill to be attained for competent practice. Its practitioners must give evidence of capacity to use that knowledge and skill. Further, the profession's programs of study demand that students, upon graduation, give evidence of possessing it and of having some capacity to use it. Thereafter, evidence will be given through the provision of competent services as judged in the field of practice. As we know, some professions, like ours, have a legally constituted authority for licensing or for certification and registration of those individuals qualified for practice. This procedure imposes a demand but, in turn, affords professional status and security to the membership, both individually and collectively.

Within this process is internship for helping the student to make the transition from learner to professional practitioner; the opportunity to develop skill in applica-

² William J. McGlothlin, *Patterns of Professional Education* (New York: G. P. Putnam's Sons, 1970), p. 7.

tion of concepts, to enhance professional identification, to increase self-awareness, and to ultimately identify with the values of the respective profession so that one grounds one's self in thinking, feeling, and acting firmly on the ethics of the profession. In other words, the goals of an internship are no different from those of other aspects of the curriculum. Like other components, internship seeks to facilitate the development of professional competence and a professional personality. The internship agency is used primarily to provide the student with an educational experience, not as a means of helping the student to render service as a staff member. Thus its major goals are to (1) contribute to the student's identification with the profession as a whole; (2) contribute to the student's self-awareness; (3) facilitate the integration of knowledge, skills, and attitudes learned in class; and (4) develop the student's skill on the level of beginning competence.

This conception of internship as oriented to educational, not service, goals underscores the importance of placing students in settings which meet stipulated educational standards. It also provides the opportunity to clearly distinguish between the role of the university department supervisor and agency supervisor. The agency supervisor helps the employee to implement the agency program on behalf of the client. The university department supervisor helps students use the agency program for their own learning in the practice of therapeutic recreation. For the employee, the agency program exists to give service; for the student, the agency program exists to help the student learn skill by engaging in appropriate professional activities. In the process, of course, service is rendered.

As important as giving evidence of competence in service is that of giving evidence of one's profession's worth as a profession. A profession has a defined scope and function. It will draw on related fields of knowledge and skill. It will have, however, a content of knowledge and method peculiarly its own, to which other professions can contribute but for which they cannot substitute. It is a professional person's right and obligation to maintain that identity. The way is eased for the person when that individual is a member of a profession which operates under a legally constituted authority, but, lacking this, it is all the more the professional person's responsibility to interpret this function and not be a party to misuse. Therapeutic recreation, by its youth and nature, has had problems articulating its place with other professions and agencies. Consequently, it has served beneath and at times beyond its capacities. Providers of therapeutic recreation education today must be concerned with developing practitioners who will intelligently and responsibly define their field of practice. However, for practitioners to do this requires them to have obtained a body of knowledge and specific skills.

Since a profession is a field of service established to serve the common good, professional education has, as its second attribute, helping its prospective practitioners develop a social conscience and a social consciousness. A profession has a philosophy by which its practitioners are guided to the extent that they are not free agents but, instead, are obligated to act in accordance with the rationale, the ethical system, of the profession. Because of this obligation, professions establish a form of group discipline through a code of ethics, as noted in the previous chapter. The ethics of the profession are learned through the acculturation process, which transforms the student from a layperson to a professional person, aware of the ethical norms in professional conduct and alert to the professional choices which reflect those ethics. The professional activities of the practitioner reflect the incorporation of both scientific knowledge and the profession's ethics.

The third attribute in professional education is the development of a capacity for establishing and sustaining purposeful working relationships. Working together characterizes all professional activity, whether the relationship be that of practitioner with recipient of services, supervisor-practitioner, administrator–staff member, or members of an interagency or intraprofessional team. In therapeutic recreation this capacity, working together, is essential in helping relationships, in collaborative working relationships, and in group-to-group relationships. Usually, the attainment of the first and second objectives will bring this one into being.

The fourth attribute focuses on developing feelings and attitudes that will make it possible for the student to continue learning, to achieve greater depth and breadth of knowledge, to reach a deeper level of self-awareness, to possess a higher sense of identification with the profession, and to offer a greater degree of skill in practice. Professional education today seeks to lay the groundwork, and no more, in preparing the student for a great variety of tasks, on a great number of levels, in a great array of settings and auspices. For these reasons, professional education must prepare the student to think about the future in a conscientious and thoughtful fashion rather than leaving the matter to chance.

The fifth and final attribute is concerned with developing in the student a capacity to think critically and analytically and to synthesize and generalize; an ability to break a concept down in order to build it up for use; a capacity to apply knowledge and a well-established habit of seeking, using, and testing it critically and formulating principles. In short, it is the objective of creating and entrenching the spirit of scientific inquiry.

The advancement of knowledge demands research. A research approach to the solution of a problem enables the practitioner to learn through experience and to convey what is learned. Certain knowledge of research and disciplined thinking will make for intelligent interpretation and the use of the work of those who are specifically engaged in it. The development within a profession of its own research both improves its service and facilitates the maturation of the field. Sound research proceeds from and contributes to sound practice.

It is evident, in summary of this introduction, that professional education seeks to provide fundamentals for professional practice. While professional education can never specify with finality what kinds of professional positions its graduates are equipped to occupy and on what level of competence they are able to perform, it can certify to the field of practice which objectives and what degree of proficiency students are expected to have attained. It is the responsibility of the specific department, through its faculty, to determine the kinds of learning, both in content and method, which will develop the student's potentialities for the fulfillment of its educational aims. However, this process cannot take place unless the field of practice also is clear as to what tasks and what levels of competency it expects of its practitioners.

HISTORICAL NOTES

Education for therapeutic recreation has moved through successive stages from apprenticeship training within various settings to its current status as a program of study within departments of parks and recreation in the university and college community. The first stage was comprised of in-service training programs which were a functional part of the agency. Such programs were taught with a focus upon agency needs only. Gradually, these early training programs were abandoned in favor of institutes or training courses for the therapeutic recreation personnel of a series of agencies. The methods of teaching and the content of the program of study very much reflected the specific concerns or problems with which these various agencies had to deal. The courses usually were not conceptual in nature, but rather were descriptive and focused on situations. Before long, however, our emerging profession was ready to act on the conviction that education for agency service to the ill and disabled should be affiliated with departments of parks and recreation in institutions of higher learning.

A philosophy of therapeutic recreation education is influenced not only by the characteristics of therapeutic recreation as a profession, but also by the history of its education. Examination of the history of therapeutic recreation education provides a preface for consideration of the problems in therapeutic recreation preparation.

In a 1969 study by Stein of park and recreation curricula, 35 programs of study indicated a therapeutic recreation option at either the undergraduate or graduate level.[3] The following year Park and Hillman identified 56 institutions (two-year through graduate level) providing programs in therapeutic recreation.[4] Martin in 1971 indicated that 80 colleges and universities were offering over 200 courses in therapeutic recreation service.[5] In 1973, the *Directory of Professional Preparation Programs in Recreation, Parks and Related Fields* listed over 350 colleges and universities reporting park and recreation curricula (two-year programs through graduate programs) and of these, 95 indicated a therapeutic recreation option.[6] While these studies did not offer evidence of quality of therapeutic recreation courses or curricula, they did give some idea of therapeutic recreation's growth in a relatively short period of time. Subsequent studies appear to indicate that today there may be as many as 150 to over 170 preparation programs in therapeutic recreation, involving over 6,000 students.[7]

[3] Thomas A. Stein, "Therapeutic Recreation Education: 1969 Survey, " *Therapeutic Recreation Journal*, 4, no. 2 (1971), 4–7, 25.

[4] David C. Park and William A. Hillman, "Therapeutic Recreation Curricula: Colleges and Universities," *Therapeutic Recreation Journal*, 4, no. 2 (1970), 13–16.

[5] Fred W. Martin, "Survey of College and University Coursework in Therapeutic Recreation Service," *Therapeutic Recreation Journal*, 5, no. 3 (1971), 123–129, 140.

[6] National Recreation and Park Association and American Alliance for Health, Physical Education, and Recreation, *Directory of Professional Preparation Programs in Recreation, Parks and Related Fields* (Washington, D.C,, 1973).

[7] Thomas A. Stein, *Report on the State of Recreation and Park Education in Canada and the United States* (Washington, D.C.: National Recreation and Park Association, 1978); Stephen C. Anderson and Morris W. Stewart, "Therapeutic Recreation Education: 1979 Survey," *Therapeutic Recreation Journal*, 14, no. 3 (1980), 4–10; Carol Ann Peterson and Peg Connolly, "Professional Preparation in Therapeutic Recreation," *Therapeutic Recreation Journal*, 15, no. 2 (1981), 40.

For many years and in a variety of ways, therapeutic recreation practitioners and educators had been attempting to systematize their knowledge. For the most part, therapeutic recreation curricula served only to introduce students to the broad scope of populations served, services provided, and activities offered. The Therapeutic Recreation Curriculum Development Conference in 1961 had as its purposes the formulation of a list of competencies needed by therapeutic recreation practitioners and the utilization of the list as a base for developing a curriculum in therapeutic recreation.[8]

Other therapeutic recreation educators in the 1960s and the early 1970s considered curriculum development and competencies.[9] In 1963, MacLean, writing in *Recreation in Treatment Centers,* posited the need for a therapeutic recreation emphasis on both the undergraduate and graduate levels and suggested competencies at both levels per the Therapeutic Recreation Curriculum Development Conference of 1961.[10] She further suggested three guiding principles of curriculum development, namely: (1) The specialization should be offered only in institutions of higher learning which are connected with or have access to medical centers or similar medical settings and a variety of clinical affiliations, (2) one department faculty member should have experience in a medical setting, and (3) institutions offering only a graduate degree in therapeutic recreation "should insist" on undergraduate therapeutic recreation competencies before admission, and those institutions offering both undergraduate and graduate programs in therapeutic recreation should provide the opportunity to make up deficiencies "while embarking upon the advanced degree"[11]

It was not until the 1973 publication by the American Association for Health, Physical Education, and Recreation of *Guidelines for Professional Preparation Programs for Personnel Involved in Physical Education and Recreation for the Handicapped* that a milestone was reached.[12] This publication was the end product of several workshops involving over one hundred therapeutic recreation practitioners and educators. Both the publication and the workshops were the result of funding provided by the United States Bureau of Education for the Handicapped (BEH). Although this publication was aimed at graduate preparation, it was the first significant effort toward organizing the knowledge base of therapeutic recreation.[13]

---

[8] Comeback, *Therapeutic Recreation Curriculum Development Conference* (New York: Comeback, Inc., February, 1961).

[9] Donald Lindley, "Relative Importance of College Courses in Therapeutic Recreation," *Therapeutic Recreation Journal,* 4, no. 2 (1970), 8–12; Doris L. Berryman, *Development of Educational Programs for the New Careers in Recreation Services for the Disabled.* Final Report, U.S. Office of Education (New York: New York University, School of Education, 1971).

[10] Janet R. MacLean, "Therapeutic Recreation Curriculums," *Recreation in Treatment Centers,* 2 (1963), 23–29.

[11] *Ibid.,* p. 25.

[12] American Association for Health, Physical Education, and Recreation, *Guidelines for Professional Preparation Programs for Personnel Involved in Physical Education and Recreation for the Handicapped* (Washington, D.C., 1973).

[13] The graduate emphasis in therapeutic recreation was the result of BEH guidelines. Because funds in 1968 were limited, and it was impossible to fund many baccalaureate programs, it was thought that funding programs at the graduate level would reach practitioners in the field quicker and result in maximum impact on programs.

The publication identified roles and functions performed by practitioners in various settings and the competencies needed by therapeutic recreators to carry out these roles and responsibilities. In addition, it offered guidelines for fieldwork experiences and practicum sites and suggestions for academic, professional, and personal qualifications for therapeutic recreation faculty. To a large degree, the guidelines suggested what a therapeutic recreator ought to know, from very basic general recreation knowledge and skills to specifics in therapeutic recreation. Moreover, this project resulted in several colleges and universities being awarded training grants to upgrade the quality of their postgraduate preparation.

Another key historical project contributing to the knowledge base of therapeutic recreation was the federally funded (BEH) Illinois Community College Project awarded to the University of Illinois in 1973. This project sought to develop a model entry level curriculum in therapeutic recreation at the community and junior college level; a curriculum based on the theory of competency-based education. The project initially focused on competency identification for entry level practitioners[14] and later on the development of a modular competency-based curriculum.[15] It also provided the first empirical analysis of competencies required by entry level practitioners. In addition, the project brought together for the first time national leaders in therapeutic recreation education to discuss educational preparation. The fallout from this experience made it possible for the field of therapeutic recreation to move more closely toward standardization of educational preparation at all levels. The curriculum goals and modules that were eventually developed are as follows:

GOALS:

— To provide the student with a basic understanding of the concepts and philosophy of therapeutic recreation.

— To assist the student in gaining a greater sense of self-awareness and the use of self as a therapeutic agent in the provision of recreation services for disabled and handicapped persons. This includes establishing effective methods of communication.

— To provide the student with basic information required in understanding normal human growth and development as well as the understanding of those conditions which affect the disabled and handicapped persons with whom they will be working.

— To provide the student with an understanding of the process employed in a therapeutic interaction in which the recreative experience is the primary modality of intervention, and acquaint the student with the implicit and explicit roles employed in the delivery of recreation services.

— To develop student leadership skills in working with individuals and groups.

— To provide the student with an understanding of the principles of therapeutic recreation programming, and develop skills in applying those principles in practical situations. This would include skill development in analyzing and adapting activities to meet specific client needs.

— To provide the student with a basic orientation to professionalism and the meaning of

[14] Jerry D. Kelley and others, *Therapeutic Recreation Education: Developing a Competency-Based Entry-Level Curriculum* (Urbana-Champaign, Ill.: Office of Recreation and Park Resources and Department of Leisure Studies, University of Illinois, 1976).

[15] Jerry D. Kelley and others, *Therapeutic Recreation Education: Guidelines for a Competency-Based Entry-Level Curriculum* (Arlington Va.: National Recreation and Park Association, n.d.).

professionalism in the enrichment of therapeutic recreation services. This would include an understanding of the roles and inter-relationships with other disciplines.

— To provide the student with opportunities to gain practical experiences in working with disabled and handicapped persons in "true-life" situations.

MODULES:

1. Philosophical and Theoretical Foundations of Therapeutic Recreation
2. Normal Human Growth and Development
3. Orientation to Disability Groups
4. Programming and Evaluation of Therapeutic Recreation Services
5. Introspection and Communication
6. Therapeutic Recreation Roles and Process
7. Group Dynamics and Leadership
8. Activity Analysis, Selection, Adaptation
9. Professionalism in Therapeutic Recreation
10. Roles and Functions of Related Disciplines and Interpersonal Relationships Field Practicum.[16]

Concurrent with this project during the mid-1970s BEH funded other competency-based education programs including paraprofessional training programs.[17] The NTRS 750-hour paraprofessional training program developed at New York University was initiated in 1975. This training scheme, when completed, allowed participants to qualify for the Technician II level registration within the NTRS registration plan. Likewise, a number of doctoral dissertations proposed competency-based curricula models in therapeutic recreation.[18] Meanwhile, the University of Illinois, within its Department of Leisure Studies, was in the process of revising its therapeutic recreation curriculum using a linear hierarchy orientation with strategies developed from Peterson's model of a systems approach to curriculum development.[19]

[16] *Ibid.*, pp. 25–26.

[17] One reason for the emphasis on competency-based education programs was the result of the federal government's adopting competency-based education "as a criteria for evaluating proposals for training grants at this time" (Kelley, *Therapeutic Recreation Education: Developing a Curriculum*, p. 12); Doris L. Berryman, *Training Professionals for New Careers in Recreation Services to the Disabled*. Final Report, U.S. Office of Education (New York: New York University, School of Education, 1971); Jerry Jordan, *A Process Analysis Approach to the Development of a Competency Based Graduate Curriculum in Therapeutic Recreation* (Philadelphia: Temple University, Department of Recreation and Leisure Studies, 1974); Doris L. Berryman and others, *A Modular Training Program for Therapeutic Recreation Technician I: the NTRS 750 Hour Curriculum* (Arlington, Va.: National Recreation and Park Association, 1975).

[18] Linda Odum, "A Curriculae Matrix for Use in the Design and Development of an Undergraduate Core Curriculum in Therapeutic Recreation" (unpublished Doctoral dissertation, The Florida State University, 1973). Robert E. Cipriano, "A Career Exploration Program with Competency-Based Mini-Courses for Entry-Level Positions in Therapeutic Recreation" (unpublished Doctoral dissertation, New York University, 1974). S. Harold Smith, "Practitioners' Evaluation of College Courses, Competencies and Functions in Therapeutic Recreation" (unpublished Doctoral dissertation, University of Utah, 1974).

[19] Scout Lee Gunn, "A Linear Modular Approach to Competency-Based Graduate Education in Therapeutic Recreation," in *Theory and Design of Competency-Based Education in Therapeutic Recreation*, eds. Jerry J. Jordan, William P. Dayton, and Kathryn A. Brill (Philadelphia: Temple University, Department of Recreation and Leisure Studies, 1978). Carol Ann Peterson, "A Systems Approach to Curriculum Development," *Therapeutic Recreation Journal*, 8 no. 3 (1974), 129–37.

The major goal of therapeutic recreation educators during the middle 1970s appeared to be helping students develop competence in three major areas: (1) conceptual and perceptual understanding; (2) skills in methods, procedures, and processes; and (3) personal professional qualities. How well the goal was reached and how well students integrated the material into service and practice is difficult to ascertain.

During this period, a number of therapeutic recreation educators criticized the preservice education of therapeutic recreation students. In 1973, Robb indicated that a crisis existed in integrating preservice education and professional functioning.[20] He commented "It is the gap or discrepancy between what is available at the college or university and the type of experiences and education needed and desired by students."[21] He further charged that many programs at the undergraduate level were "anachronisms" and that program specialization does not exist at the undergraduate level, but workforce needs are for those having the bachelor's degree. Thus students are grossly underprepared in entering therapeutic recreation service and practice. A year later, Austin commented that there needed to be a better relationship between field placement agencies and universities. He suggested that therapeutic recreation training centers be established within various university-affiliated agencies wherein students, agency staff, and faculty could work closely together and provide client services jointly, and where faculty could offer formal instruction so as to quickly apply theory to practice. With faculty spending time in the agency, it would also provide the opportunity for them to revise and improve curriculum on a consistent basis.[22] Lastly, Smith, in a study of practitioners and their views concerning undergraduate training in therapeutic recreation, concluded that preservice education did not appear to prepare practitioners for their job requirements nor did the programs provide an adequate philosophical base for their work.[23] Specifically, as related to the study, he commented:

> Overall, the findings tended to support the premise that the undergraduate training experience had not, in many cases, properly trained the bachelor level practitioner to meet the requirements of the job situation or give him/her a strong philosophical base from which to work. Indeed, it appears that, in general, training at the undergraduate level perpetuated some confusion and a lack of professional identity. . . . Taking . . . the . . . facts into consideration, it would seem that a long and serious appraisal of the undergraduate professional training program in therapeutic recreation needs to be done. Such an appraisal comprising not only the type of courses being offered but also the type of opportunities being provided in the clinical experience as well.[24]

The proliferation of therapeutic recreation curricula at various academic levels, coupled with workforce demands by the mid-1970s, created a problem center-

[20] Gary Robb, "Integrating Preservice Education and Professional Functioning," *Therapeutic Recreation Journal*, no. 2 (1973), 44–46.

[21] Ibid., p. 41.

[22] David R. Austin, "The University Can't Train Therapeutic Recreators," *Therapeutic Recreation Journal*, 8, no. 1 (1974), 22–24.

[23] S. Harold Smith, "Practitioners' Evaluation of College Courses, Competencies, and Functions in Therapeutic Recreation," *Therapeutic Recreation Journal*, 10, no. 4 (1976), 152–156.

[24] *Ibid.*, p. 156.

ing on the identification of the role of educational institutions in the preparation of therapeutic recreators. As a result, BEH funded the Community College Miniconference in conjunction with the 1975 Midwest Symposium on Therapeutic Recreation. The focus of the conference was on developing better communication and strategy between and among those responsible for the 750-hour training program; the two-year, four-year, and masters programs; and the professions. Although the conference produced guidelines[25] to further communication efforts among its participants, subsequent action was limited. However, the conference did yield a number of interesting recommendations; namely to (1) determine the existing manpower need, (2) identify skills required for various employment positions, (3) convert existing four-year and masters therapeutic recreation curricula and compare, (4) evaluate competency-based curricula with follow-up studies, and (5) establish field placement standards and develop a procedure to accredit practicum sites.[26] These recommendations were similar in nature to what other educators had been saying for a number of years.

Since the early 1960s, various park and recreation organizations at the national level had been working together to develop and establish standards and evaluative criteria for recreation education. In 1975, the National Council on Accreditation sponsored by the NRPA in cooperation with the American Association for Leisure and Recreation was established. Since 1974, the NTRS had worked with the council in developing therapeutic recreation standards. During the mid-year meeting (1976), the NTRS officially approved, and the council sanctioned, on an interim basis, undergraduate and graduate therapeutic recreation standards as recommended by NTRS.[27] In the same year, during the Congress for Recreation and Parks at Boston, the standards received final approval from the council and were subsequently added to the National Council on Accreditation's standards and evaluative criteria document.[28]

As indicated in an earlier chapter, one of the items considered by the Presidential Commission on Assessment of Critical Issues was accreditation. To accomplish the objectives associated with accreditation, the committee, under the direction of Carol A. Peterson, undertook two substudies which they felt were imperative to generate background and foundation information for the accreditation investigation. One study was concerned with the identification and validation of entry level competencies for practice, and the other focused on describing the current status of therapeutic recreation preparation programs at both the undergraduate and graduate levels. In the former study, the investigators identified and validated eighty-nine competencies thought to be appropriate and necessary educational

[25] Marcia Carter, "Articulation of Therapeutic Recreation Curricula," in *Expanding Horizons in Therapeutic Recreation III*, eds. Gary Robb and Gerald Hitzhusen (Columbia, Mo.: University of Missouri, Department of Recreation and Park Administration, 1976), 45–48.

[26] *Ibid.*, pp. 46–47.

[27] Gerald S. O'Morrow, "Therapeutic Recreation Program Accreditation, *Therapeutic Recreation Journal*, 10, no. 3 (1976), 86–87.

[28] National Council on Accreditation, *Standards and Evaluative Criteria for Recreation, Leisure Services, and Resources Curricula Baccalaureate and Masters Degree Program* (Arlington, Va.: National Recreation and Park Association, March 1977).

prerequisites for entry level personnel.[29] The committee recommended to NTRS that the competencies identified "serve as a starting point" in "the adoption of a set of minimum competencies or define areas of knowledge, skills and abilities."[30]

While some findings of the curricula study concerned with the current status of therapeutic recreation preparation will be reported later in this chapter, it is important to note the investigators' conclusions as they related to the various programs of study ($N = 51$).

> The results of this study verify the incredible variety and diversity that exists in Therapeutic Recreation curricula. This finding is understandable with the absence of a comprehensive set of curricula guidelines or standards provided by NTRS. Although it was not the purpose of this study to make judgements about any specific program, it is safe to say that many programs are extremely weak in their content and resources related to Therapeutic Recreation preparation. It is indeed difficult to establish credibility as a profession with such diversity and variety of depth in the preparation programs.[31]

During the next several years, feedback was occurring concerning the standards and evaluative criteria as applied to recreation education including therapeutic recreation education. Standards can be useful only if they can be realistically applied to the phenomena being evaluated and if they have general acceptance by those using them. Although the standards were generally accepted, there were a number of legitimate problems within the document which needed attention if the standards were to guide the further professional development of the park and recreation field. As related to therapeutic recreation, there were specific concerns about strengthening the knowledge and skill base of therapeutic recreation service and practice. A review and revision would certainly lead to (1) providing a better foundation for credentialling and program and personnel standards; (2) enhancing credibility of NTRS with other health-related organizations, disciplines, and federal and state agencies; (3) improving quality of services and practices to individuals in various types of settings; (4) standardizing course content and giving direction to the body of knowledge that was developing; and (5) enhancing the credibility of therapeutic recreation as a profession.

Therapeutic recreation, like other professional occupations, seeks to rise within the professional hierarchy, so that it, too, may enjoy maximum prestige, authority, and monopoly, which presently belong to a few professions. Therapeutic recreators want to rise in the professional hierarchy both for personal gain (status and financial) and for consumer benefit. Some of the reasons are the ability to recruit qualified people to the field, the opportunity to secure better pay and fringe benefits, and the possiblity of obtaining more intellectually creative members who can improve on knowledge and service delivery methods.

[29] Carol Ann Peterson, *Accreditation Committee Report* (Report submitted to the National Therapeutic Recreation Society Board of Directors and Past Presidents Council, September 30, 1978, personal copy), Appendix B.

[30] *Ibid.*, p. 3.

[31] *Ibid.*, p. 5.

In 1980 the council embarked on a major review and revision of the accreditation standards with national input from educators and practitioners. New accreditation standards were approved by the council in 1981. Therapeutic recreation standards adopted and approved by NTRS and incorporated into the new document were treated from the standpoint of what the therapeutic recreation practitioner should know. In 1983 the council discontinued accrediting preparation programs at the master's level. The practice of the therapeutic recreator is seen as typically guided by knowledge of the therapeutic recreation standards which follow:

— Knowledge of human anatomy and physiology.
— Understanding of the nature and etiology of illness and disability.
— Understanding and ability to use basic medical and psychiatric terminology.
— Understanding of the attitudes and self-concepts of disabled persons towards themselves and towards their illness or disability.
— Understanding of the societal attitudes towards illness and disability.
— Understanding of the bio-psycho-social limitation imposed by illness and disability as related to leisure involvement.
— Knowledge of various assistive techniques related to specific illness or disabilities: including, but not limited to, transfer techniques, ambulation, self-help skills, signing, orientation and mobility.
— Knowledge of the health care delivery systems.
— Understanding of the role of therapeutic recreation as a component of health care systems.
— Knowledge of the legal issues in delivering services for special populations.
— Knowledge of local, state and federal (national) laws, regulations and standards regarding recreation services for special populations.
— Knowledge of appropriate inter-agency and intra-agency referral procedures to meet individual client needs.
— Understanding of a variety of treatment approaches and their implications for therapeutic recreation programming.
— Understanding of the concept of habilitation, rehabilitation, maintenance and prevention as related to therapeutic programs.
— Understanding of the concept of a continuum of therapeutic recreation service.
— Ability to conceptualize and plan appropriate therapeutic recreation programs for diverse special need populations.
— Ability to conduct client assessment procedures, analyze and interpret results for programming.
— Ability to design individual treatment and program plans.
— Knowledge of the theory and technique of therapeutic intervention including, but not limited to, reflective listening, reality therapy, nondirective therapy, transactional analysis and behavior modification.
— Knowledge of various adaptive devices and equipment.
— Ability to demonstrate and translate medical record charting techniques.
— Knowledge of the credentialling process related to therapeutic recreation.
— Understanding of ethical and professional behavior related to therapeutic recreation.
— Understanding the role of the therapeutic recreation professional as an advocate for services for special populations.[32]

[32] National Council on Accreditation, *Standards and Evaluative Criteria for Recreation, Park Resources and Leisure Services Baccalaureate Curricula* (Arlington, Va.: National Recreation and Park Association, October 1981, Rev.), pp. 9–10.

PROBLEMS IN
THERAPEUTIC RECREATION
PREPARATION

In an earlier chapter, reference was made to Goode's core characteristics of professionalization—body of knowledge and service orientation.[33] Therapeutic recreation would certainly rank high on the variable of service orientation, but where would it rank among the allied health or other professions in relation to a body of knowledge? All professions draw on a well-defined and well-organized body of knowledge that serves as their basic foundation of practice. A profession's body of knowledge is a basis for claiming that its practitioners, and no others, have the theoretical and technical skill to do what it is they profess to do. Further, the substantiation of such a claim requires the profession to identify the theoretical basis for action, to validate its postulates through research, and to demonstrate their effectiveness through application and refinement of technique. Lastly, the degree to which this attribute—body of knowledge—is achieved will establish the limits of achievement for the other attributes of professionalism. [34]

Therapeutic recreation is only beginning to develop its theoretical base and to recognize the usefulness of practice theory. In that respect, therapeutic recreation is to some degree like other emerging professions. Its knowledge is incomplete. Thus therapeutic recreation finds itself in a situation familiar to other professions: much of our knowledge is tentative and, as is true in so many other professional fields, a good part of it is borrowed for use in our field. But there is no question at all that a body of specialized knowledge for effective education or practice is needed and that such a body of knowledge, indeed, underlies practice.

Today there appears to be no uniformity in therapeutic recreation curricula, although the number of institutions adding a therapeutic recreation option are increasing. In addition, there is a limited knowledge base for developing theoretical and technical competence. As Peterson and Connolly commented "The result is hundreds of students graduating annually with diverse knowledge, skills and abilities of unknown quality. . . . Therapeutic recreation, because of its emerging status has even more reason to be concerned with its entering practitioners."[35]

Therapeutic recreation education has, as its central task, the preparation of students to assume professional roles and responsibilities for improving the quality of life of individuals with physical, emotional, mental and social problems through recreative experiences. The task is an enormous one. It is a mission which challenges the adequacy of our knowledge, skills, and abilities.

Knowledge, skills, and abilities are all used in the therapeutic recreation endeavor. In fact, the first two elements make up the body of knowledge which is sytematically applied to achieve a particular purpose or a socially desirable goal; to bring about a change in the consumer. Knowledge is that part of reality that is

[33] William J. Goode, "Encroachment, Charlatanism, and the Emerging Profession: Psychology, Sociology, and Medicine," *American Sociological Review*, 25, no. 12 (1960), 903.

[34] Lee E. Meyer, "Philosophical Alternatives and the Professionalization of Therapeutic Recreation" (Arlington, Va.: National Recreation and Park Association, 1980), p. 45.

[35] Peterson and Connolly, "Professional Preparation," p. 45.

confirmable; that which is known about people and their social systems. It includes cognizance of human development, human diversity, and social system theory. It is knowledge that directs the response to need, including information concerning assessment, relationships, and the therapeutic recreation process. It is insight gained from practical experience. It is used to conceptualize practice. Knowledge is complex, requiring more than superficial understanding.

Skill is seen as technical expertise, the ability to use knowledge effectively in the execution of performance competence. For example, in relation to a social-functioning problem, it is necessary to make choices from a variety of possibilities based on knowledge. Skill may be defined from a sociological perspective as "a complex organization of behavior (physical or verbal) developed through learning and directed toward a particular goal or centered on a particular activity."[36] In practice, three types of skills are needed by all therapeutic recreators: activity skills, cognitive skills, and interactive or relationship skills. Activity skills are those used in conducting, directing, or teaching an activity. Cognitive skills are those used in thinking about the consumer in situations, in developing understanding about the person and the situation, in identifying the knowledge to be used, in planning for intervention, in decision making, and in performance evaluation. Interactive skills are those used in working jointly with client or consumer, in communicating and developing understanding, in joint planning, and in carrying out the plan of action. In essence, the interactive skills incorporate basic helping skills, engagement skills, observation skills, and communication skills. Therapeutic recreation does not have one skill but a wide variety of skills useful for many different situations.

The practice of therapeutic recreation is based not only on knowledge, skills, and abilities, but also on attitudes or values, as noted in the previous chapter. The therapeutic recreation specialist's attitudes reflect the professional values and ethical commitments to which one adheres; they are preferred behavioral guides. Values and ethics, therefore, also need to be learned. In problem-solving activities the therapeutic recreation specialist applies not only specific cognitive knowledge, but also values and ethical judgements, to the situation. Knowledge, values, and ethics are reflected in professional skills, and values and ethics are revealed as attitudes in the behavior of professional persons. Figure 6-1 depicts the relationship of these elements in therapeutic recreation professional preparation.

As we begin to explore some of the problems associated with therapeutic recreation preparation, it seems appropriate to consider a major barrier related to professional preparation and professionalization. Wilensky has pointed out this obstacle:

> If the technical base of an occupation consists of a vocabulary that sounds familiar to everyone . . . or if the base is scientific but so narrow it can be learned as a set of rules by most people, then the occupation will have difficulty claiming a monopoly of skill or even a roughly exclusive jurisdiction. In short, there may be an optimal base for professional practice—neither too vague nor too precise, too broad nor too narrow.[37]

[36] George Theodorson and Achilles Theodorson, *A Modern Dictionary of Sociology* (New York: Thomas Y. Crowell Company, Inc., 1969), p. 382.

[37] Harold L. Wilensky, "The Professionalization of Everyone?" *American Journal of Sociology*, 70, no. 2 (1964), 148.

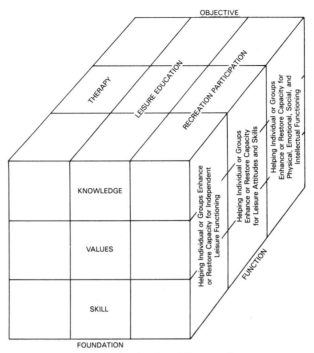

FIGURE 6-1 Therapeutic Recreation Professional Preparation

He goes on to say:

> . . . the optimal base of knowledge or doctrine for a profession is a combination of intellectual and practical knowing, some of which is explicit (classification and generalizations learned from books, lectures, and demonstrations), some implicit ("understanding" acquired from supervised practice and observation).[38]

The problems associated with therapeutic recreation preparation at the undergraduate level are many and varied. The low visibility and fragmentation of therapeutic recreation's body of knowledge is certainly the result of a lack of in-depth research. In fact, therapeutic recreation research, except in a few instances, has been of limited value in advancing our body of knowledge. Although Chapter 8 considers therapeutic recreation research problems in depth, it is important here to highlight in brief the concern because it has a direct relationship to therapeutic recreation's body of knowledge and professional preparation.

A profession can only hope to enlarge its body of knowledge through the use of the scientific method rather than the jury method of ascertaining truths. Therapeutic recreation is beginning to place, in a very small way, increasing emphasis on knowledge that is scientific as opposed to beliefs in unconfirmed ideas. Although attempts are being made to develop a body of knowledge that begins to move toward the hardness characteristic of the sciences, more information is needed. Therapeutic recreation needs to continue to search for the acceptance of common concepts and shared frames of reference and to test hypotheses about the nature

[38] *Ibid.*, p. 149.

of practice in the effort to become more scientific. In fact, the base of therapeutic recreation should consist of three types of knowledge: (1) tested knowledge, (2) hypothetical knowledge that requires transformation into tested knowledge, and (3) assumptive knowledge (or practical knowledge) that requires transformation into hypothetical and then tested knowledge. The practitioner uses all three types of knowledge and carries a professional responsibility for knowing at any time which type of knowledge he or she is using and what degree of scientific certainty should be attached to it. However, the search for common concepts and frames of reference will not be without its problems, some of which include:

1. Problems that come from borrowing knowledge from another discipline. Mobily has suggested that no progress will be made in the development of our body of knowledge "until recognition of applicable areas of knowledge from other fields are considered."[39] However, this borrowing may provide yesterday's knowledge rather than the current thinking of the disciplines developing the knowledge. Often, borrowed knowledge is given much more credence than that knowledge generated by the developing discipline. Also, borrowing tends to be of a simplified nature. Questionable assumptions may result when knowledge appropriated from other fields is improperly used.

   On the other hand, Mobily's point has merit. It is recognized that for any profession with aspirations to being a learned profession it is necessary to draw on available knowledge from other academic disciplines. But a problem may arise in doing so. To make knowledge useful for the purpose of therapeutic recreation, for example, relevant parts from the information available or potentially available in the social and biological sciences must first be selected, then transplanted and organized into appropriate bodies of knowledge pertinent to the professional context of therapeutic recreation. In order to achieve selection of appropriate content and to organize it in a fashion useful to therapeutic recreation, a process must be initiated to determine what is appropriate for therapeutic recreation. A means for the selection of pertinent knowledge has to be available. This selecting mechanism, as it were, is yet to be found. In time, perhaps, the recently adopted position statement may provide clues.

2. Problems that develop because therapeutic recreation practice has often been conceptualized insufficiently to separate fact, perception, ideas, and skills. Practice has often not been tested by applying it in different situations in a controlled manner. Its validity and reliability with respect to the nature of people, specific settings, and human relationships has not been examined. Thus it is difficult to determine if knowledge gained from practice is appropriate in a given situation. Kennedy found, relative to expectations of competencies between educators and practitioners regarding therapeutic recreation graduates, a need for more dialogue "in order to understand the different expectations that are held in regard to the performance levels of . . . graduates."[40]

3. Problems that develop because of the many variables involved in the "human situation" and in the "therapeutic recreator–consumer interaction." This makes it difficult to generalize knowledge for use in determining interventive possibilities.

[39] Kenneth E. Mobily, "Quality Analysis in Therapeutic Recreation Curricula," *Therapeutic Recreation Journal*, 17, no. 1 (1983), 20.

[40] Dan W. Kennedy, "Congruence of Expectations of Competencies for Therapeutic Recreation Graduates Between Recreation Educators and Practitioners," in *Directions in Health, Physical Education, and Recreation—Therapeutic Recreation Curriculum: Philosophy, Strategy, and Concepts.* Monograph Series 1, ed. David R. Austin (Bloomington, Ind.: Indiana University, School of Health, Physical Education, and Recreation, 1980), pp. 26–32.

4. Problems that result from a tendency to use terms and concepts without sufficient definition or without agreement as to definition. Without agreement, terms and concepts are sometimes used with different meanings. For example, our field for some years debated *therapeutic recreation, therapeutic recreation process*, and *therapeutic recreation service*. Now that we have a philosophical position statement with new terms, will a new series of debates develop? Sessoms speaks of an uniqueness in our occupation,[41] but uniqueness is not always that easily communicated or recognized by other professions, or ours in particular. What is this uniqueness?

5. Problems that result from a tendency not to develop sufficient relationships among terms and concepts. Social systems theory has given a framework for doing this, at least in part. However, practice-theory knowledge is very difficult to place in an organized framework except at an abstract level.

6. Problems associated with the nature of our speciality, which is concerned with the complex phenomenon of the human being in the social environment, tend to give an impression of possible "softness" to the development of our body of knowledge.

It is hoped that, as a result of the acceptance of the philosophical statement, NTRS will adopt a long-term research emphasis which will stimulate efforts by therapeutic recreators to identify and enlarge the scientific principles upon which therapeutic recreation rests and will encourage research by them in the application of these principles to therapeutic recreation.

Another particularly vexing problem is that of specialization including the subquestions of how much content to incorporate within the specialization, the quality and number of therapeutic recreation faculty to teach the specialization, and the specialist versus generalist approach to preparation. A pendulumlike trend is seen regarding specialization. As noted earlier, the tendency a decade or more ago was for specialization in therapeutic recreation to come primarily at the graduate level. At present, as a result of growth, development, and recognition, it occurs more at the undergraduate level. Growth brings with it new demands, and challenges. Responding to these demands and challenges often requires that we do things in different ways, consider other approaches, and revise concepts and beliefs. Determining what a student must take in general within a park and recreation curriculum, plus specialized therapeutic recreation courses and those courses to support the therapeutic recreation specialization poses problems in the preparation used to meet minimum competence.

Given the philosophical statement adopted by NTRS, can therapeutic recreators obtain sufficient knowledge and techniques in present therapeutic recreation programs of study to engage successfully in therapeutic recreation practice? This is not only a question which the profession must answer to satisfy its own claim to technical competency and exclusive jurisdiction within society, but it is one the public at large will ask before granting recognition and possibly legal sanction. The curriculum implications of the adopted NTRS position relative to a body of knowledge suggest that equal attention would have to be given to the three service areas or

---

[41] H. Douglas Sessoms, "Therapeutic Recreation Service: The Past and Challenging Present," in *Exetra Perspectives: Concepts in Therapeutic Recreation*, eds. Larry L. Neal and Christopher R. Edginton (Eugene, Ore.: University of Oregon, Center of Leisure Studies, 1982), pp. 12–13.

continuum care model (therapy, leisure education, recreation participation) so that students would have "equal" abilities in all three areas.[42] Broadening the body of knowledge "would intensify the need to broaden the course offerings and to expand the criteria for accreditation of the therapeutic recreation option."[43] This would require the continued efforts of NTRS toward gaining more influence over the accreditation of this option, since Meyer reminds us that "there is evidence to suggest that NTRS does not determine or control the training of persons being prepared to practice therapeutic recreation . . ."[44]

In Chapter 2 we discussed the process of professionalization. It was noted that the profession, in this case NTRS, determines and controls the standardized training for entry into the profession. But where is NTRS located organizationally? It is a branch within NRPA. Consequently, changes in therapeutic recreation competency standards associated with accreditation must eventually be approved by the National Council on Accreditation. Further, the accreditation of specializations comes after general accreditation. Thus there are specific general recreation requirements that must be met initially before consideration of the specialization. Because NTRS is a branch within NRPA, the specialization must be compatible with the purposes of NRPA. Such an arrangement makes it difficult to develop an in-depth, successful specialization. In a recently completed job analysis study of entry level professionals by NRPA, it was found that therapeutic recreation specialists, as a group, were substantially different from the other three groups—recreation programmers, park management–recreation resource specialists, and commercial recreationists in a matrix schema analysis of *importance* versus *performance* tasks. The study found that the therapeutic recreation group had a large number of *high performance–high importance* tasks and concluded that this was attributed to the more "unique and specialized nature of their positions."[45]

In turning our attention to the topics of specialization content and faculty qualifications and ratios, we find as much variance within one as we do within the other. A number of therapeutic recreation educators have investigated course work in therapeutic recreation since the 1970s, as has been noted. Of relevance here is the Peterson and Connolly investigation of undergraduate therapeutic recreation courses offered within curricula in institutions. These authors found a range of from 1 to 2 to 7 to 9 courses.[46] Such a range raises serious questions about our therapeutic recreation program of study; its educational objectives and its content and quality. As Humphrey and Reynolds commented regarding the study;

> While the limited offering of 1–2 courses raises serious questions concerning the quality of professional preparation, we may be opening the door to legitimate ridicule

[42] National Therapeutic Recreation Society, *Alternative Positions and Their Implications to Professionalism* (Arlington, Va.: National Recreation and Park Association, 1981), pp. 13, 20.

[43] *Ibid.*, p. 14.

[44] Meyer, *Philosophical Alternatives*, p. 47.

[45] National Recreation and Park Association, National Certification Board, *Report on Job Analysis Study of Entry-Level Professionals in Park and Recreation Occupation*, Final Report (Alexandria, Va.: the Association, June 1982), p. 16.

[46] Peterson, *Accreditation Report*, Appendix B; Peterson and Connolly, "Professional Preparation," pp. 40–41.

through the claim that our unique body of knowledge is so extensive it takes 7–9 courses to adequately complete the professional preparation process.[47]

Although the Peterson and Connolly study did not offer an underlying rationale for the amazing variety of courses with therapeutic recreation content, one cannot help but speculate that the lack of therapeutic recreation educational objectives might very well be the cause for the extensive range of courses. Responding to educational objectives requires answering two preliminary questions: What is the nature of therapeutic recreation? What is the nature of therapeutic recreation education?

The development of a curriculum for any profession naturally requires clarity about the nature of that profession. The NTRS position paper has tried to make explicit the views and assumptions about therapeutic recreation. In the light of these assumptions and values, it stated the nature of therapeutic recreation in terms of its ultimate goal and its functions and activities. The ultimate goal of therapeutic recreation is seen as the enhancement of leisure functioning for disabled people through leisure experiences. The method of achievement of this goal, as conceptually viewed within the position paper, can be grouped into four categories: assessment of the problem, planning for the resolution of the problem, implementation of the plan, and evaluation of the outcome. Thus the position paper serves as one tool for the identification of educational objectives.

A response to the other question about the nature of therapeutic recreation education is difficult at this time. The range of courses leads one to believe that we have no educational philosophy. A therapeutic recreation philosophy of education, in its development, cannot ignore the past nor be unaware of the requirements of the present and the foreseeable future. Further, the philosophy must evolve in the light of an examination of whether or not therapeutic recreation meets the criteria of a profession. It is a pertinent question for study. Still further, therapeutic recreation education needs to develop an educational philosophy that centers around providing the student with the basic body of knowledge, skills, and attitudes necessary to develop a generalized mode of approach, a way of problem solving. It should not seek to provide all the facts, concepts and techniques required to deal effectively with every professional problem the student may encounter throughout a career. It is immaterial how many courses are offered. Rather, the important consideration is that the courses that comprise the concentration should include the concepts that are germane to professional growth. Such a philosophy would incorporate class and field learning and be governed by the three principles of continuity, sequence, and integration. Thus the second question, when eventually clarified, will provide a second tool for the identification of desirable educational aims, their organization, and their distribution within the curriculum. One may again suggest that the program of therapeutic recreation education should be thought of as encompassing the following components: (1) study of relevant content in the basic disciplines, (2)

---

[47] Fred Humphrey and Ronald Reynolds, "The Editors' Viewpoint," *Therapeutic Recreation Journal*, 15, no. 2 (1981), 5.

study of related content from the professions, and (3) study of therapeutic recreation content.

Professional service requires mastery of a body of knowledge as well as skills and abilities. But the question as to what to emphasize has had almost a pendulumlike quality. Currently there is evidence that a number of programs have moved far in the direction of theory and others have erred in the direction of overemphasis on practice, ending up with a how-to-do-it procedure which limits students and graduates in adapting to changing conditions. The effective practice of therapeutic recreation requires both the appropriate selection of techniques for a particular situation and the ability to use techniques effectively. This selection is based on a conscious use of knowledge. The ability to appropriately combine the elements of knowledge and skills and apply them to the helping situation is indeed a major characteristic of the therapeutic recreator. It is toward this blending of knowledge and skill that therapeutic recreation as an emerging profession should be aspiring.

The apparent confusion as to what to emphasize and how course offerings and their content should be organized may reflect, in part, the prevailing uncertainty as to therapeutic recreation educational objectives and the proper function of undergraduate therapeutic recreation programs. A brief study of catalogs and other printed materials concerning the number of courses or hours offered in therapeutic recreation curricula reflects a certain pattern of regularly recurring courses. These are (1) a descriptive introduction to therapeutic recreation including history, (2) an introduction to programming methods and techniques used in therapeutic recreation practice, and (3) some experience in an agency either through observation or a supervised internship. From these minimums (a surprising number of catalogs reflected only the introductory descriptive course and an internship) there is a proliferation in some colleges and universities of therapeutic recreation courses which suggest almost certain duplication of courses offered at the graduate level. It is small wonder that some students entering graduate therapeutic recreation programs have complained of repetition of work taken in their junior and senior years in college. The discontinuity between educational levels (undergraduate and graduate) may be another factor making it difficult to develop a coherent program of therapeutic recreation education. But more than likely the confusion is the result of fortuitous circumstances, historical "drift," or the demands of expediency.

The issue of faculty, its quality and number within therapeutic recreation professional preparation programs, has been debated for some years. At the time that therapeutic recreation standards were proposed for incorporation within the accreditation document, a recommendation was made concerning the number and experience of therapeutic recreation faculty by the NTRS. However, the recommendation was not acted upon by the Council on Accreditation. This fact would appear to support Meyer's view that the NTRS does not determine, like the training of persons to practice therapeutic recreation, the qualifications of faculty responsible for therapeutic recreation programs.[48] The advent of such activities as training

---

[48] Meyer, *Philosophical Alternatives*, p. 47.

would require the approval and support of existing structures within NRPA.

Although many programs taught by well-qualified faculty exist, there is also reason to believe that there are programs at the opposite end of the spectrum. In 1982, Smith and McGowan reported that in a study of sixty-six faculty responsible for teaching therapeutic recreation courses, 17 percent had no formal degree training in therapeutic recreation. Further, while 44 percent of the teachers had seven or more years of practical experience, the authors concluded that consultation, teaching, workshops, and intern supervision were included within the respective responses to practical experiences. Lastly, they found that 49 percent of the teachers had no "face-to-face" client experience, rather, their experience was as a program supervisor or director of services.[49] No amount of change in curriculum structure and stated content will achieve therapeutic recreation educational objectives unless the faculty engaged in teaching the program is highly skilled, knowledgeable, and enthusiastic. Care must be exercised to avoid employing some nondescript therapeutic recreation specialist who has neither fundamental scholarship nor a professional understanding of what therapeutic recreation is. The importance of insuring the presence on the faculty of knowledgeable personnel cannot be overemphasized. Rich and stimulating teaching comes only from those who are themselves vitally involved in the subject matter.

Regarding the number of faculty, the Peterson and Connolly study of 1979 found that of forty-nine institutions reporting an undergraduate therapeutic recreation program of study, "therapeutic recreation faculty members represented only 19 percent of the total, full-time recreation and leisure studies faculty."[50] When this was correlated with the number of students enrolled in the therapeutic recreation program within these institutions, the average full-time therapeutic recreation faculty was 1.4 to an average of seventy-four students.[51]

It is difficult to ascertain the reason for the high student-faculty ratio. There can be little question that a problem does exist and that it appears to be chronic. It may very well be the result of university department economics or the inability to recruit adequately prepared therapeutic recreation faculty. On the other hand, it may be an attitudinal problem. In certain instances, a program of therapeutic recreation may not be consistent in philosophy with other department options.

Before moving on, it seems important to briefly touch upon the subject of where therapeutic recreation programs of study are located within a university or college department of parks and recreation. Although not a specific problem which has been highlighted in the literature, it has been discussed informally. The traditional placement of therapeutic recreation programs in departments of parks and recreation in the past was not questioned. Recent developments in therapeutic

---

[49] S. Harold Smith and Robert W. McGowan, "A Study to Determine the Educational Level and Practical Experience of College Teachers in Therapeutic Recreation: 1980," in *Exetra Perspectives: Concepts in Therapeutic Recreation*, pp. 99–108, eds. Larry L. Neal and Christopher R. Edginton (Eugene, Ore.: Center of Leisure Studies, University of Oregon, 1982).

[50] Peterson, *Accreditation Report*, Appendix B; Peterson and Connolly, "Professional Preparation," p. 41.

[51] *Ibid.*

recreation (therapy concept, employment patterns, independent certification, etc.) raise the question of whether affiliation with a department of parks and recreation is always the most desirable arrangement. Plans whereby therapeutic recreation is aligned with allied health or established as a separate department justify careful consideration. There are therapeutic recreation programs today operating both within allied health structures and independently. What factors might lead to such an organizational structure? Requirements causing therapeutic recreation majors to be overloaded with general park and recreation courses are one factor. The number of therapeutic recreation offerings may also be sufficiently limited so that the full-time therapeutic recreation faculty member would be expected to teach certain park and recreation courses. As a result of this, the teacher may lose touch with therapeutic courses. On the other hand, what might prevent such a division? Funding is certainly a major concern in considering an independent department. In an allied health setting, one might also encounter different professional ideologies and a lack of common prerequisite content. In general, any arrangement is not free of disadvantages and each has desirable features. However, although difficulties are commonly associated with the various types of administrative structure and need to be guarded against, they do not appear to be inevitable concomitants of any given organizational schema.

The specialist approach in contrast to the generalist orientation has been an issue associated with therapeutic recreation educational preparation for some years. There has always been a general acceptance that there is a common recreational base resulting in an unitary conception of therapeutic recreation regarding both health and community. The guidelines for accreditation clearly emphasize this approach. However, over the past few years, a specialist or clinical path in preparation has emerged. A quick content analysis of therapeutic recreation articles published during this past decade in the *Therapeutic Recreation Journal* and elsewhere supports this view. Further, a study conducted by Fain, Champion, and Scully found that in a random sample of individuals registered with the NTRS in 1977, nearly 92 percent of the 147 individuals completing the questionnaire work in institutional or clinical settings.[52] Humphrey and Reynolds have commented that "professional preparation and registration are presently moving toward a greater emphasis on specialization and a conceptual orientation toward the therapeutic model."[53]

With the movement toward a specialist track has come a backlash from some educators about the failure to give more attention to preparation for community service to special populations.[54] On the other hand, health care agencies which employ specialists dictate, directly and indirectly, the form and substance of education programs. If too much time is spent on a generalist approach, the highly technical competency the young therapeutic recreator needs to fulfill the expecta-

[52] Gerald S. Fain, Lynn Champion, and Daniel G. Scully, "Employment Status Study of Therapeutic Recreation Personnel" (unpublished study, Boston University, Department of Movement, Health and Leisure, n.d.).

[53] Humphrey and Reynolds, "The Editors' Viewpoint," p. 5.

[54] *Ibid.*, pp. 4–6; Peter A. Witt, "Therapeutic Recreation: The Outmoded Label," *Therapeutic Recreation Journal*, 11, no. 2 (1977), 39–41.

tions of his or her first employer may not be met. This situation is further compounded by the question of whether our programs should concentrate on either preparing for initial job competence or providing students with a broad base of principles to facilitate long-range growth and development.

One last issue needs to be addressed regarding our professional preparation programs of study; specifically, the association with higher education in general. The mythology of higher education holds the university to be a critic of society and an agent of social change. However, universities have not generally performed this function, nor will they do so in the foreseeable future, as the result of present economic ills. It is this problem which gives an air of unreality to any attempted innovation within our programs. Further is the apparent eternal problem of those university requirements relating to liberal arts. As we know, the university generally maintains that a reasonable portion of a liberal arts education should be part of the experience of each graduate. Such course work reduces time for purely professional study.

This particular problem is not unusual to therapeutic recreation; it is encountered by all disciplines which consider themselves to be offering professional education at the undergraduate level. It is a problem that will have to be answered by each program of study. Each situation depends on what the general institutional requirements are, what the particular emphasis is in a given course, and similar variables. It can only be recommended that the program faculty analyze the content of the therapeutic recreation offerings and then determine what courses in the general education requirements best serve as a basis for, or in support of, these therapeutic recreation courses. In the final analysis, the sources of knowledge used by the therapeutic recreator are wide and varied, coming from a number of disciplines of diverse natures. For example, study of the natural sciences provides tools for scientific thinking and an understanding of the physical aspects of the human condition. Study of the humanities aids in the development of the creative and critical thought processes. It also provides an understanding of the nature of the human condition through the examination of creative endeavors. If it is any consolation, a 1982 survey of students at ten institutions participating in the Project on General Education Models found students do value a broad general education but at the same time value equally as high knowledge and skills directly related to their careers and mastering of a specialized body of knowledge.[55]

The focus of this section for the most part has been on the undergraduate preparation of therapeutic recreators. Admittedly, therapeutic recreation education is a cohesive whole, with an undergraduate and graduate layer which are both integral to it. However, there appears to be little planned continuity between undergraduate and graduate therapeutic recreation training. One is inclined to assume that this is the result of a lack of universally accepted undergraduate therapeutic recreation educational objectives. Further, the discontinuity between undergraduate and graduate programs of therapeutic recreation study is the result of a vagueness concerning what the profession wants practitioners to do with additional training, coupled with an uncertainty as to the function of graduate therapeutic recreation

---

[55] "Student-Watching," *National On-Campus Report* (1983), p. 4.

programs. Until further research provides a validated basis for a systematic differentiation of practice which can be widely related to different educational levels (excluding doctoral preparation for teaching and research), we can consider at this time only undergraduate preparation.

SUMMARY

If thereapeutic recreators are to provide consumers with competent service, they must be equipped with a substantial body of knowledge. Therapeutic recreation's body of knowledge is eclectic, interdisciplinary, tentative, complex, and often subjective. Therapeutic recreation however, continues to search for the acceptance of common concepts and frames of reference. The body of knowledge used to guide the therapeutic recreator's interactions with consumers has, for the most part, been developed by therapeutic recreators. Much of this information is in the form of insights gained from practical experiences. However, to achieve a substantial level of recognition from society, the occupation must strive to develop a more convincing body of applied knowledge.

The many issues identified in this chapter, especially those concerned with course content and method, appear to indicate that little consideration on the part of those responsible for a therapeutic recreation program of study has been given to a systematic approach to curriculum building. Curriculum construction requires three steps: selection and formulation of educational objectives, design and organization of learning experiences to attain those objectives, and evaluation of whether or not the students actually have attained the desired objectives. The steps of choosing and formulating educational objectives and the selection and organization of learning experiences to attain objectives yield goals toward which to aim the education program and outline means by which therapeutic recreation goals will be achieved. In following these steps, learning experiences are developed that have been checked against various criteria derived from practical experience.

Although a universally accepted therapeutic recreation educational philosophy does not exist, the authors suggest that academic education for therapeutic recreation should have the following characteristics and goals:

1. Develop in the student the kinds of behavior which cannot readily or effectively be acquired on the job. Give priority to teaching concepts as opposed to isolated facts, principles as opposed to techniques, broad problem-solving approaches as opposed to specific procedures.
2. Place greater emphasis on development in the student of changes in thinking, feeling, and doing, particularly the facilitation of understanding, critical thinking, analysis, self-awareness, and empathy and relationship skills.
3. Be concerned with developing in the student a scientific and attitudinal base for therapeutic recreatin practice, for awareness of new problems, for addition of knowledge now unused or unavailable, and for creation of better methods of solving problems in therapeutic recreation practice. This implies that appropriate scientific content should constantly be sought for introduction into the curriculum. Alertness to changing conditions should be developed, and critical thinking should be stimulated to test old solutions and arrive at new ones. Further, the profession must develop a body of skills

which are the result of the fusion of attitudes and knowledges. Skills reflect the application of general concepts and principles which are characteristic of the methods of the profession. The practice of a method meets the criteria of systematic procedures and seeks to add to the body of theory on which professional practice rests. It achieves this by distilling, from professional practice and related disciplines, concepts which add to professional knowledge, and it therefore furthers the evaluation of the effectiveness of professional practice.

4. Develop and impart knowledge, not for the sake of knowledge, but for use in problem-solving activities. Skill in the use of the profession's problem-solving methods is the hallmark of the professional practitioner. Therapeutic recreation education should possess a relatively coherent, systematic, and transmissible body of knowledge rooted in scientific theories, which enables therapeutic recreation practitioners to utilize concepts and principles and to apply them to specific situations. In other words, the therapeutic recreation practitioner must know why as well as how.

5. Include learning experiences in both class and field. As a result of this practice, the agency should have a significant part in the education process.

6. Select students equipped to meet the intellectual and emotional demands made by the education process. This implies that the prerequisite knowledge, skills, and attitudes should be made explicit.

7. Require appropriate adaptive behavior on the part of students, in order for them to function in their respective roles. The student seeks to master the expected professional tasks which are perceived as necessary in order to become a therapeutic recreator.

8. Develop a study program that considers the following principles relative to course content: continuity, sequence, and integration. *Continuity* refers to the reiteration of important concepts, skills, abilities, and attitudes in a series of experiences. For example, the development of problem-solving skills is an important objective in several areas. To develop these skills it is necessary to see that there is recurring and continuing opportunity for them to be practiced. This means that, over time, the same kinds of skills will be brought into continuing operation. *Sequence* is related to continuity but goes beyond it. It is possible for a concept, skill, ability, or attitude to recur again and again merely at the same level, so that there is no progressive development of it. Sequence as a criterion emphasizes the importance of having each successive experience build upon the preceding one, but goes more broadly and deeply into the matter. Lastly, *integration* refers to the horizontal relationship of curriculum experiences. The organization of these experiences should be such that they help the student obtain a comprehensive view of, and consistent behavior in relation to, the concepts, skills, abilities, and so on that he or she learns in various areas of the curriculum. In developing communication skills in working with clients, it is also important to consider the ways in which these skills can be utilized effectively in working with staff and members of other professions.

9. Create objectives of therapeutic recreation education that are attainable within the undergraduate level of preparation. It is essential to select objectives that can actually be achieved to a significant degree in the time available. Furthermore, the objectives which are finally selected should be highly consistent, grouped into homogeneous wholes, and arranged appropriately. In light of therapeutic recreation educational objectives, the authors further suggest that educational objectives should have the following characteristics:

   a. Each educational objective should make explicit a behavioral and a content aspect.

   b. The educational objectives selected should be limited to those that are crucial and best developed through professional education. This is in keeping with the view that the function of formal professional education is to provide basic, or fundamental, education for professional practice and to achieve the learning of generalized modes or approaches to problem solving.

c. The content areas of the educational objectives should be primarily framed as concepts but need to be illustrated by situations and phenomena.

d. The concepts which comprise the content dimension of educational objectives should be couched on a level of abstraction sufficiently specific to enable the student to see the relationship between the concept and the practice. At the same time, the concept should be sufficiently general to enable the student to see its relationship to other ideas.

10. Be constantly alert to changing needs and personnel requirements and realize that findings relative to trends, needs, and recommendations can be valid only for a limited period of time.

The suggestions offered are only recommendations. It is hoped, however, that they will be given serious consideration. If implemented, they will be gradual rather than abrupt. If implementation is initiated, it will be important to be wise and judicious. We have known for a long time that factual education without concepts is poor education, but we must recognize that conceptual education without facts is also poor education. Concepts are no more than abstractions describing a series of phenomena. Lest the pendulum swing too far, let us remember that concepts cannot be learned unless they are illustrated and supported by facts.

In conclusion, if therapeutic recreators are to receive the acclaim associated with professionalization, they must find ways to resolve some, if not all, of the issues discussed within this chapter. Without recognition, the occupation cannot perform its essential services and select qualified potential members. The place of therapeutic recreation programs of study in institutions is jeopardized, because financial support is hard to acquire and hold. Without acknowledgement, therapeutic recreation as a service field and as an emerging profession will not be recognized nor will it exist. Therapeutic recreation finds itself in a challenging position. What it does relative to its programs of study within the next few years may determine its future. Whether it will continue on its emerging professional path is within its power to determine. The decision as to how this will occur is in the hands of its educators and practitioners.

STUDY GUIDE QUESTIONS

1. From your perspective as a student, develop a 2,000-word paper about the knowledge, skills, and values you expect to attain in your therapeutic recreation professional education.

2. Conduct a survey among your fellow students concerning courses necessary for therapeutic recreation practice. Discuss your results in class.

3. Prepare a four-year curriculum with an option in therapeutic recreation. Justify your rationale for each therapeutic recreation course offered and provide course objectives.

4. Trace the major influences on undergraduate therapeutic recreation preparation, beginning with the 1961 Therapeutic Recreation Curriculum Development Conference (Comeback, Inc., February 16–18, 1961).

5. Compare earlier (pre-1961) and modern curricula in therapeutic recreation. What common strands and marked differences do you find?

6. Your instructor plays a central role in your professional preparation. Explain how the instructor helps you by:

     a.   Serving as a role model
     b.   Clarifying the program of study
     c.   Guiding you in fieldwork experiences
     d.   Integrating theory with practice

7. Does therapeutic recreation have a well-defined function, the nature of which can be identified? If so, describe in a 1,000-word paper. If not, indicate why, in the same number of words.

8. Discuss in class the current status of the subject matter of therapeutic recreation. In what areas of therapeutic recreation do we possess a systematic body of knowledge, skills, and attitudes? In what domains, from your perspective, do we need further identification and systematization of knowledge, skills, and attitudes? In what instances are there lags between available knowledge and translation into skills? Conversely, in what areas are skills not sufficiently buttressed by knowledge?

9. Develop a paper around the following question: Is the subject matter of therapeutic recreation sufficiently developed that it can be transmitted as a regimen of professional education? If not, why not?

10. Consider the following for debate or as a paper: Is the nature of therapeutic recreation education such that it can be viewed as an integrated whole which comprises an undergraduate liberal arts foundation and an undergraduate professional sequence? If not, why not?

11. From your perspective: What should be the equipment of the therapeutic recreation specialist in knowledge, skills, and attitudes that would enable the specialist to perform therapeutic recreation tasks in a variety of agency settings? Would the acquisition of such equipment require both undergraduate and graduate training, and, if so, what should be the distribution of curriculum content over the undergraduate-graduate continuum?

12. Can undergraduate and graduate content of a therapeutic recreation curriculum be of a kind to avoid gaps and duplications and foster continuity of learning? If so, why? If not, why not?

13. Does your curriculum facilitate further professional development on the job, so that you can keep attuned to the differing demands for service and practice?

14. What objectives are appropriate for the undergraduate phase of a program of therapeutic recreation education? In answering, consider these questions: (1) What content drawn from the basic sciences and humanities should be incorporated into therapeutic recreation content areas in undergraduate therapeutic recreation education? (2) What therapeutic recreation content should be incorporated into the therapeutic recreation content areas in undergraduate therapeutic recreation education?

15. Discuss in 1,000 words the sources of therapeutic recreation knowledge. Does it come from basic sciences conceived as underlying therapeutic recreation practice, from therapeutic recreation practice itself, or from both?

ANNOTATED BIBLIOGRAPHY

AMERICAN ASSOCIATION FOR HEALTH, PHYSICAL EDUCATION, AND RECREATION, *Guidelines for Professional Preparation Programs for Personnel Involved in Physical Education and Recreation for the Handicapped.* Washington, D.C., February 1973. Provides early guidelines to assist in initiating, developing, expanding, or evaluating programs of graduate preparation in adapted physical education and therapeutic recreation, highlighting competencies needed by students to assume various roles.

AUSTIN, DAVID R., "The University Can't Train Therapeutic Recreators," *Therapeutic Recreation Journal,* 8, no. 1 (1974), 22–24. Offers ideas and suggestions to correct the problem of universities not directing their internship programs to prepare students to assume responsibility in establishing new therapeutic recreation services.

COUNCIL ON ACCREDITATION, *Standards and Evaluative Criteria for Recreation, Leisure Services and Resources Curricula Baccalaureate Degree Programs*. Alexandria, Va.: National Recreation and Park Association, 1981. Outlines the standards by which recreation, leisure services, and resources curricula are evaluated for accreditation by the National Council on Accreditation.

HUMPHREY, FRED and RONALD REYNOLDS, "The Editors' Viewpoint," *Therapeutic Recreation Journal*, 15, no. 2 (1981), 4–6. Seeks to stimulate readers about the articles appearing in this issue on professional preparation, professional standards, etc.

KENNEDY, DAN W., "Competency Based Education: Its Relationship to Therapeutic Recreation Curricula," in *Directions in Health, Physical Education, and Recreation— Therapeutic Recreation Curriculum: Philosophy, Strategy, and Concepts*. Monograph Series 1, pp. 20–25, ed. David R. Austin. Bloomington, Ind.: Indiana University, School of Health, Physical Education, and Recreation, 1980. Provides an overview of competency based education (CBE), its characteristics and its values, to assist educators in the development of CBE in therapeutic recreation.

MEYER, LEE E., *Philosophical Alternatives and the Professionalization of Therapeutic Recreation*, pp. 44–48. Arlington, Va.: National Recreation and Park Association, 1980. Offers the results of an extensive study of philosophical issues related to therapeutic recreation, incorporating a comprehensive analysis of the historical antecedents of therapeutic recreation and outlining three alternative positions advanced by various segments of the therapeutic recreation field.

MOBILY, KENNETH, E., "Quality Analysis in Therapeutic Recreation Curricula," *Therapeutic Recreation Journal*, 17, no. 1 (1983), 18–25. Suggests ways to improve the quality of therapeutic recreation curricula through use of a "competency cluster" procedure.

O'MORROW, GERALD S., "Therapeutic Recreation Accreditation: Its Problems and Future," *Therapeutic Recreation Journal*, 15, no. 2 (1981), 31–38. Surveys the historical development and the purpose of accreditation in therapeutic recreation education and its program accreditation.

PETERSON, CAROL A. and PEG CONNOLLY, "Professional Preparation in Therapeutic Recreation," *Therapeutic Recreation Journal*, 15, no. 2 (1981), 39–45. Provides the results of a 1978 state-of-the-art study, discusses the relationship of therapeutic recreation programs of study to credentialling, and examines the issues relating to further development of therapeutic recreation preparation programs, all of which reflect upon therapeutic recreation professionalization.

ROBB, GARY, "Integrating Preservice Education and Professional Functioning," *Therapeutic Recreation Journal*, 7, no. 2 (1973), 40–46. Reacts to major discrepancies in therapeutic recreation curricula and suggests that universities develop more appropriate and relevant curricula and experiences for students majoring in therapeutic recreation, with examples of new programs and alternatives.

SMITH, S. HAROLD, "Practitioners' Evaluation of College Courses, Competencies, and Functions in Therapeutic Recreation," *Therapeutic Recreation Journal*, 10, no. 4 (1976), 152–56. A report of a study by the author that suggests that undergraduate training may not prepare students for entry level positions or give them a strong philosophical base from which to work.

BIBLIOGRAPHY

ANDERSON, STEPHEN C., and HELEN A. FINCH, "Systematic Curriculum Development," in *Exetra Perspectives: Concepts in Therapeutic Recreation*, pp. 109–20, eds. Larry L. Neal and Christopher R. Edginton, Eugene, Ore.: University of Oregon, Center of Leisure Studies, 1982.

_____ and MICHAEL J. LEITNER, "Course Sequencing in Recreation Curricula," *Therapeutic Recreation Journal*, 12, no. 2 (1978), 15–34.

_____ and MORRIS W. STEWART, "Therapeutic Recreation Education: 1979 Survey," *Therapeutic Recreation Journal*, 14, no. 3 (1980), 4–10.

AUSTIN, DAVID R., and DAVID F. LEITZMAN, "Systematic Curriculum Design," in *Directions in Health, Physical Education, and Recreation—Therapeutic Recreation Curriculum: Philosophy, Strategy, and Concepts.* Monograph Series 1, pp. 13–19, ed. David R. Austin. Bloomington, Ind.: Indiana University, School of Health, Physical Education and Recreation, 1980.

_____ and LOU G. POWELL, "Competencies Needed by Community Recreators to Serve Special Populations," in *Directions in Health, Physical Education, and Recreation—Therapeutic Recreation Curriculum: Philosophy, Strategy, and Concepts*, Monograph Series 1, pp. 33–34, ed. David R. Austin, Bloomington, Ind.: Indiana University, School of Health, Physical Education and Recreation, 1980.

BERGER, PETER, and THOMAS LUCKMAN. *The Social Construction of Reality.* New York: Doubleday & Company, Inc., 1967.

BERRYMAN, DORIS L., and others, *A Modular Training Program for Therapeutic Recreation Technician I: The NTRS 750 Hour Curriculum.* Arlington, Va.: National Recreation and Park Association, 1975.

CORWIN, RONALD G., *A Sociology of Education.* Englewood Cliffs, N.J.: Prentice-Hall, Inc., Appleton-Century-Crofts, 1965.

HENKEL, DONALD, "Accreditation," *Parks and Recreation*, 15, no. 8 (1980), 53–54.

HOWE, CHRISTINE J., "Some Uses of the Multi-Modal Model of Curriculum Evaluation in Therapeutic Recreation," in *Exetra Perspectives: Concepts in Therapeutic Recreation*, pp. 87–98, eds. Larry L. Neal and Christopher R. Edginton. Eugene, Ore.: University of Oregon, Center of Leisure Studies, 1982.

LEGGE, DAVID, ed., *Skills.* Baltimore: Penguin Books, 1970.

SESSOMS, H. DOUGLAS, "Education in the Eighties—Forecast—Change," *Parks and Recreation*, 16, no. 5 (1981), 48–50, 70.

SHULMAN, LAWRENCE, *The Skills of Helping: Individuals and Groups.* Itasca, Ill.: F.E. Peacock Publishers, Inc., 1979.

"THERAPEUTIC RECREATION SERVICE CURRICULUM TODAY AND THE NEED FOR CHANGE," Editorial in *Therapeutic Recreation Journal*, 4, no. 2 (1970), 2–3.

CHAPTER SEVEN
THE NORMALIZATION-INTEGRATION ISSUE

If we integrate the ill, the disabled, the handicapped, into normative settings, we remove them from the therapeutic and rehabilitative milieu. We are in effect saying that such persons do not need therapeutic milieu. They have gone about as far as they can go in the treatment milieu, and that the main objective should be fun. In most instances, however, the ill, the disabled, the handicapped (in their ever changing needs at each age level, etc.) can best be served in a clinical setting. That is, where they can have access to many rehabilitative services in one setting, and where the recreation is therapeutic; that is, addressed to the amelioration of the changing aspects of the disease or disability.[1]

These words, challenging the principle of normalization and its related tenet of integration in recreation services for the disabled, appeared in the *Therapeutic Recreation Journal* in 1967. Since then, the concept of normalization has become recognized as a major ideology guiding the provision of human services (including leisure) to all groups of disabled persons. Although few recreators would challenge this concept so directly (or vehemently) today, it continues to be widely misunderstood, misinterpreted, and misapplied. How did this principle come into being?

[1] Jack M. Goodzeit, "Therapeutic Recreation vs. Recreation for the Handicapped," *Therapeutic Recreation Journal*, 1, no. 2 (1967), 31.

What are its origins and major tenets? What is its relevance and concern to the field of therapeutic recreation? This chapter attempts to shed light on these questions while providing a learning plan and strategy for applying normalization to therapeutic recreation practice.

THE CONCEPT: ORIGIN
AND MEANING

The term *normalization* owes its origin to the head of the Danish Mental Retardation Service, Bank Mikkelsen, who coined the word to mean "letting the mentally retarded obtain an existence as close to the normal as possible." Following a series of translations and retranslations, Wolf Wolfensberger publicized and popularized this concept in North America through his 1972 text, *The Principle of Normalization in Human Services.* Wolfensberger's classic definition of the concept is "Utilization of means which are as culturally normative as possible in order to establish and/or maintain personal behaviors and characteristics which are as culturally normative as possible."[2]

Recently, Wolfensberger has altered (and expanded) this original definition to an informal instructional definition.

> Use of culturally normative means (familiar, valued techniques, tools, methods) in order to enable persons' life conditions (income, housing, health services, etc.) which are at least as good as average citizens, and to as much as possible, enhance or support their behavior (skills, competencies, etc.) appearances (clothes, grooming, etc.) experiences (adjustment, feelings, etc.) and status and reputation (labels, attitudes of others, etc.).[3]

Most simply stated, it can mean "The use of culturally valued means in order to enable people to live culturally valued lives."[4]

The concept of normalization is appearing with increasing frequency in therapeutic recreation literature. In most cases it appears as a synonym for mainstreaming, which is an educational term describing the practice of integrating disabled children into regular classroom environments. Although such physical integration is one corollary or practice of the principle of normalization, the concept has much broader and more profound implications for the field of therapeutic recreation and human services. The following section describes and examines several factors and trends which make the concept of normalization of vital interest to therapeutic recreation professionals.

[2] Wolf Wolfensberger, *The Principle of Normalization in Human Services* (Toronto, Canada: National Institute on Mental Retardation, 1972), p. 26.

[3] Robert J. Flynn and Kathleen E. Nitsch, eds., *Normalization, Social Integration and Community Services* (Baltimore, Md.: University Park Press, 1980), p. 80.

[4] *Ibid.*

NORMALIZATION
AND THERAPEUTIC
RECREATION

The principle of normalization is a comprehensive theory concerning the way services (including recreation and leisure) are provided to and for all groups of disabled individuals. As such, it applies to persons with physical, mental, social, and emotional deficits; in short, persons who make up the clientel of therapeutic recreation specialists.

Because of its ability to transcend various handicapping conditions, the principle is becoming more widely embraced and practiced by a variety of human-service professionals in clinical and community settings. Thus, to be able to communicate with other health care service providers, therapeutic recreation personnel must understand the application of this concept to their field.

Recent practices such as leisure education have stressed the preparation of clients for self-sustained leisure participation in community settings. The concept and practice of normalization is entirely consistent with this goal and, as such, can provide a viable tool for its attainment.

Therapeutic recreation specialists are increasingly assuming direct advocacy roles with clients, are working with parent groups or voluntary advocate associations, or both. Normalization is fast becoming a guiding principle in the advocacy movement. Therefore, the therapeutic recreation professional must be familiar with the movement's basic tenets and ideologies. Furthermore, as disabled persons and advocate groups obtain more influence over the types of recreational services provided, therapeutic recreation personnel must be able to design, implement, and evaluate programs which are compatible with the theory of normalization.

AN EXAMINATION
OF THE CONCEPT
OF NORMALIZATION

While this notion may appear to be relatively simple, in reality it represents a comprehensive theory with several complex axioms and corollaries. Following are descriptions of some of the major tenets of the normalization principle and discussions of the implications which each may have for therapeutic recreation service. While reading these principles, the reader should keep in mind that these concepts are highly interrelated and must not be viewed as being separate or distinct components of the theory. Figure 7-1 illustrates the concept and its related principles and terminology.

Principle 1—Integration

The most widely recognized (and misunderstood) feature of normalization is the corollary of integration.[5] Historically, this principle is a reaction to the concept

[5] Unless otherwise indicated, these concepts appear and are described in depth in Wolfensberger's, *The Principle of Normalization in Human Services*, 1972.

TABLE FIGURE 7-1 Model of the Relationship of Normalization to its Major Principles and Tenets. Cited directly or parapharsed from Wolf Wolfensberger, *The Principle of Normalization in Human Services*, chaps. 1–5.

THE PHILOSOPHY
(Normalization)

The utilization of means which are as culturally normative as possible, in order to establish or maintain personal behaviors or characteristics which are as culturally normative as possible.

Leads to the Practice of
INTEGRATION

The process consisting of those practices and measures which maximize a person's (potential) participation in the mainstream of his/her culture.

Which Takes Place in
GENERIC AGENCIES
(MUNICIPAL AND PUBLIC RECREATION)

Agencies not oriented toward a single condition such as mental retardation, visual impairment, etc., and are utilized by typical citizens.

	Which Provides for INTEGRATION	
PHYSICAL	SOCIAL
Location	Program Features
Physical Context	Labelling
Access	Building Perception
Size or Dispersal	Dignity of Risk

of *segregated*, or "special," services which have been traditionally provided to groups of disabled individuals. It is a departure from the theory that segregated services can better meet the needs of disabled persons and that individuals with handicapping conditions "ought" to be isolated from the mainstream of society. In describing the process of integrating an individual, Wolfensberger stated that:

> . . . integration is achieved when he lives in a culturally normative community setting in ordinary community housing, can move and communicate in ways typical for his age, and is able to utilize in typical ways, typical community resources, developmental, social, *recreational** and facilities. . . .[6] (Italics are the authors'.)

There are two basic components of this process, *physical* and *social* integration. Social integration involves the interaction of individuals, while physical integration relates to settings, which can promote or inhibit social interaction. Each has its own set of important, related tenets.

The following four concepts are included in this notion:

[6] Wolfensberger, *Normalization*, p. 48.

153

Physical integration   *Location*—This variable relates to the proximity of the service to other community resources and to the general public. It is particularly important because it influences the degree to which disabled people may become part of the larger society. It is usually undesirable to isolate disabled individuals. Therefore separate therapeutic recreation programs, such as remedial swimming instruction for youngsters with cerebral palsy at an out-of-the-way pool, should be avoided.

Physical Context—This refers to the relationship of the facility or service to other programs or facilities which surround it. Physical context influences the degree to which disabled persons can be integrated into other nearby services. In general, areas with a large number and variety of resources will be better able to accommodate disabled individuals.[7] For example, it would be more desirable to hold a leisure education course in a section of the city which had a number of stores, movies, libraries, churches, and other public places.

Access—The idea of access relates to the relative ease with which disabled persons can utilize a program or service. A number of factors can influence access. Therapeutic recreation programs and services should be offered in areas which have good transportation available.

Size or Dispersal—These notions refer to the degree to which services for disabled individuals are distributed within a given area. It is important to spread services throughout a community. In this fashion, disabled people have an ample opportunity to become absorbed in the mainstream of society. As an illustration, therapeutic recreation programs should not be concentrated in one center, residential facility, or camp setting.

Social integration   As defined by Wolfensberger, social integration has three major considerations:

Program Features—Central to this factor is the idea that, whenever possible, disabled individuals should be involved in programs or services which are generic (used by the general public) in nature. This is crucial in allowing persons with special needs to interact with their nondisabled peers. Specifically, it is more desirable to schedule an aerobics course for paraplegic persons at the local health club than at a special rehabilitation facility.

Labeling—This concept refers to the fashion in which clients, services, and facilities are identified. Care should be taken to avoid images which are deleterious to the disabled person. For example, it is not desirable to label participants as being *retarded* or *patients*. Programs and classes should also not be labeled with terms which are different from those offered to the public, for instance, "The New Hope Recreation Program" for substance abuse clients.

Building Perception—The physical design of the facility is important in this concept. Specifically, buildings which have an undesirable external appearance will negatively affect the public's perception of individuals utilizing the setting and the types of services provided. Therefore, recreation activities should not be scheduled in reconverted prisons, orphanages, and the like.

[7] *Ibid.*

Application of integration to therapeutic recreation service provision The principle of integration and its related corollaries have both obvious and subtle implications for the provision of therapeutic recreation service. The following two examples may prove useful in illustrating the application of integration to leisure service provision. These two contrasting situations are indicative of varying degrees of normalization in therapeutic recreation service. Both are based upon such service being provided in a transitional living center for individuals who have been treated for problems related to substance abuse.

Center A—The Integrated Approach

This residence is centrally located on a major bus route in a residential section of the city. It is near a shopping mall, a post office, a library, and a community recreation center. It has no external signs or other identifying features, and it does not differ from other housing in the area. The therapeutic recreation specialist conducts leisure education sessions at the residence, yet utilizes the surrounding community for most activities with residents. The participants are encouraged to walk or use public transportation to nearby recreational resources and travel individually or in groups of twos and threes.

Center B—The Nonintegrated Approach

This facility is located in an isolated area two miles from the city, in a large facility which served as a home for incurables for several years. It has been remodeled inside and boasts a sign "Sunflower Home" on the front porch. The therapeutic recreation specialist concentrates on conducting large group activities within the residence or transports all the participants in the home's labeled van into town to various spectator events. Many residents sport T-shirts with the home's logo at these activities.

It is important to note that the concept of integration represents a *continuum* of services. In fact, in the above examples, Center A provides leisure services partway between highly prescriptive, clinically based recreation and self-sustained leisure participation in the community. The continuum of leisure services has been described by Hutchison and Lord and includes the following stages:

1. Upgrading experiences in institutions.
2. Segregated upgrading experiences in associations or settings used by disabled persons.
3. Segregated upgrading experiences in the community.
4. Homebound and individualized upgrading experiences in the community.
5. Integrated experiences in the community with advocacy and support.
6. Integrated experiences in the community with little or no advocacy.
7. On-going community involvement.[8]

[8] Peggy Hutchison and John Lord, *Recreation Integration: Issues and Alternatives in Leisure Services and Community Involvement* (Ottawa, Canada: Leisurability Publications, Inc., 1979), p. 112.

Principle 2—Avoidance
of Deviancy Juxtaposition

The concept of deviancy juxtaposition as described by Wolfensberger is highly related to the previously outlined concept of integration.[9] Basically, the idea centers around the avoidance of mixing various groups of disadvantaged or "devalued" people, providing inappropriate role models for disabled individuals, or both. This principle holds that the pairing of various disabilities or disadvantaging conditions results in the learning of inappropriate responses and behaviors and leads to negative perceptions of disabilities on the part of the public. For example, the operation of a summer camp catering to separate groups of persons who are mentally retarded, emotionally disturbed, and physically disabled is contrary to this principle.

Principle 3—Dignity of Risk

Perske pointed out that many individuals who work with disabled persons have a tendency to be overzealous in their efforts to "protect," "comfort," "keep safe," "take care of," and "watch out for." He further stated that when these responses are taken to extreme, the result may be a stifling of the disabled individual's growth potential and, ultimately, the human dignity which can only result from the ordinary risk-taking activities of daily life.[10] Simply stated, disabled persons also have the "right to fail." This author has identified four major areas where disabled persons should be allowed to experience challenges similar to those faced by society in general. A summary of these four major areas and examples of risk-taking activities in each follows. A complete description of these areas may be found in Wolfensberger.[11]

Normal risk in community experiences   Mentally retarded adults were given the opportunity to travel to a special event in a nearby community and later to find their own way home by using public transportation and asking directions.

Normal risk in industry   After proper training, disabled workers were allowed to operate machinery with no special modifications or atypical safety devices.

Normal risk in heterosexual relationships   A reduction in the number of men's and women's "only" dormitories is taking place in many residential facilities for disabled adults.

[9] Wolfensberger, *Normalization*, p. 115.

[10] Robert Perske, "The Dignity of Risk," in *The Principle of Normalization in Human Services*, (ed. Wolf Wolfensberger Toronto, Canada: National Institute on Mental Retardation, 1972), pp. 194–200.

[11] Wolfensberger, *Normalization*, pp. 196–98.

Normal risk in building design Architects in Scandinavian countries are beginning to design residences which have hanging fixtures, lightweight doors, and large amounts of glass.

The concept of dignity of risk has direct implications for therapeutic recreation professionals in the areas of both facility design and program implementation. For example, there may be a movement away from sites and equipment which are overly protective and, hence, unduly restrictive. There already appears to be a shift from activities which are totally "safe" and of "guaranteed success" to programs of adventure, wilderness survival, and high-risk ventures.

Principle 4—Behavioral Techniques

Behavior modification and its related techniques and practices represent powerful tools for the therapeutic recreation specialist to use to engender desired responses in clients. Behavioral procedures, including operant conditioning, have grown in popularity through the 1970s and continue to be used with a variety of disabled clients in numerous settings. Examples of the use of behavioral techniques in therapeutic recreation settings include controlling disruptive behavior in individuals and groups,[12] promoting social skills in camp settings,[13] and increasing play skills of the mentally retarded.[14]

Because of the power and popularity of behavior modification techniques and principles, it is fortunate that this learning theory, *when properly applied,* is compatible with the ideology of normalization. Indeed, according to Roos, behavioral therapy may be contrasted favorably with other approaches to "treatment" such as the medical model, which presumes an "illness," or "pathology," on the part of the client.[15] This author outlined several common criticisms of behavior modification. These included the beliefs that a behavioral approach is superficial and does not affect the underlying cause of behavior, that the approach is devoid of human warmth and understanding, and that the approach "controls" the recipient of such an intervention. Roos took exception to these criticisms and pointed out that most normative, cultural means for maintaining and developing behavior are actually principles of behavior modification.[16] In fact, behavioral-learning theory may be

[12] E. William Volger, George Fenstermacher, and Paul Bishop, "Group Oriented Management Systems to Control Disruptive Behavior in Therapeutic Recreation Settings," *Therapeutic Recreation Journal*, 16, no. 1 (1982), 20–24.

[13] Harve E. Rawson, "Short-Term Residential Therapeutic Camping for Behaviorally Disordered Children, Aged 6–12; An Academic Remediation and Behavior Modification Approach," *Therapeutic Recreation Journal*, 12, no. 4 (1978), 17–23.

[14] Paul Wehman, "Applications of Behavior Modification Techniques to Play Problems of the Severely and Profoundly Retarded," *Therapeutic Recreation Journal*, 11, no. 1 (1977), 16–23.

[15] Phillip Roos, "Reconciling Behavior Modification Procedures with the Normalization Principle," in *The Principle of Normalization in Human Services*, (ed. Wolf Wolfensberger Toronto, Canada: National Institute on Mental Retardation, 1972), pp. 136–48.

[16] *Ibid.*, p. 144.

viewed merely as a more specific and systematic application of real-life learning. Behavioral techniques, then, can be valuable tools in promoting normative behavior.

In selecting and applying behavior modification approaches such as operant conditioning and modeling, the therapeutic recreation specialist must be judicious in insuring that the strategies selected are consistent with the principle of normalization. The following suggestions are made for reconciling behavior modification and normalization in therapeutic recreation practice:

1. Target behaviors should be chosen which are desirable and typical of those exhibited by peers in everyday settings. As an illustration, it is far more appropriate to teach adult mentally retarded persons to identify numbers and suits of playing cards than pictures on a deck of Old Maid playing cards.
2. Whenever possible, "normal" reinforcers should be utilized. For example, everyday social reinforcement such as verbal praise, rather than artificial tangible or token reinforcers, should be administered to emotionally disturbed children in game settings. If tangible reinforcers are necessary at first, they should gradually be replaced by social praise.
3. Appropriate role models should be used in demonstrating desired behaviors. For example, it may be highly effective to integrate "nondisturbed" adolescents into sports and game situations to demonstrate appropriate social skills to emotionally disturbed youth.
4. Clients should be consulted in determining target behavior, behavior strategies, reinforcement schedules, and goals. This is crucial to insuring client autonomy and commitment to the intervention. In attempting to improve the social skills of a psychiatric patient, the therapeutic recreation specialist should work closely with the client in identifying which skills need improvement, what reinforcers will be administered to engender these skills, and what activities will most likely provide these rewards.

Principle 5—Advocacy

Consumer advocacy is a cornerstone of the normalization ideology. Fortunately, the "process directed toward improving the quality of goods and services rendered to consumers and an advocate as a person who generates and sustains the advocacy process"[17] has long been identified and encouraged as an essential activity of therapeutic recreation specialists. Edginton and Compton[18] identified the following advocacy roles which therapeutic recreation professionals may assume relative to working with disabled clients:

Initiator or organizer—This role may be played by a disabled individual or an "outsider." This function centers around designing strategies for improving the recreational services the disability group currently receives.

[17] John A. Nesbitt and Christopher R. Edginton, "A Conceptual Framework for Consumerism and Advocacy in Parks, Recreation, Leisure and Cultural Services" (Paper delivered at the Urban Recreation Conference, Montclair State College, Upper Montclair, New Jersey, 1973).

[18] Christopher R. Edginton and David M. Compton, "Consumerism and Advocacy: A Conceptual Framework for the Therapeutic Recreator," *Therapeutic Recreation Journal*, 9, no. 1 (1975), 26–32.

Investigator or ombudsman—The practitioner becomes involved in fact finding, data gathering, and identification of the current status of recreation services received.

Mediator or negotiator—The professional deals with situations in which no response has been received from the recreation service delivery system.

Lobbyist—The lobbyist gains attention for the leisure concerns of the group and persuades appropriate decision makers.

Counselor—In this role, the professional offers guidance regarding the quality of leisure and recreation services to the group.

Resource assistant—The professional is responsible for coordinating logistics associated with the process of improving the quality of recreational services.

Educator—This calls for improving the level of societal awareness of the recreational needs of the disabled.

Critic or evaluator—The professional assists the organization in determining whether or not they have met the goal of improving the quality of leisure services received.

Weiner has defined the roles of the therapeutic recreation specialist in integrating disabled clients into community-based, leisure services.[19] These major responsibilities include placement of the client in the appropriate program, systematic monitoring of client progress, assistance to the client in managing "red tape" associated with participation, evaluation of the program through feedback from agency and client, and education of the public and other groups as to clients' needs.

A most effective and interesting technique of advocacy in therapeutic recreation settings has been described by Hunt and Wyatt.[20] These authors detailed the process of utilizing parents as evaluators of the effects of a residential camping program for mentally retarded children. This procedure apparently resulted in increased accountability, improved understanding of the nature of the program, and knowledge of the likes and dislikes of the individual participants.

In summary, the therapeutic recreation specialist must be knowledgeable of the advocacy process and capable of performing the previously outlined roles when assisting in the integration of disabled persons into generic recreation services.

[19] Andrew Weiner, "The Recreation Advocate: Your Leisure Insurance Agent," *Therapeutic Recreation Journal*, 9, no. 2 (1975), 63–68.

[20] Sharon K. Hunt and William J. Wyatt, "Using Parents as Evaluators of a Therapeutic Recreational Camping Program for the Retarded," *Therapeutic Recreation Journal*, 10, no. 4 (1976), 143–48.

FACTS AND FALLACIES
ABOUT NORMALIZATION

Despite the widespread application of the previously outlined principles of normalization, several misconceptions concerning its practices abound. The following discussion of the problems associated with this process in the provision of therapeutic recreation service is based on previous work outlining common misunderstandings related to the normalization process.[21]

Fact #1

Integration is both a process and an ultimate goal for disabled persons. The therapeutic recreation professional must work with the client to outline and achieve the various steps leading to integration. As an illustration, the client may be assisted to become involved in a number of "special" and "semi-integrated" disabled sports programs before being able to participate independently in a community bowling league.

Fallacy

The normalization principle is applicable only to mentally retarded individuals. Although developed in conjunction with the provision of services to mentally retarded persons, the principle, as previously discussed, is comprehensive and has wide potential applicability to a variety of disabling and disadvantaging conditions. Other individuals served by therapeutic recreation professionals who could profit from the application of this theory include incarcerated offenders, the economically disadvantaged, blind and visually impaired persons, emotionally disturbed youth, adults with functional mental disorders, the hearing impaired, and the orthopedically handicapped.

Fact #2

Being integrated precludes being involved in special (segregated) programs. It is quite conceivable and appropriate that a client served by a therapeutic recreation specialist could be involved simultaneously or longitudinally in several different activities, of varying degrees of integration. For example, a visually impaired client could be a member of a blind bowling league and a fitness class for visually impaired adults and enjoy concerts at a local community center. The important point, however, is that all segregated programs should be viewed as *stepping-stones* to mainstream involvement. The therapeutic recreation specialist must continually evaluate the client's progress in terms of his or her ability to become involved in community-based programs of choice.

[21] Ronald P. Reynolds, "Normalization: A Guideline to Leisure Skills Programming for Handicapped Individuals," in *Leisure and Handicapped Individuals: Adaptations, Techniques, and Curriculum* (Baltimore, Md.: University Park Press, 1981), pp. 1–13.

Fallacy

All disabled persons would benefit from immediate inclusion and participation in fully integrated leisure services. Because of differing physical, social, and emotional levels of development, all disabled individuals are not ready (or able) to successfully take part in self-sustained participation in generic leisure services. However, the therapeutic recreation specialist should not lose sight of the fact that integration is an ultimate goal. It is relatively easy to decide for the client that participation in integrated recreation settings is not a feasible or realistic possibility. However, this attitude can, unfortunately, result in severe limiting of the client's development.

Fact #3

Successful integration depends upon the involvement of small groups or individuals in existing programs or services. Attempts at the integration of disabled persons into recreational programs and settings are frequently doomed to failure by the size of the group which is to be involved. In attempts at integration, it is important that the number of disabled persons entering a regular recreation program be kept small so as not to create an atypical situation and therefore insure easy access and dispersal. It is the responsibility of the therapeutic recreation professional to adhere to this practice in structuring recreational programs and experiences. For example, it is far more desirable in an open bowling situation at a community facility to disperse individuals or dyads of mentally retarded persons throughout the various lanes. Similarly, at a public campsite, small numbers of physically disabled campers should be scattered at various sites, rather than congregated en masse at a central location.

Fallacy

Operating an integrated program means grouping people with various disabilities together in the same setting. Occasionally one learns of recreational programs described as being examples of integrated efforts which contain two or more groups of disabled individuals. For example, some summer camps boast of "integrating" physically handicapped and mentally retarded youngsters. Claims concerning the alleged benefits of this arrangement include the theory that disabled individuals feel more comfortable around other persons with limitations, and that each group can help the other group by utilizing their residual functional abilities. In actuality, such arrangements fall short of the goals of normalization for several reasons. *First,* because of the lack of nondisabled persons, typical role models are not present. *Second,* such endeavors provide little opportunity for public education, awareness, and the hoped-for acceptance of disabilities. *Third,* the deviancy juxtaposition situation created may result in a negative image on the part of the public. *Finally,* due to the size and concentration of large numbers of disabled persons, opportunities for access and dispersal are extremely limited.

The therapeutic recreation specialist should be aware of these limitations and develop truly integrated recreational opportunities.

Fact #4

Integration requires careful and systematic planning, not merely "dumping" disabled clients into regular programs.   Because of the complexity of the normalization theory and process, it is critical that therapeutic recreation professionals closely assess each opportunity to integrate their clients before the involvement process is begun. Hutchison and Lord have described the essential phases of the recreation-integration process:

> *Upgrading*— Developing the skills of the client which are necessary to participate in the activity. Processes and techniques available to the therapeutic recreation professional in this phase might include activity analysis, perceptual motor training, behavioral therapy, etc.
> *Education*— This procedure should impact on the client and all other individuals who will be involved in the integration process. Such persons might include: other participants, staff, parents, volunteers, members of advocate associations, etc. The therapeutic recreation professional would employ a leisure education approach in this phase.
> *Participation*— This final phase involves the actual inclusion of the disabled person in the regular program or service. The therapeutic recreation specialist should carefully monitor and assess the client's level of leisure functioning and provide any remedial assistance necessary to ensure success.[22]

Fallacy

It makes little difference what types of recreational pursuits are undertaken by the disabled client.   The selection of *appropriate* activities is extremely important in the normalization process. To illustrate: mentally retarded adults should be given the opportunity to become involved in age-appropriate activities such as chess, checkers, and backgammon, rather than children's games such as Candy Land and Go Fish. Similarly, the therapeutic recreation professional must be skilled in techniques of activity modification, so as to avoid unduly simplifying sports for disabled persons.

Fact #5

Integration can best be achieved by a cooperative approach.   In examining the best way to facilitate the integration process, one discovers that a great number of individuals and agencies are in a potential position to impact on the disabled client. For example, a single attempt at involving a person in a residential-clinical setting in a community-based activity might include the following persons:

---

[22] Margaret L. Hutchison and John C. Lord, "Recreation Integration: A Model for Integrating Persons with Disabilities into Community Recreation Programs," *Recreation Canada*, 33, no. 3 (Fall 1975), 60–64.

ward staff and personnel, treatment team members (nurses, etc.), community recreation staff, trained volunteers, public transportation personnel, advocate association members, and the disabled person. It is obvious that the therapeutic recreation professional involved in the integration process must function in the role of a coordinator or facilitator in marshalling the efforts of the aforementioned resources.

Fallacy

Integration is reached and guaranteed by physical proximity. True integration is achieved only when *social* interaction takes place between disabled and nondisabled persons in a recreational setting. Therefore, the therapeutic recreation specialist cannot be satisfied with merely having his or her clients "co-act" in the same setting with the public. For example, while a first and enviable effort may be the enrollment of two former psychiatric patients in a crafts class in a community recreation center, true integration will not be achieved until these persons can interact comfortably and appropriately with other members of the class.

NORMALIZATION IN-CLASS LEARNING EXERCISES

The following situations depict a number of hypothetical and real-world instances in which various tenets of the normalization principle are threatened. In each case study, certain information concerning the particulars is provided. Learners may want to go beyond the specifics of each case by adding their own details or altering the facts presented. Readers are also encouraged to modify and add to the study guide questions provided. It may be beneficial, in certain instances, to try to achieve group consensus.

Situation 1—The "Vets" versus the Recreation Department

You are a recreation specialist employed in a rehabilitation facility which provides therapeutic recreation services to a large number of physically disabled veterans. For the past several weeks, you have run skill-upgrading, instructional swimming classes for your orthopedically disabled clients. Twelve veterans, all amputees, with varying levels of swimming ability, have decided as a group to attend a free swimming session at the local municipal recreation department. They have asked you to contact personnel at the community center to work out logistical details. Upon contacting the aquatics director, you find this person is reluctant to admit the "vets" to the free swim. When you pursue this decision, the director states that the lifeguard cannot adequately supervise twelve additional swimmers. When further pushed, the director explains that the guard is hesitant to deal with individuals who require special assistance. Finally, the director admits concern that the able-bodied participants who frequent the free swims may feel uncomfortable in the presence of physically disabled persons. As a solution, the director offers to set aside a special one-hour swimming session just for the vets on a regular, weekly basis, suggesting that your rehabilitation agency provide a qualified lifeguard for this activity. You report this information back to your clients. They find this suggestion unacceptable and reinforce their right to attend any and all tax-supported recreation programs.

DISCUSSION QUESTIONS

1. Which principle(s) of normalization come into play in this situation?[23]
2. Which of the following strategies or combination of strategies would you adopt?
   a. Accepting the suggestion of the aquatics director
   b. "Wheeling in" to protest the recreation department, publicizing the situation at hand
   c. Going above the aquatics director to the program supervisor or center director to receive satisfaction
   d. Suggesting to the vets that small numbers (e.g., dyads and triads) of clients be integrated into several free swims throughout the week
   e. Offering to run a training session for the recreation department's pool staff on "adapted aquatics"
   f. Suggesting to the vets that they first become involved in other recreation department activities to insure their acceptance in the free swim
3. Would this situation be altered if you were representing a different client group such as mentally retarded children or emotionally disturbed adults? Would the situation change if there were fewer vets wishing to become involved?
4. Should you have initially attempted to enroll the vets in instuctional swims at the local recreation center?

Situation 2—The Saturday Matinee

You are a therapeutic recreation specialist in a large residential center for mentally retarded adults. For the past six weeks, you have been conducting a leisure education course for eight male residents. Last week, as part of the leisure education class, the residents were given the assignment of selecting from the entertainment section of the newspaper a movie to attend next Saturday afternoon. They have unanimously chosen the cartoon version of *Pinocchio* and have notified you of their decision. You had previously agreed to drive them to the theater in the facility's van. The day before the show, the administrator of the residence calls you into the office, ostensibly to discuss your next year's activity budget and "other matters." In the course of the meeting, your administrator makes the following statement:

> I understand that eight of our residents want to see *Pinocchio* at the Palace Theatre downtown tomorrow afternoon. I also have heard that you intend to take a van—the one with our logo and name on it—to escort them. I'm all for recreation, and have supported your department in the past. This time however, I must intervene. I'm afraid

---

[23] This and other discussion questions concerning principles pertain to the material previously presented under the five principles of normalization and facts and fallacies headings.

that the local association for retarded citizens will see our people at this movie and object. They are a powerful group in town and could influence our future funding. I don't object to your plan *personally*, but please don't proceed with this activity.

DISCUSSION QUESTIONS

1. What principle(s) of normalization are in question in this situation?
2. Following the meeting with your administrator, which of the following strategies or combination of strategies would you undertake?
   a. Ignore the position taken by the administrator and go to the movie as planned.
   b. Notify the residents of the administrator's position and tell them to select another film.
   c. Rent or borrow the *Pinocchio* film from a local library and show it in the residence.
   d. Schedule the outing for the evening show, so that the residents will be "less conspicuous."
   e. Suggest that the residents each escort a child from a local foster-home residence to the movie.
3. Suppose that the residents had selected an x-rated film to attend. Would you allow them to view it and accompany them in the van?
4. In the future, would you avoid similar situations by giving your clients a specific list of movies to choose from?

Situation 3—The Donation

You are a therapeutic recreation specialist in a municipal recreation department. A wealthy local resident, Mrs. Goodwill, has approached the city council with an offer. She would be willing to donate a large sum of money for the construction of a recreation activity center for orthopedically disabled adults and children. Once completed, the center would be run by your department. The conditions she proposes are as follows:

— The facility is to be called "The New Hope Haven for Crippled Persons."
— The center is to be for the *exclusive* use of physically disabled individuals.
— The site for the construction of the facility is to be an isolated section of a large urban park system.
— The adivsory board for the center is to be largely composed of Mrs. Goodwill's "church friends" and "business acquaintances."

Over the past several years, your department has operated under a philosophy of normalization in its approach to serving disabled persons. The city council has asked the director of the recreation and parks department for the department's input on this proposal. The director, in turn, has asked you to prepare a written position paper to be shared with the mayor, the city council, and Mrs. Goodwill.

Learning task   Draft a two- or three-page letter reacting to the donation proposal, focusing on the following points:

1. The impact of the proposal (pro and con) on the physically disabled residents of your city.

2. The impact of the proposal on the recreation department's current approach to serving disabled persons.

3. Mrs. Goodwill's conditions for donation and whether they are acceptable, unacceptable, or negotiable.

4. Suggestions you may have for an alternate project or proposal which Mrs. Goodwill might be inclined to fund.

Situation 4—The Field Day

You are a therapeutic recreation specialist working in a rural municipal recreation department. You have been approached by a well-known high school coach in the area. He would like the support of you and your department in staging a one-day Field Day Competition for mentally retarded children. According to the coach, he has already solicited the support of the local association for the mentally retarded, who will provide transportation, several merchants who will donate prizes and refreshments, and a scout troop who will help to run and judge the track and field events. The coach feels the event will be extremely successful in demonstrating the abilities of mentally retarded persons to the public and improving the self-concept and fitness of the mentally retarded children who participate. He will even feature an "everyone wins" atmosphere by giving ribbons and medals to all participants. The coach also points out that this high visibility event will be good publicity for your department and program, as local media coverage will be heavy. You have agreed to take the matter under advisement.

While considering the coach's proposal, you are contacted by a small but concerned group of parents of mentally retarded children. They encourage you to reject the coach's offer in lieu of providing more opportunities for children to participate in regular recreation programs. They offer the following arguments to defend their position:

— The segregated nature of the event will tend to isolate the mentally retarded children in the eyes of the public.

— The concept of "everyone wins" is an unrealistic one which is not adhered to in sport and in the rest of our culture. Therefore, the mentally retarded children should not be indoctrinated with this idea.

— This one-shot event will not encourage the participants to train or achieve physical fitness on a regular schedule. Furthermore, the fact that this event is scheduled may cause school officials and recreation personnel to deemphasize or ignore other leisure services which should be provided to mentally retarded children.

DISCUSSION QUESTIONS

1. Which principle(s) of normalization are the focal points of controversy between the coach's and the parents' perceptions?

2. Would you assist in the provision of the Field Day Competition as proposed by the coach, favor not becoming affiliated with the event, or favor staging the event in a modified form?

3. If the Field Day were being planned for physically disabled adults, would the same principles (and controversy) apply?

4. In the future, do you feel that special, one-shot events for disabled people will increase or decrease?

Situation 5—The Rebellion in the Nursing Home!

You are a recreation professional employed in a large (250-bed) nursing home and convalescent hospital complex. Your clients range in age from 62 years old to 95 and above. They also vary greatly in degree of alertness, functional ability, and orientation to reality. A recently formed coalition of twelve alert, ambulatory (and very vocal) residents has met regularly over the past several weeks with the chief administrator of the facility. Their major concern centers around "having to associate with other residents who are 'out of it,' 'messy,' 'loud,' and 'whiney.'" One of their demands is for a separate recreational program of their own where they can avoid less alert residents. They want a separate recreational schedule which would feature organized parties, outings, special events, and a "diner's club" where they would take meals in isolation from the rest of the residents. The administrator has assured them that their requests will be considered and refers their recreational "suggestions" to you. You have a limited staff and would have to assign one of your therapeutic recreation assistants on a full-time basis to comply with the resident's proposal.

DISCUSSION QUESTIONS

1. What principle(s) of normalization are involved in the situation?
2. How far would you go in complying with the demands of the residents' group?
3. What (if any) rights of the rest of the residents in the facility are at issue in this scenario?
4. As a principle, should separate programs be offered for geriatric (or psychiatric) patients of differing functional levels of mental ability?

Situation 6—The Dance

You have been hired recently as a therapeutic recreation specialist at a local rehabilitation center for the blind. One of your objectives is to involve the participants at the center in more community-based activities. The participants and administration at the rehabilitation center have agreed with this philosophy and goal. For years, the center has sponsored a regular Friday evening dance for members of the center. It has been consistently well received and attended by young adults who are visually impaired. Last week, you received a phone call from the program director of a nearby YWCA, who invited the members of the center to a dance the YWCA is sponsoring. She indicated that participants will be the same age as your clients and that they come from the community at large. You relay this information to the visually impaired clients at the weekly consumer meeting, and it is met with hesitation. When probed, members of the rehabilitation center state that they are comfortable at their dances because of the structured environment. Specifically, men and women position themselves along opposite ends of the room between dances. Additionally, the area in which the dance is held is brightly lighted. Both of these practices allow maximum mobility and prevent the embarrassment which could occur if members chose partners of the same sex.

DISCUSSION QUESTIONS

1. Which principle(s) of normalization are of concern in this example?
2. Which of the following actions or combination of actions would you take in this situation?
   a. Politely thank the director for her offer, but decline the invitation.
   b. Urge the clients to accept the invitation without further discussion or preparation.
   c. Explain the clients' concern to the director and ask her to increase the lighting, remove any potential obstacles, and arrange for males and females to sit at opposite ends of the room.
   d. Obtain several sighted volunteers to escort the clients to the YWCA dance and assist them in locating dance partners, and so on.
   e. Call the director and suggest that the dance be scheduled at the rehabilitation center and that she urge her participants to attend.
3. What barriers to participation would other disabled clients (i.e., mentally retarded or auditorially impaired adults) encounter in a similar situation? How would you deal with these obstacles?

Situation 7—The Doll

You are a therapeutic recreation specialist in an extended-care facility. An elderly confused resident has acquired a large doll which she has adopted as her "baby." She and the doll are inseparable, and she wanders around the facility during meals and visiting hours talking to the doll and "feeding" it. There have been numerous complaints by residents and their families who find the woman's actions "silly" and "disturbing." Because the resident relates well to you in her lucid moments, the administrator of the facility has asked you to take the doll from the woman.

DISCUSSION QUESTIONS

1. What principle(s) of normalization are involved in this situation?
2. Which of the following actions or combination of actions would you undertake?
   a. Ask the woman for the doll or remove it from her grasp at the earliest time possible.
   b. Ask the nursing staff to remove the doll from the woman's bed when she is asleep.
   c. Insist that the client only play with her doll in her room.
   d. Explain to the other residents and visitors that the client is "senile" and not responsible for her actions.
   e. Let the woman keep the doll and hope that she finds an interest in other activities.
3. If the situation were the same, and the client were a young mentally retarded male or female, would the principle(s) be the same? What action(s) would you take?

Situation 8—The Camp
Rivalry

You are a therapeutic recreation specialist employed in a residential summer camp. This camp has successfully integrated several physically disabled and mentally retarded children with children with no disabilities. The age range of the campers is 12–16 years old. The athlethic director of another nearby camp, unaware of the fact that you have several disabled youngsters, has challenged your entire camp to a full Campers' Field Day competition. This event would consist of several strenuous physical activities such as a 10-mile relay race, a 3-mile canoe paddle, and a ropes challenge course. The conditions of the competition are that each camper must participate in at least one event. You are certain that many of the disabled campers would not be able to successfully compete in the activities outlined. Your staff and campers have learned of this challenge.

DISCUSSION QUESTIONS

1. Which principle(s) of normalization are involved in this situation?
2. Which of the following action(s) would you adopt?
   a. Contact the athletic director of the "rival" camp and explain that you have several disabled campers and cannot participate.
   b. Explain the situation to the athletic director and arrange for competition to take place between the nondisabled campers from each camp.
   c. Explain the situation to the athletic director and suggest that, instead of competition, both camps get together for a cookout.
   d. Suggest that more passive activities, such as checkers and fishing tournaments, be substituted in the competition.
   e. Accept the athletic director's challenge, but suggest that the disabled children assume roles such as timers, judges, and equipment managers.

Situation 9—The Inmates'
Offer

You are a therapeutic recreation specialist in a private residential center for emotionally disturbed adolescents. You receive a phone call from a group of inmates at a local, minimum security correctional facility. They are interested in starting a Big Brother program in which an inmate would "adopt" an adolescent from your center and interact with him in recreational activities over a period of time. Most of this programming would take place either at your facility or at the correctional center. You agree to consider the inmates' offer and get back to them.

DISCUSSION QUESTIONS

1. What principle(s) of normalization are being violated in the proposed scenario?
2. What image do you think this type of endeavor would have on the public?
3. What pros and cons could you see resulting from this arrangement?
4. What would your reply be to the inmate group?

Situation 10—Positive? Reinforcement

You are a therapeutic recreation specialist employed at a residential center for mentally retarded adolescents. For several weeks, you have been stressing the concept of personal fitness and a positive life-style as a means to achieving mental and physical well-being. One of the objectives of this program is to have each member of the residence embark upon a regularly scheduled program of exercise. Pam, an obese adolescent, is a particular challenge. She appears to abhor any type of physical activity. She will, however, occasionally ride a stationary exercise bike with prompting. The director of the center approaches you with the suggestion that you should initiate a token behavior modification program with Pam in which she could "earn" coupons redeemable for food at a local fast food chain. The director feels that this is probably the only method of motivating Pam which would be effective, and Pam has agreed to undertake this arrangement on a trial basis, if you think it is appropriate.

DISCUSSION QUESTIONS

1. Which principle(s) of normalization appears to be compromised in this setting?
2. Would you proceed with this arrangement? Defend your response.
3. If there were no other techniques which would motivate this client's participation, would you proceed with the arrangement?
4. List several behavioral management techniques and processes which would be compatible with normalization. List others which would not be.

Situation 11—The 10-Mile Wheel

You are a therapeutic recreation specialist employed in the outpatient service department of a large rehabilitation center for orthopedic disabilities. Several months ago, four adult clients who are confined to wheelchairs asked your advice and assistance in undertaking a program of wheelchair sports. Since then, their chief activity has been training for road races. This week, announcements were made for a first annual 10-mile "fun run" to benefit the cancer fund. It is being sponsored by several community service groups and is expected to draw some 1,000 participants. The race itself will be run through the streets of the city and along part of a 2-mile footpath in a park. Your clients have come to you and asked you to assist them with entry forms and other particulars. They are extremely excited about the prospect of entering this event. When you inquire as to their training to date, they reply that their longest training "wheel" has been eight miles, but they feel "pretty sure" they can make ten miles. Also, all their training so far has been on asphalt, not on surfaces like the footpath in the park. When asked about this potential problem, they feel certain they can traverse the path.

DISCUSSION QUESTIONS

1. What principle(s) of normalization are applicable in this situation?
2. Which of the following action(s) would you undertake relative to the upcoming race?

    a.   Encourage your clients to continue training until they have achieved the full 10-mile distance and are certain that they can replicate this feat in a race.

    b.   Encourage your clients to enter the race, but to attempt only the 8-mile distance by eliminating the footpath.

    c.   Have the clients enter the race, but station several volunteers at the park to assit them through the footpath area.

    d.   Encourage the clients to enter the race for the full distance. However, arrange for them to be accompanied by a motor scooter escort *or* to start half an hour before or after the rest of the participants.

    e.   Let them enter with no further consideration and wish them luck.

3. What would the effects on your clients be if they did not complete the course? What would the impact be on the public? On your agency?

4. List and discuss a number of other actual and hypothetical activities and programs which contain a high degree of risk for disabled participants.

5. What percentage of risk of failure do you think is acceptable to disabled participants in an activity? Should this probability be the same as for the general public?

STUDY GUIDE QUESTIONS

1. How do you personally feel about the theory and practice of normalization in human services?

2. To what extent is the concept of normalization and its various principles compatible with the goals and practices of the field of therapeutic recreation?

3. To what extent do you feel the field of therapeutic recreation has embraced and applied the idea of normalization?

4. Do you predict that the concept of normalization in therapeutic recreation will receive wider attention and application in the future?

5. Which principles of normalization are most compatible with the field of therapeutic recreation? Which are least compatible?

6. Is the term *therapeutic recreation* compatible with the notion of normalization?

7. Can normalized recreation ever take place in clinical and institutional settings?

8. Elaborate on this statement: Normalization in therapeutic recreation is both a process and a goal.

9. Classify your agency (or another facility) in terms of its position on Hutchison and Lord's continuum of recreation services. Defend your position.

10. Identify the major barriers which therapeutic recreation professionals would encounter when attempting to implement normalized recreation programs.

11. Identify several therapeutic recreation programs which are in basic accord with the principle of normalization. Identify others which are not.

12. Design a questionnaire which would assess an individual's basic knowledge of normalization and its application to recreation services for disabled persons. Administer this instrument to several practicing therapeutic recreation professionals.

ANNOTATED BIBLIOGRAPHY

BARKLEY, ALLEN L., and PAMELA ROBINSON, "Ticket to Re-Integration," *Leisurability*, 2, no. 3 (1975), 3–10. Describes a systematic, nonprofit hospital service designed to aid in the re-integration of adult psychiatric patients into community recreational events. The approach could serve as the basis for discussion of the merits of segregated versus integrated programs and the responsibility of clinical therapeutic recreation workers to encourage community involvement.

BOYD, WALTER, and FRANCES HARTNETT, "Normalization and Its Implication for Recreation Services," *Leisurability*, 2, no. 1 (1975), 22–27. Imparts the weaknesses of the medical model and the "do-gooder" approaches to recreation service provision for disabled persons, encouraging readers to compare current recreation service delivery practices to the model orientations outlined.

BULLOCK, CHARLES C., "Mainstreaming—In Recreation Too!?" *Therapeutic Recreation Journal*, 13, no. 4 (1979), 5–11. Sets forth the initial difficulties the author encountered when mainstreaming was applied to a recreational program, and therefore is useful in promoting discussion concerning problems and mechanics of implementing normalization in leisure service settings. Provides brief, but thorough, overview of the philosophical and legislative mandate for normalization.

FLYNN, ROBERT J., and KATHLEEN E. NITSCH, eds., *Normalization, Social Integration and Community Services*. Baltimore, Md.: University Park Press, 1980. A vital 425-page sequel to the 1972 normalization work of Wolfensberger. Composed of three major sections, featuring contributions from over twenty-five primary authors, the book modifies and clarifies the concept of normalization and extends its application into several community-based service areas related to recreation. Of special interest to therapeutic recreation personnel are sections on empirical research into the efficacy of the application of the principle and its relevance to special education and vocational habilitation settings. It also includes, in appendix form, approximately three hundred bibliographic entries related to the principle and practice of normalization in a variety of settings, probably the most current and comprehensive index in existence and an excellent source for term papers and classroom discussion.

HUTCHISON, MARGARET L., and JOHN C. LORD, "Recreation Integration: A Model for Integrating Persons with Disabilities into Community Recreation Programs," *Recreation Canada*, 33, no. 3 (Fall 1975), 60–64. Describes the concept of integration and a three-phase approach to achieving this goal; outlines the procedures of skill upgrading, education, and recreational involvement; details continuum of leisure services, from segregated programs in institutional settings to self-sustained participation in leisure activities. All invaluable to students in planning the progression of actual or hypothetical clients through the various levels of programming in therapeutic recreation settings.

HUTCHISON, PEGGY, and JOHN LORD, *Recreation Integration: Issues and Alternatives in Leisure Services and Community Involvement*. Ottawa, Canada: Leisurability Publications, Inc., 1979. Based on the previous reference by these authors, an extremely comprehensive theoretical and practical 152-page guide to normalization in recreational settings that overviews the need for play, leisure, and recreation and examines societies' reactions and commitment to disabled individuals. Contains excellent sources for designing in-depth classroom discussion learning experiences and a reference useful in aiding therapeutic recreation professionals to define their roles and the responsibilities of others in working with disabled persons.

"Mentally Retarded Persons and Integration—Two Recent Studies," *Leisurability*, 3, no. 4 (1976), 31–38. Presents two brief studies: "Community Recreation Opportunities for Retarded Persons," and "Retarded Children and Integrated Camping," both focusing on the *process* of the integration of disabled persons into regular recreation programs and activities. Useful in identifying barriers to participation in therapeutic recreation settings in brainstorming strategies for their elimination.

REYNOLDS, RONALD P., "Normalization: A Guideline to Leisure Skills Programming for Handicapped Individuals," in *Leisure and Handicapped Individuals: Adaptation, Techniques, and Curriculum*, eds. Paul Wehman and Stuart Schleien. Baltimore, Md.: University Park Press, 1981. Surveys historical, philosophical, empirical, and legislative support for normalization in recreation services, and details the relationship between normalization and leisure, pointing out myths associated with integrating disabled persons into less restrictive programs. Helps students devise appropriate program techniques for the development of clients' leisure skills.

Therapeutic Recreation Journal, 13, no. 4 (1979). Special Issue on Mainstreaming Handicapped Individuals in the Community. Includes the following articles: "Mainstreaming—In Recreation Too!?" "A Conceptual Basis for Mainstreaming Recreation and Leisure Services: Focus on Humanism," "A Systematic Approach to Mainstreaming in a Public Recreation Department," "A Catalyst to Change," "Is Mainstreaming for Everyone? Concepts and Issues as Experienced in One Program," "Mainstreaming: Social Ramifications of Integrating Physically Handicapped and the General Population," and "Mainstreaming in a Municipal Recreation Department Utilizing a Continuum Method."

THRONE, JOHN M., "Normalization Through the Normalization Principle: Right Ends, Wrong Means," *Mental Retardation,* 13, no. 5 (1975), 23–25. Argues that the normalization principle ignores the fact that the mentally retarded do not develop normally when utilizing regular procedures, providing a desirable and necessary contrast to literature which tends to be pro the normalization concept. Easily applied to recreational settings and techniques such as activity analysis and equipment modification.

WHITE, MARY ELLEN, "Children's Games for the Adult Mentally Retarded," *Leisurability,* 1, no. 2 (1974), 4–7. Identifies and criticizes such common programming practices as preconceived activities, inappropriate scheduling, unrealistic awards and refreshments, and selection of media offerings. Pleads with therapeutic recreation professionals to reexamine their roles in relation to mentally retarded adults. A powerful introduction to the complex issue of normalization that helps students pinpoint everyday examples of the violation of normalization in therapeutic recreation settings.

WOLFENSBERGER, WOLF, *The Principle of Normalization in Human Services.* Toronto, Canada: National Institute on Mental Retardation, 1972. Two-hundred-and-sixty page classic traces the origin and practice of the normalization principle from its Scandinavian inception in the late 1950s applying it to leisure and recreation in several instances. Many examples illustrate the relationship of therapeutic recreation service to the human-service concept of normalization and its related tenets.

ZIPPERLAN, HELEN R., "Normalization," in *Mental Retardation and Developmental Disabilities, Annual,* pp. 265–87. New York: Brunner/Mazel, Inc., 1975. Examines the sources of dispute and controversy relative to the concept of normalization and mentally retarded adults. Although theoretical, contains several real-world situations with which the therapeutic recreation student and practitioner can identify and is excellent for learning and discussion when paired with the Throne and the Hutchison and Lord references.

CHAPTER EIGHT
SCIENTIFIC INQUIRY: THE FOUNDATION FOR PROFESSIONAL DEVELOPMENT

Research investigations generate the body of knowledge from which a profession draws. As such, they are a critical bench mark of its development. A field's research efforts provide the knowledge and tools which its practitioners use to effect direct service to their clients. A profession's research may also be scrutinized and evaluated by related professions. Thus its journals and other publications become standards by which its claim to competence (and legitimacy) is judged. Finally, research is basic to providing information related to resolving issues concerning the professional development of a field such as preparation, credentialling, normalization, and the use of technologies. It is critical to note that research, in fact, holds the key to the solution of many of the problems outlined in this text. Research, in its broadest sense, is the responsibility of all professionals in the therapeutic recreation field. As Mobley pointed out:

> The scientific method is not the private domain of the scientist or researcher. Every administrator, supervisor, program leader, and so forth should use a sound scientific approach to all problem solving. In assessment, evaluation and decision making, research is the only way to make rational choices between alternative practices, to validate improvements, and to build a stable foundation of effective practices as a safeguard against faddish but inferior innovations.[1]

[1] Tony A. Mobley, "Practitioner/Researcher: A Team," *Parks and Recreation Magazine,* 15, no. 4 (April 1980), 40.

This chapter examines several aspects of research in therapeutic recreation. After a brief overview of the global nature of research and a defintion of the areas encompassed by this term, the reader is presented with a review of the literature related to the status of research in the field. A series of study guide questions follows this segment of the chapter. These points of discussion will, it is hoped, enable students to reflect upon past, present, and future trends in the overall direction of research related to leisure and disabled persons. The next portion of the chapter takes a more ''microscopic'' perspective and examines the challenges to empirical investigation faced by researchers in this area. Two hypothetical studies and related study guide questions conclude this discussion.A series of learning tasks related to practitioner settings follows this segment of the chapter and is designed to help students gain expertise in applying research methodology to problems encountered in clinical and community-oriented therapeutic recreation settings. An annotated instructional bibliography, facilitating further study, concludes the chapter.

DEFINITION OF TERMS

In this text, the term *research* is used in its broadest sense as the ''systematic, controlled, empirical and critical investigation of hypothetical propositions about the presumed relations among natural phenomena.''[2] This definition encompasses the following types of data gathering, which are addressed throughout this chapter:

— *Micro research*   Investigations designed to discover and test the relationship(s) between variables which have the potential for immediate application in therapeutic recreation settings. For example, studying the relationship between participation in a specific camp program and changes in the self-concept of participants.

— *Macro research*   Investigations or series of investigations designed to answer complex questions concerning major factors affecting the delivery of leisure services to disabled individuals. For example, determining how attitudes toward handicapped persons might be improved in recreational settings.

— *Assessment*   ''The process of gathering decision-making information relative to individualized program planning.''[3]

— *Evaluation*   ''Evaluation research measures the results of programs in relation to their goals. It assesses the degree to which the program fulfills identified goals, and thereby provides the basis for deciding whether to continue, modify, or stop the program.''[4]

In examining research efforts and trends in therapeutic recreation, four ''indicators'' of the status of scientific inquiry in the field are available. According to McLellan, these sources are academic journals which devote space to research,

[2] Fred N. Kerlinger, *Foundations of Behavioral Research* (New York: Holt, Rinehart & Winston, General Book, 1973), p. 11.

[3] Scout L. Gunn and Carol Ann Peterson, *Therapeutic Recreation Program Design: Principles and Practices* (Englewood Cliffs, N.J.: Prentice-Hall, Inc., 1978), p. 75.

[4] Kurt Finsterbusch and Annabelle Motz, *Social Research for Policy Decisions* (Belmont, Calif.: Wadsworth Publishing Co., 1980), p. 119.

information systems which reveal research which is underway but unreported, conference proceedings wherein research papers are presented, and available funding and federal interest for research.[5] The following discussion of the state of the art of therapeutic recreation research is based upon these sources.

RESEARCH IN THERAPEUTIC RECREATION: PAST TRENDS AND CURRENT STATUS

Because of the newness of the therapeutic recreation profession, its research efforts have yet to become fully defined in terms of methodology, content, and philosophical direction.[6] This indeed is not surprising, or a cause for alarm, as disciplines with hundreds of years of development have yet to reach consensus concerning the parameters of their empirical investigations. As would be the case with any profession scarcely three decades old, the field of therapeutic recreation finds itself at a critical crossroads in terms of its attempt to add to its body of knowledge. The following discussion attempts to overview the past and present status of research in the field and to identify specific trends which have become focal points for various issues today.

Because of its nature, the field of therapeutic recreation is a challenging area in which to launch empirical inquiry. Its boundaries are broad with respect to client populations served, service delivery settings, and treatment or intervention modalities. To illustrate the complexity of the field, and the problems it poses to research efforts, one might adopt the following conceptual model. First, arbitrarily select any three "levels of research," or *Treatment,* as one major dimension of interest. For example, "Direct Client Intervention" might be level 1 of this dimension. "Program" (clusters of service for groups of clients) could serve as level 2. Level 3 could be categorized as "Service Delivery Systems." A second dimension of this matrix could conceivably be *Type of Disability,* with various handicapping conditions comprising it. A third dimension could be *Basic versus Applied* investigation, in which one could differentiate between active field studies and more theoretical investigations designed to establish fundamental relationships between variables. Immediately, a three-dimensional, multilevel, matrix of potential research topics is created. If one were to further (and legitimately) add topical areas such as the professional concerns, techniques, and issues dealt with in this text, the possible number of cells would become astronomical! As the following overview suggests, this situation may, in fact, be partially responsible for the diversity of our past and current research efforts.

In a neophytic profession such as therapeutic recreation, it is arbitrary and perhaps artificial to distinguish between past and present research. Nevertheless,

---

[5] Robert McLellan, "Research," *Parks and Recreation Magazine,* 15, no. 7 (July 1980), 62–67, 90.

[6] Some of this material originally appeared in Reynolds, R.P. "Research in Therapeutic Recreation: Past, Present and Future Trends" (Paper delivered at 1982 S.P.R.E. Research Symposium, National Recreation and Park Association, Congress, Louisville, Kentucky, October 1982).

some *ex post facto* insights are necessary to provide an adequate background for discussion and debate. The methodologies, statistics, and other techniques used by researchers in investigating problems and topics germane to therapeutic recreation are not unique. Indeed, the survey techniques, between- and within-groups designs, inferential comparisons, and even referencing format have been appropriated from or modeled after disciplines and professions such as psychology, sociology, or education. Studies with titles such as *A Bio-Socio-Psycho Approach to _____ in Therapeutic Recreation* attest to the fact that therapeutic recreation is an eclectic field.

As a profession, we have also related strongly to longer-established areas, for example, practices such as leisure counseling, leisure education, and the area of study designated as the sociology of leisure. Although the discipline of therapeutic recreation has drawn from, and in certain cases emulated, the research of longer-established professions, the uniqueness of its investigations appears to lie in the fashion in which it has applied behavioral and social science research methods to the study of leisure service delivery to disabled persons.

It is definitely safe to state that the vast majority of research in the field of therapeutic recreation has taken place during the last three decades. As Frye and Peters pointed out, "From 1950 to 1970 more than four times as many studies were completed concerning therapeutic recreation and closely related topics than were done in the previous thirty years. One third of all such studies in the last fifty years have been completed since 1963."[7] It seems reasonable to assume that this exponential rate of growth in the number of completed research investigations has continued, and it may well be that the vast bulk of inquiry has occurred in the last decade. When reflecting upon this situation, it is easy to draw a parallel to the snowballing, post–Industrial Revolution generation of technical knowledge, in which the preponderance of technical information generated in a few decades surpassed the information accumulated in the previous 200 years!

This rapid growth in research and technical knowledge, however, has not occurred without corresponding introspection and, at times, discomfort and discouragement. In a special issue of the *Therapeutic Recreation Journal* devoted to research, Linford and Kennedy questioned the current level of research conducted in therapeutic recreation with this statement:

> In our opinion, there isn't anyone trained specifically in therapeutic recreation who has sufficient backgound in quantitative methods to guide any but the most simplistic doctorial dissertations. Similarly, the ability of university faculty to instigate and direct research studies which involve the more modern statistical designs is severely limited.[8]

As a solution to this situation as perceived by these authors, the following suggestions and strategies were put forth:

[7] Virginia Frye and Martha Peters, *Therapeutic Recreation: Its Theory, Philosophy and Practice* (Harrisburg, Pa.: Stackpole Books, 1972), p. 180.

[8] Anthony G. Linford and Dan W. Kennedy, "Research: The State of the Art in Therapeutic Recreation," *Therapeutic Recreation Journal*, 5, no. 4 (1971), 168.

— The employment of full-time research specialists in all university recreation curriculums granting terminal degrees.

— That concentration be placed on developing and evaluating demonstration programs based on existing literature to test hypotheses in therapeutic recreation.

— That grant funds be made available to enable post-doctoral study of modern research technology for therapeutic recreation faculty.

— The implementation of regional workshops on program evaluation for therapeutic recreation practitioners.

— That college instructors be chiefly responsible for interpreting research to students in classroom settings.[9]

In addition to this philosophical (and controversial) view of the status of research with respect to higher education in therapeutic recreation, the early 1970s brought forth the first empirical attempts to analyze the existing body of knowledge in the field. Lewko applied a content analysis technique to a sample of literature in therapeutic recreation for the purpose of determining the extent to which therapeutic recreation was a service as contrasted to a theoretical model of delivery of service.[10] Although the ultimate purpose of the investigation was to determine if the therapeutic recreation field fit a conceptualized paradigm for service, several subquestions related directly to the type and quality of therapeutic recreation research in the early 1970s. Specifically, inquiry into the development of specialized knowledge and the primary source, utilization, and users of such knowledge provided valuable information concerning the state of the art of therapeutic recreation research. The following findings are extracted from discussion centering around these questions, as presented by Lewko. It should be noted that the literature analyzed was limited to 1972 issues of the *Therapeutic Recreation Journal, Annual,* and *Parks and Recreation Magazine.*

— Scientist-researchers were virtually nonrepresented as contributors to the body of knowledge.

— Communications from sources other than individuals in the recreation field was extremely limited.

— Consumer and applied research and development situations accounted for 12 percent of the items of communication.

— No "basic research" was found in this sample. Likewise, theory-building and review articles were nonexistent.

— Psychology and social psychology accounted heavily for a majority of knowledge base identification items, in articles where the identification of a knowledge base was possible.

— No common theme was prevalent in the applied research endeavors which appeared in the publications during this year.

— Variation existed concerning the format of research reports. However, the most consistent procedure was the use of the headings "Introduction," "Method," "Results," and "Discussion" to organize the information. There was also great variability in stating the purpose of the study or describing research hypotheses. Statistical treat-

[9] *Ibid.,* pp. 168–170.

[10] John Henry Lewko, "The Analysis of Therapeutic Recreation as a Service," (unpublished Doctoral dissertation, University of Illinois at Champaign-Urbana, 1974).

ments and data reporting techniques also varied greatly. In some studies, no indication was given concerning the actual statistical analysis. Data summary techniques, such as the use of tables, appeared inadequate.

— Few research-oriented individuals produced research in the field. Few of these individuals were therapeutic recreators.

— Apparent difference in content of writings produced by individuals in practice-oriented and academic environments, possibly indicating a "researcher-practitioner gap."

In short, "the development of knowledge through research was minimal and random in orientation toward research problems."[11]

Concern over such random fact-gathering activities was partially responsible for prompting the U.S. Bureau of Education for the Handicapped to sponsor a conference to establish research priorities related to leisure and disabled persons in 1974. At this conference, the following critical areas for research or demonstration projects were identified, although not rank ordered:

1. Social Psychology and Leisure Behavior
2. Leisure Activity Analysis and Programming
3. Barrier Reduction and Environmental Design
4. Dissemination and Utilization of Research
5. Service Delivery[12]

Noting that these priority areas did not necessarily reflect the current activities of researchers in therapeutic recreation or relate to perceived future needs of researchers, Lewko and Crandall undertook two investigations designed to determine research trends for leisure with special populations.[13]

The first study found four different areas of *current* interest, based upon open-ended responses from researchers. These categories were: leisure patterns-needs of clients, use of leisure-recreation activities as a treatment tool, development and validation of programs and tests, and counseling-therapy approaches to leisure. In terms of *future* proposed research areas, the respondents indicated the following five priorities: antecedents (needs and consequences) of leisure behavior, descriptive studies of leisure needs-patterns, teaching-therapy methods, measurement and methodology, and theory building. The second study, a content analysis of all articles published pertaining to leisure and recreation and special populations during 1976, found that only one-fourth of the articles were communicating specific "tested" information which could be integrated into a reader's current activities.

In discussing these and other results, these authors noted:

— The fact that it might be beneficial to shift from a multidisciplinary to a more integrated interdisciplinary approach to knowledge development in the field.

---

[11] *Ibid.*, p. 221.

[12] Regional Rehabilitation Institute on Attitudinal, Legal and Leisure Barriers, *Focus on Research: Recreation for Disabled Individuals* (Washington, D.C.: The George Washington University, April 1980), p. 18.

[13] John Lewko and Rick Crandall, "Research Trends in Leisure and Special Populations," *Journal of Leisure Research*, 12, no. 1 (1980), 69–79.

— A strong interest among researchers in determining the basic leisure needs of special populations.

— A discrepancy between the large number of individuals engaged in validating therapeutic approaches to the use of leisure and the small number of persons identifying this process as a future need, possibly indicating methodological problems, such as inadequacy of control groups, subjectivity in activity analysis, difficulty in selecting target behaviors.

They concluded, "In general, it would appear that one major thrust for researchers in leisure and special populations should be a more careful delineation of the antecedents and consequences of leisure for the populations with whom they are concerned."[14]

In 1980 two national conferences were held which attempted to determine the state of the art of therapeutic recreation research and to set future directions for the development of knowledge in the field. The first of these symposiums held by the Regional Rehabilitation Research Institute on Attitudinal, Legal and Leisure Barriers of George Washington University, identified several major areas of research.

A sample of these categories and individual research topics within these areas follows:

Consumer Input

— What techniques exist to increase consumer involvement in recreation planning, decision making, operation, and so on?

— What strategies or techniques are used by service providers who have effectively involved consumers in the development of leisure and recreation services and programs?

— How can policies and procedures of commerical leisure service providers be affected relative to consumer involvement?

— What are the effects of recreational involvement on the self-esteem of disabled individuals?

— What barriers exist to implementing integrated recreation programs?

— What attitudes held by disabled persons prevent them from using available recreation facilities and program resources?

Treatment Implications

— Using case study methodology, can it be established that participation in therapeutic recreation has contributed to adequate lifelong leisure functioning of disabled persons?

— Is there a relationship between leisure education and vocational success?

— What is the effect of therapeutic recreation on the recidivism rate and adjustment to the community?

Personnel Preparation

— What information should be included about disabled persons in degree programs for community recreation personnel?

— What are the factors affecting job choices of trained recreation therapists?

— What is preventing disabled persons from working in leisure occupations?

[14] *Ibid.*, p. 78.

Accessibility

— How can information on accessibility be effectively disseminated to disabled and able-bodied groups?
— How do attitudes and stereotypes create segregated recreation facilities?
— How do disabled individuals or groups feel about accessibility modifications?[15]

The National Consortium on Physical Education and Recreation for the Handicapped was the second forum on therapeutic recreation research held in 1980. Participants at this congress suggested several measures to stimulate therapeutic recreation research, including:

— The initiation of small grants programs to fund research projects.
— Polling practitioners as to research needs in the field.
— The formation of a long-range plan for research action to stimulate topical areas.
— The creation of a research journal for therapeutic recreation and adapted physical education.
— Strengthening accreditation requirements to reflect higher research standards within college curricula.
— The provision of post-doctoral workshops on research methodology.[16]

A recent empirical study, ''Sources of Articles Published in the *Therapeutic Recreation Journal*'' during the 1970s, provides a comprehensive insight into trends and problems associated with research in therapeutic recreation.[17] In contrast to the previous studies, the content of research articles was not the primary focus for analysis. Several interesting trends, however, were discovered relative to the authorship, quantity, and methodology of research investigations. Although there are understandable differences from the Lewko and Crandall reports in the data reported and their interpretations, several similar trends emerge. The summary of findings concerning research in the 1970s that was reported in this study follows:

— Almost two-thirds of the articles appearing in the journal from 1975 to 1980 were written by university personnel. (This proportion includes both research and non-research articles.)
— Non-research articles outnumbered research articles consistently across the decade by a ratio of approximately three to one.
— Of the 67 research articles published over the decade, approximately 58 percent were authored by university affiliated personnel, while about 36 percent of the articles were contributed by agency-based authors.

[15] Regional Rehabilitation Research Institute on Attitudinal, Legal, and Leisure Barriers, "Focus on Research," pp. 10, 101, 126, 142.

[16] John L. Taylor, David M. Compton, and Terri M. Johnson, eds., *Directions for the 80's— 1979–80 Proceedings. The National Consortium on Physical Education and Recreation for the Handicapped* (Rochester, N.Y., 1980), pp. 37–38.

[17] David R. Austin and Dan W. Kennedy, "Sources of Articles Published in the *Therapeutic Recreation Journal* during the 1970's," *Therapeutic Recreation Journal*, 16, no. 3 (1982), 35–42.

— Over 70 percent of the articles did not explicitly state an hypothesis.
— Less than 36 percent of the research studies employed any inferential statistics. In those articles using statistics, correlation was the most frequently utilized technique.

The authors concluded that:

> Even though a call was made for "more and better" research in a special issue of the *TRJ* early in the 1970's . . . it is now apparent that research did not show obvious gains in quality and quantity during the decade. At least, if change occurred, it is not reflected in the examination of *TRJ*. The number of research articles were relatively the same during the first and last halves of the decade. Neither were there detected any leaps forward in the sophistication of the research which did appear.[18]

In a recent attempt to correct this situation and to foster cooperation and an integrated, interdisciplinary approach to research in therapeutic recreation, Bullock, McGuire, and Barch sought to answer the following questions:

1. What research topics do therapeutic recreation professionals perceive as important?
2. To what extent are therapeutic recreators doing research?
3. What barriers exist to doing research?
4. What do therapeutic recreators perceive as their role in the research process?[19]

In this investigation, a survey listing seventeen potential research areas, based upon the previously reviewed studies and conference proceedings, was mailed to therapeutic recreation professionals in the southeastern United States. Interestingly, the top five priority research needs identified by these respondents revealed a marked similarity to the "future" research needs identified by subjects in the 1976 study by Lewko and Crandall. These areas were: identifying techniques to motivate individuals to participate in activities, identifying effective teaching and therapy strategies to use with individuals, determining needs that can be met through leisure, evaluating program effectiveness, and studying the role of recreation in treatment. Concerning the number of therapeutic recreation professionals conducting research, only 15 percent reported research activity in the past twelve months. However, nearly 25 percent of these respondents were educators. Lack of time was overwhelmingly identified as the chief obstacle in undertaking research, followed by lack of training and cost barriers. When asked what the role of the recreator was in the research process, a majority of the respondents indicated that "keeping up to date on research in the field" and "incorporating research findings into their jobs" were of chief importance. "Doing research" and "working cooperatively with researchers," although perceived as less important, were nonetheless listed as either somewhat or very important.

Despite the previously outlined problems with and barriers to conducting research in therapeutic recreation, there were several positive trends in research

---

[18] *Ibid.*, p. 40.

[19] Charles C. Bullock, Francis A. McGuire, and Elizabeth M. Barch, "Research Needs of Therapeutic Recreators" (unpublished paper, University of North Carolina at Chapel Hill, 1983).

which one of the authors observed during his editorship of the *Therapeutic Recreation Journal* in the first three years of the 1980s. Some of these changes are obvious, others more subtle. For example, the average overall length of research articles submitted appears to have increased. Whether this is an attempt to comply with more rigid editorial policy standards or a reflection of the depth of research investigations undertaken may be open to debate. There also appeared to be an increase in the proportion of research versus nonresearch articles submitted. This trend manifested itself in several mini research themes. Research sections also became regular features of the journal.

When the content of research endeavors is examined, one is struck by the increased application of research topical issues in our profession including programming, curriculum and academic preparation, standards, continuing professional development, and even the generation of a philosophical position statement! Of particular note is the increase in articles related to research methodology, instrumentation, design, and analysis. There has, in fact, been so much interest in the area of client assessment, that an entire issue of the 1980 volume was devoted to this topic. Also apparent in recent issues is a decline in the number of status (state-of-the-art) surveys in favor of more conceptual and hypothesis-testing research. Due to this trend, it has become possible to initiate an editorial policy excluding statewide surveys from publication. Although Austin and Kennedy (1982) reported that approximately 33 percent of the articles submitted to the *Therapeutic Recreation Journal* were of a research nature, an informal sampling of the manuscripts submitted in 1981 and 1982 revealed a much higher proportion (40–45 percent) using some type of research technique. Again, academics continued to be greatly overrepresented as authors of research studies. As Lewko indicated in 1974, the range of topics which have been investigated using the scientific technique is vast and includes a range of subjects from the efficacy of wilderness survival programs to surveys of collective bargaining at universities offering therapeutic recreation curricula.

STUDY GUIDE QUESTIONS

The following points of inquiry are based upon the previous discussion of state-of-the-art facts and trends in research in therapeutic recreation. These questions ask the reader to project or speculate beyond the information at hand. Many require from the reader additional research, completion of a learning task, or both. It is hoped that all are provocative in terms of stimulating interest and discussion related to this crucial area of professional development.

1. In the introduction to this chapter, it was stated that a profession's research efforts may be used to substantiate its claim to competence and its reason for being. How do current research efforts compare to those of other professions in general? To other disciplines within the allied health care professions, such as occupational therapy, physical therapy, and nursing? After which disciplines has the field of therapeutic recreation modeled itself in its research endeavors? What change(s) in the direction of therapeutic recreation would you suggest to better enable it to articulate with other related fields?

2. Research was described as a primary means of obtaining information to aid in making decisions related to professional issues. How successful has the field of therapeutic recreation been in applying research techniques to issues such as professional preparation, credentialling, the development of a philosophical position? Identify several other issues which you feel need to be addressed through research in therapeutic recreation. Suggest some specific strategies or plans of action to attack each of these problems or issues.

3. In general, do you feel that the research competencies exhibited by practitioners and educators within the field of therapeutic recreation are less than, equal to or greater than should be expected at this stage of the profession's development? Defend your position!

4. It was stated that the field of therapeutic recreation was a particularly challenging area for research. Are the challenges we as a profession face in research any greater than or different from, those in the fields of occupational therapy or medicine? What unique challenges would be faced by individuals conducting research in therapeutic recreation settings?

5. The authors stated that the field of therapeutic recreation was eclectic in drawing from methodologies and research designs of other professions. Do you agree with this point? Just how different and unique is research in therapeutic recreation from other areas of the recreation profession? From other disciplines such as psychology, biology, and sociology? From research conducted in the allied health care professions?

6. It was noted that research in therapeutic recreation has increased in an almost geometric fashion over the past decades. Would you predict that this trend will continue at the current rate? When would you anticipate a leveling off, or reduction, in research activity in the field?

7. In an earlier chapter, it was stated that educators teaching in graduate curricula in therapeutic recreation in the early 1970s lacked basic research competencies. Do you feel this was an accurate assessment? If so, has this situation improved? What specific recommendations would you make for improving the research knowledge of educators teaching at the undergraduate and graduate levels in therapeutic recreation professional preparation programs?

8. It was previously reported that very few individuals who could be described as full-time scientist-researchers were active in producing research in therapeutic recreation. Does this come as a surprise to you? Do you view this as a detriment to the development of the body of knowledge in our field? Should universities employ more individuals who are directly and totally involved in conducting research in therapeutic recreation? Should our professional organization attempt to employ a specialist or specialists for this purpose?

9. It was also noted that persons within the recreation field generated most of the research in the discipline of therapeutic recreation. Are you surprised by this finding? Do you feel this is a problem or a shortcoming? If so, how could research from outside the profession be encouraged? Do you feel that most professions (including the allied health care fields) draw largely from their own members in terms of research? What could the field of therapeutic recreation gain (or lose) by encouraging interdisciplinary approaches to research investigations?

10. Consumer and applied research accounted for approximately one-eighth of the content of the *Therapeutic Recreation Journal* in the sample analyzed by Lewko. It appears that this proportion is currently increasing. What percentage (or proportion) of the field's professional publications do you feel should be devoted to applied research on a regular basis?

11. The previously described sample also revealed no basic research investigations. How do you feel about the necessity for such theoretical investigations? What should the

ratio of basic versus applied research in therapeutic recreation be now? In five years? In fifteen years?

12. In a previously reviewed article by Linford and Kennedy, several suggestions were made for improving the quality of research in therapeutic recreation in colleges and universities. Review these proposed strategies. Which do you feel would be most effective on a short- and long-term basis? Suggest several of your own ideas for improving the quality and quantity of research training in advanced degree study in therapeutic recreation.

13. Psychology and social psychology were identified as heavily contributing to the knowledge base in therapeutic recreation. Do you think these disciplines are a logical basis for investigation in the field of therapeutic recreation? What other fields do you feel would bring potentially rich contributions to the knowledge base in therapeutic recreation?

14. In the 1972 sampling of applied research articles which appeared in the *Therapeutic Recreation Journal,* no common theme was found. Do you feel that research in therapeutic recreation in general is devoid of identifiable trends? Can you list a central theme or themes of applied study which have appeared in therapeutic recreation over the past few years? Can you suggest some topical areas which would be particularly valuable to pursue with applied research?

15. The early content analysis by Lewko in 1972 found great variation in the format of research reports in therapeutic recreation studies, and in the statement of purpose, hypothesis, inferential statistics, and reporting procedures. Has this situation changed in today's research? Can you identify trends in statistics, reporting procedures, and hypothesis testing in recent research in therapeutic recreation? Can you suggest some practices that therapeutic recreation researchers should follow relative to these areas?

16. The topics of social psychology and leisure behavior, activity analysis, barrier reduction, research dissemination, and service delivery were identified as critical areas for research in the mid 1970s. Do you feel that these issues were and are of top priority in therapeutic recreation? What other subjects do you feel are important to investigate in the next five years? In the next fifteen years?

17. Brainstrom strategies to investigate the research questions generated by the Regional Rehabilitation Institute in 1980.

18. University personnel appear to be largely responsible for conducting research investigations in therapeutic recreation. Does this come as a surprise to you? Is this situation common in other fields? Do you feel that this balance is appropriate and beneficial to the field of therapeutic recreation?

19. In relation to the previous question—Does a researcher-practitioner gap exists in the field of therapeutic recreation? If so, what specific actions or strategies would you suggest to eradicate or reduce this rift? Do you feel that other disciplines in the allied health care professions suffer from a research-practice communication problem?

20. In general, do you think therapeutic recreation agency-based personnel have contributed adequately to the research body of knowledge in the field? If not, what barriers prevent them from contributing more heavily? What strategies would you suggest for removing or reducing these obstacles?

21. Do you agree with Austin and Kennedy's statement that research in therapeutic recreation has not become more sophisticated over the past decade? Defend your position! What specific indices do you feel should be employed to judge the level of sophistication or efficacy of research in general, and in therapeutic recreation? What suggestion(s) would you make to researchers in the field of therapeutic recreation concerning practices which would improve the quality of current investigations?

22. Do you feel that the application of research to professional issues and concerns in the

field of therapeutic recreation is an indication that the discipline is becoming more research conscious and research oriented? What professional issues do you feel merit immediate and long-term investigation?

23. Is the distinction between *researchers* and *practitioners* in therapeutic recreation an artificial one? Shouldn't all persons in the field of therapeutic recreation be responsible for undertaking research?

24. It has been suggested that the field of therapeutic recreation develop "intermediary journals" or publications which explain or interpret the implications of research findings to practitioners. What are the potential benefits and drawbacks of this idea? Would you favor the creation of such journals?

25. Much research in therapeutic recreation has been funded by outside sources such as governmental agencies, and in some cases, private foundations. To what extent have funding recipients been accountable to sponsoring agencies? To what degree have such agencies encouraged researchers to undertake projects which transcend and impact beyond their programs? To what extent have both sponsors and recipients attempted to coordinate research efforts with other governmental, university, and agency-based personnel? If you feel past efforts havs been lacking in this area, what future changes would you suggest?

26. Although there appears to have been an increase in the number of special research issues of our professional journal and in mini research themes, there is currently no professional journal devoted specifically and entirely to research in therapeutic recreation. Would you favor the creation of such an organ? What would the pros and cons of such a periodical be? Has the field of therapeutic recreation evolved to a stage of development where it warrants (and would benefit from) such a publication?

27. As a professional organization, what has the Research Committee of the NTRS done to improve the quality of research in the field? What are some of its major roles and accomplishments to date? What strategies or actions could NTRS take in the future to encourage productive research activity?

28. In general, are graduates of four-year colleges with curricula in therapeutic recreation adequately prepared to interpret, critique, and apply the research which exists in the field today? What academic preparation should bachelor's degree students receive relative to research and methods of research? What form should this preparation take in terms of course work? What research competencies is it reasonable and appropriate to expect from graduates of four-year colleges with curricula in therapeutic recreation? List and outline these knowledges and skills.

29. Respond to the previous question in terms of academic preparation at the master's and doctoral levels.

30. Do you feel your own academic educational preparation is, or was, adequate in preparing you to undertake, interpret, and critique research in therapeutic recreation? What specific recommendation(s) would you make for its improvement?

31. In general, do you feel that agency-based personnel in therapeutic recreation engage in adequate continuing professional development relative to research? Identify the means of continuing educational activities which are (or will be) available to you. Design a personal plan of continuing education which you could employ to keep yourself up to date concerning current research and research practices.

32. Identify a minimum of ten journals or research publications from the allied health care professions with which therapeutic recreation professionals should be familiar.

33. Researchers in the field of therapeutic recreation have been criticized for the use of overly simplistic research designs. In view of the complex nature of the field, as previously described, is this a valid observation? Is it necessary to design future studies

which test for multiple interactions among variables and which are high in external validity? Have our current research efforts achieved this need? How generalizable and transferable are findings in therapeutic recreation research studies in general? Have we emphasized microscopic studies of program and treatment intervention to the exclusion of macroscopic studies related to barrier reduction and service delivery investigations?

34.   What suggestions would you have for moving the field from a multidisciplinary approach to an interdisciplinary orientation to research as suggested by Lewko and Crandall?

THE RESEARCH PROCESSS IN THERAPEUTIC RECREATION

Before examining and critiquing the actual mechanics of research investigations in therapeutic recreation, it may be helpful to delineate some of the common problems faced by researchers in the field today. The major difficulties associated with conducting research in therapeutic recreation can be categorized under the headings of lack of existing knowledge base, setting factors, and the therapeutic experience.

Knowledge Base

Because of the breadth and newness of the field and the lack of previous investigations, today's researcher in therapeutic recreation does not have an extensive knowledge base from which to draw. Indeed, it is not uncommon for researchers to report that "no prior studies have taken place" with a given population of subjects under a certain set of conditions. As a result of this situation, those conducting research studies in the field have frequently drawn from data bases which exist in sociology, psychology, special education, counseling, and related disciplines. Although the extrapolation of findings and methodologies from these fields have proved productive in many instances, it may have detracted from establishing basic sets of relationships between variables of interest to therapeutic recreators. This, in turn, has frequently left investigators in therapeutic recreation isolated in their efforts and prone to random fact-gathering activities. The dearth of review articles and replication studies in therapeutic recreation research is evidence of this situation.

One manifestation of the lack of research in the field to date, which has been a particular hindrance to researchers, is the scarcity of available measurement instruments. This paucity of valid and reliable measurement and assessment tools is particularly frustrating when investigators attempt to determine the outcomes or effects (dependent variables) of their interventions or treatments. A common result of this dilemma has been a borrowing of established instruments, including scales, questionnaires, tests, and inventories, from related disciplines in an attempt to monitor the impact of experiences in therapeutic settings.

Setting Factors

A meeting of two or more individuals who have conducted, or attempted to conduct, research in therapeutic recreation agency settings would likely produce a lively discussion concerning the difficulties inherent in such an endeavor. These obstacles, although present in any study of a "field" nature, are particularly pronounced in actual agency-based investigations. The first problem faced by a researcher implementing an investigation in a real-world recreation setting is that of *control*. Because of the complexity of events constantly taking place in an agency, it is very difficult to prevent external occurrences from entering the investigation and contaminating the results. Anyone who has experienced the well-intentioned "extra assistance" given by aides to subjects taking a posttest fitness program assessment can empathize with this situation!

A second obstacle faced by researchers in therapeutic recreation is the proverbial *small n,* or lack of an adequate numbers of subjects for between-groups comparisons. This becomes particularly problematic in studies containing several levels of treatment, types of disability groups, and so forth. It is rare that enough subjects meeting the criterion of the study can be found in one agency or setting. Even when sufficient subjects are available, discharges, movements from units, medical procedures, and everyday interruptions frequently result in a loss of participants. Fortunately, idiographic, within-subjects research designs allowing the use of small numbers of subjects are beginning to become popular in therapeutic recreation research.

Logistical considerations represent a third obstacle to conducting field investigations in therapeutic recreation settings. Program interventions frequently have to be superimposed or integrated into existing agency routines. This often requires large amounts of agency support and cooperation and removes the ultimate control of the experiment from the researcher. A particularly useful approach which can prevent this situation is the formation of a multidisciplinary research team composed of agency therapeutic recreation personnel and staff members and others with research expertise from outside the facility. This strategy appears to be a growing trend in the literature.

A final consideration related to research in therapeutic recreation concerns the *right to treatment*. This concept, which has been the basis of recent litigation, has as a corollary the principle that it is unethical to deny or withhold beneficial treatment. The possible implications for therapeutic recreation research are interesting and complex. If a researcher "feels" that participation in a certain activity, program, or process is therapeutic, can he or she deny a group of clients participation in this activity by assigning them to a control group receiving a different intervention, or no intervention at all?

The Therapeutic Experience

A final consideration in therapeutic recreation research relates to the structuring, preserving, and assessment of the recreative experience. Because of the fragile nature of leisure, several questions arise. What blend of therapy and recreation can an experiementer maintain in an intervention without destroying the elements which cause it to be perceived as recreation or leisure on the part of the participant? Do obstrusive measures such as external observers, testing devices, and special equipment change a recreational activity into a therapy session? Can an individual be informed that he or she is taking part in a research study and still perceive the process as recreational? At what point does therapeutic recreation become recreation participation? Are "diversional" activities appropriate avenues of investigation for therapeutic recreation specialists?

The following two exercises exemplify some of the obstacles inherent in undertaking research investigations in therapeutic recreation and challenge the reader to react to these problems and suggest alternate strategies for their resolution. *It should be noted that these research studies are hypothetical and do not represent actual empirical investigations in the field. The data and literature review sections are for purposes of illustration only. All references cited are fictitious.*

STUDY A—THE EFFECTS OF SELECTED RECREATIONAL ACTIVITIES UPON ENDOGENOUS AND REACTIVE DEPRESSION

Abstract

This study sought to determine (1) if recreational activities could be used to elevate the self-concept of depressed psychiatric patients, and (2) if selected recreational activities would exert differential effects upon the self-concept of patients with endogenous and reactive depressions. To achieve this end, twenty-four (24) patients were assigned to groups receiving either internal locus-of-control activities for the treatment of endogenous depression or external locus-of-control activities to ameliorate reactive depression. Although all groups scored significantly higher on the Feelgood Self-Concept Scale, no group varied significantly from any other. It was concluded that any program of activities would be successful in the treatment of depression.

Review of Literature

Endogenous and reactive depression have been common forms of psychiatric diagnosis for the past several years (Dudley and Maskell, 1982; Fieldman, 1976; Kearns and Bates, 1972). In attempting to provide remediation for these conditions, clinicians have utilized various drugs and electroconvulsive shock treatment. In recent investigations, various forms of recreational programming have apparently shown promise as a treatment for these diagnoses (Lockwood, 1982; Smith & Tucker, 1981; Thomas, 1979), although the direct relationship between recreation and depression is unclear. Recreation is a promising treatment modality, as it utilizes activity directly in motivating individuals to improve their psychological well-being. The purpose of this study was to attempt to substantiate the link between recreation and the remediation of depression and to determine if particular types of depression were differentially amenable to specific types of recreational treatment.

Past researchers (Bryson, 1981, Dean, 1982, Morgan, 1980), have stated that the endogenous-reactive conceptualization is particularly relevant for viewing and treating depression. This view posits that endogenous depressions are caused internally, while reactive depressions are a response to external environmental events. Based on this theory, it is logical to assume that persons with these diagnoses would respond differentially to all types of treatment, including recreational therapy. Specifically, since endogenous depression results from a loss of internal control in the individual, it is postulated that individuals with this condition would respond most favorably to individual activities which allowed them to exert a maximum degree of individual control. Conversely, it was reasoned that persons with reactive depression, resulting from external factors, would respond favorably by participating in group activities which encouraged them to interact with other individuals and conditions in the environment.

Method

Subjects   Twelve (12) subjects (ten females and two males) with diagnoses of endogenous depression and twelve (12) subjects (eight females and four males) with diagnoses of reactive depression were utilized in the study. All were inpatients of a large medical center hospital and were referred by a psychiatrist who suggested that they could benefit from additional treatment. The subjects ranged in age from 14 to 61 years old. Their average length of stay at the facility was three months, with a range of residence from two weeks to eight-and-a-half months.

Treatment groups   Twenty-four (24) subjects were placed in four groups of equal size (six subjects per group) on the basis of diagnoses and type of treatment. Group 1 consisted of endogenous depression subjects who received individual control activities. Group 2 was comprised of endogenous depression subjects who received group interaction activities. Group 3 (reactive depression subjects) received individual control activities, while group 4 (reactive depression) subjects received group interaction activities. Definitions of *individual-control* and *group interaction* activities are as follows:

> *Individual-Control*   These were activities upon which success was determined solely by participant's skill level, for example, individual performance in archery, bowling, darts, and pool.
>
> *Group Interaction*   These were games and sports of a team cooperative effort, where outcome was determined by combined effort, such as basketball, soccer, and softball.

Procedures   Following assignments to treatment groups, the following procedures were initiated. Groups 1 and 3 (endogenous depression and reactive depression) received a four-week activity program consisting entirely of individual control activities such as those described above. Groups 2 and 4 (endogenous and reactive depression) received a program of group interaction activities for an identical four-week period. Because of the previously outlined theory of depression and selected activity type, it was hypothesized that groups 1 and 4 would show the greatest rate of improvement, and groups 2 and 3 the least.

Instruments and Data Collection

The Feelgood Self-Concept Scale was administered to all subjects in a pretest and posttest immediately before and after the four-week activity program. This instrument has an overall test-retest reliability of .64 and correlates .73 and .47 respectively with the Otis and Jones self-concept measures. The scale was designed specifically to determine the self-concept of emotionally disturbed adolescents in correctional facilities and was pilot tested and validated in such settings. It contains fifty items related to self-concept and produces a range of scores from 0 to 100, with 100 indicating the highest degree of self-concept possible.

Results

Table 8-1 represents the mean pretest and posttest scores of the four treatment groups on the Feelgood scale. A two-way analysis of variance (ANOVA) was performed to determine if significant differences existed between treatment groups

TABLE 8-1   Mean ($\overline{X}$) and Variance ($\sqrt{2}$) Scores of Four Treatment Groups on Feelgood Self-Concept Scale

$\overline{X}$	GROUP 1 (n = 5) (ENDOGENOUS-INDIVIDUAL ACTIVITIES)	GROUP 2 (n = 4) (ENDOGENOUS-GROUP ACTIVITIES)
Pre	$\overline{X}$ = 61.8 $\sqrt{2}$ = 6.2	$\overline{X}$ = 59.3 $\sqrt{2}$ = 4.7
$\overline{X}$ Post	$\overline{X}$ = 72.1 $\sqrt{2}$ = 7.1	$\overline{X}$ = 69.2 $\sqrt{2}$ = 5.2

$\overline{X}$	GROUP 3 (n = 5) (REACTIVE-INDIVIDUAL ACTIVITIES)	GROUP 4 (n = 6) (REACTIVE-GROUP ACTIVITIES)
Pre	$\overline{X}$ = 57.5 $\sqrt{2}$ = 4.2	$\overline{X}$ = 58.0 $\sqrt{2}$ = 6.0
$\overline{X}$ Post	$\overline{X}$ = 67.2 $\sqrt{2}$ = 3.9	$\overline{X}$ = 69.3 $\sqrt{2}$ = 5.3

NOTE: Due to discharges and drop-outs from the experiment, four subjects did not complete both the pretest and the posttest.

or levels of treatment. Results indicated that significant differences existed between pretest and posttest scores on the Feelgood scale in each of the four groups (F = 2.87, df. = 3, P < .05), indicating an overall improvement in the self-concept of all four groups. Interaction effects of individual treatments between groups, however, were not significant (F = .67, df. = 3, P > .05), indicating that no overall differences existed between the four treatment groups.

Discussion and Conclusion

It was originally hypothesized that the greatest differences in improvement in self-concept would be evident in treatment groups 1 and 4, in which the types of activity programs were matched with the corresponding etiologies of depression. Specifically, it was postulated that those with endogenous depression would benefit most from individual control activities, and that reactive depression clients would show the greatest improvement while engaging in group activity programs. Furthermore, it was postualted that recreation programs in general would result in improvements in self-concept. In this experiment, only the latter hypothesis was supported. Although all groups in the program revealed significant differences in self-concept after participating in four-week activity programs, no group (or groups) demonstrated significantly greater improvements than other groups. From this data, it appears that prescribing specific types of activities for various classifications of depressed patients will not result in gains in self-concept beyond what could be reasonably expected from participation in general recreational programs. Therefore, it is recommended that therapeutic recreation professionals working in psychiatric settings need only provide an adequate program of general recreational activities for their depressed clients.

STUDY A—DISCUSSION QUESTIONS

1. Do you agree with the authors' basic theory and subsequent hypotheses concerning the etiology of depression and the differential effects which individual-control and group interaction activities might produce in the treatment of depression?

2. Do you feel that the sample of subjects utilized in this study was adequate in size, properly selected, and possessed of appropriate demographic characteristics to be of use in testing the theory? Would a control group have been a useful addition to this study?

3. Do you feel that the four treatment conditions in this study were suitable for testing the hypothesis under study? Were the individual-control and group interaction activities explained in enough detail to be replicated?

4. Did the Feelgood Self-Concept Scale appear to be an appropriate instrument to use in this study? Were its reliability and validity adequate? Was it described in sufficient detail?

5. If this were an actual experiment, would the reported results surprise you? What effect(s), if any, would the reported variances have had in the analysis? Was the statistical technique utilized appropriate for this design?

6. Do you agree with the conclusion of the authors that the specific treatments used had no greater effects than any type of general recreation program had or would have? Identify several variables or factors which might have biased or influenced the out-

come of this experiment. Do you feel that the overall improvement in self-concept of the four treatment groups can be directly attributed to the four-week activity program?

7. Would you support the publication of this study in therapeutic recreation literature? If not, could methodological, or conceptual revisions be made to the investigation to make it suitable for publication?

8. Design a hypothetical study which adequately tests the efficacy of two or more recreation therapy programs on a specific disability or handicapping condition. Present the investigation in research report form including an abstract; brief hypothetical review of literature; problem statement and hypothesis; method section including specifics on subjects, treatments, instruments, and data collection procedures; results; and discussion. Invite other learners to analyze and critique your research "study."

STUDY B—A COMPARISON OF THE ATTITUDES OF THERAPEUTIC RECREATION AND ALLIED HEALTH CARE PERSONNEL TOWARD HANDICAPPED PERSONS

Abstract

This study sought to determine if therapeutic recreation personnel varied significantly from other allied health care professionals in their attitudes toward persons with disabilities. To answer this question, the Attitude Toward Handicapped Individuals Scale (ATHIS) was administered to four groups of allied health care specialists—medical students, occupational therapists, nurses, and therapeutic recreation specialists. Results indicated that nurses scored significantly higher than medical students and occupational therapists, while therapeutic recreation personnel scored significantly below these two groups. All groups scored significantly higher than the general public. It was concluded that, while therapeutic recreation personnel were generally more empathetic toward disabled persons, they were less so than more "traditional" members of the caring professions.

Review of Literature

Attitudes toward disabled individuals have long been a source of inquiry to those in the social sciences (Henry, 1972; Longfellow, 1946; Stedley, 1981). Recently there has been considerable attention focused upon the attitudes of those professionals in the "caring fields" toward their clients and handicapped individuals in general. Although few studies have been done to date in this area, those available appear to indicate that people in the allied health care professions score significantly higher on instruments measuring degrees of positive attitudes toward handicapped persons (Bass et al., 1982, Franklin and Connors, 1976; Hanks and Barlow, 1981). This study sought to replicate the previous investigations by comparing attitudes of allied health care personnel to the general public and to each other. It was hypothesized that individuals in the health care professions would reveal significantly more empathetic attitudes toward the handicapped than people in general, yet would not differ significantly from each other.

Method

Subjects   All subjects in this investigation were selected from programs of study at a large university medical center in a metropolitan area. Group 1 consisted of forty (40) first-year medical students (31 males and 9 females). Group 2 was comprised of thirty-five (35) occupational therapy students completing senior internships following a four-year course of study (28 females and 7 males). Group 3 was made up of twenty-seven (27) female nurses with bachelor's degrees who had returned to the university to complete an advanced course of study in health care management. The fourth group (therapeutic recreation specialists) consisted of thirty-two (32) freshmen (14 males and 18 females) enrolled in a four-year therapeutic recreation curriculum.

Instrument   The ATHIS was selected for use in this investigation. This instrument consists of twenty statements about handicapped persons with which respondents are asked to indicate various degrees of agreement. The range of scores possible on this test goes from -1.00 to $+1.00$. Although this scale has not been compared to other instruments in a formal fashion, it appears, from other administrations, to have excellent face validity. Pilot testing on the general population has resulted in producing a mean ($\bar{X}$) score of $+ .42$.

Procedures   The instrument (ATHIS) was administered to respondents in the following fashion. A notice was posted on departmental bulletin boards of the respective programs, asking for volunteers to "take a brief, nongraded test." This procedure produced the previously described number of respondents. Due to problems in scheduling, the subjects were given the ATHIS at various times throughout the 1980–81 academic year. Whenever possible, the test was administered in group fashion. In one case (the graduate healthcare students), however, the test had to be administered individually by the experimenter to the subjects.

Results

Table 8-2 contains the average scores of each of the groups on the ATHIS. A subsequent one-way analysis of variance (ANOVA) and selected planned comparisons (Smith, 1981) revealed significant differences between the nursing group and the three other cohorts and the therapeutic recreation personnel and the three other groups (t = 1.58, df. = 24, P < .05 and t = 2.57, df. = 24, P < .05 respectively). An identical comparison of the four subject groups to the general population mean indicated that all four groups scored significantly higher than the public at large.

TABLE 8-2 Mean Scores of Respondent Groups on Attitude Toward Handicapped Individuals Scale

MEDICAL PERSONNEL	OCCUPATIONAL THERAPISTS
$\overline{X}$ = .74 $\sqrt{2}$ = .072	$\overline{X}$ = .72 $\sqrt{2}$ = .045
NURSES	THERAPEUTIC RECREATION PERSONNEL
$\overline{X}$ = .81 $\sqrt{2}$ = .061	$\overline{X}$ = .62 $\sqrt{2}$ = .054

Discussion and Conclusion

The results strongly support the notion that allied health care professionals, as a group, are more empathetic in their feelings toward disabled individuals. This is not surprising, as the groups in this experiment had preselected themselves into courses of study deisgned to prepare them to work directly with individuals exhibiting special needs. The variation between the groups in this study, however, is more difficult to explain. From examination of the data, it is obvious that nurses scored significantly higher, and the therapeutic recreation personnel significantly lower, than the other two groups. It is highly probable that nursing, as an established profession, is highly likely to attract more empathetic personnel than the relatively new profession of therapeutic recreation. Secondly, nurses generally meet the daily-living needs of disabled persons on an around-the-clock basis, while physicians, occupational therapists, and recreation personnel tend to deal with clients in a highly specialized and segmented fashion. Thus the nursing field attracts more empathetic individuals.

While these findings must be viewed as preliminary and tenuous due to the small sample size, they provide support for the notion that those in the "caring professions" have more positive attitudes toward disabled persons as a whole. The results also indicate that there may be a wide variation among groups of allied health care personnel in the way they perceive disabilities and react to handicapped persons.

STUDY B—DISCUSSION QUESTIONS

1. Concerning the relevance of the study, do you feel that this topic is germane to the field of therapeutic recreation and worthy of investigation?
2. Were there any specific problems associated with subject selection in this study? Were the groups of subjects utilized appropriate for testing the hypothesis under investigation?
3. Was sufficient justification presented concerning the use of the ATHIS instrument? Based on its description, do you feel that the scale was appropriate for this investiga-

tion? Are you satisfied that the experimenters carried out this testing in an unbiased fashion?

4. Do the reported results justify the conclusions drawn by the researchers? Do the statistical analyses seem adequate?

5. Do you agree with the conclusions drawn by the experiementers? Are there any other "rival explanations" which could explain the results found? Do you concur with the investigators' reasoning about the nature of the field of nursing as compared to other allied health professions? Is the conclusion regarding the lower scores of the therapeutic recreation specialists warranted?

6. Design a study which may more accurately investigate the questions outlined in the abstract. Develop alternative sampling plans, testing procedures, and so on which could be used.

LEARNING TASKS RELATED TO RESEARCH IN THERAPEUTIC RECREATION

Imagine yourself in each of the following situations, with the outlined tasks confronting you. Drawing upon your educational background and experience, design a detailed research strategy to accomplish the stated goals. Be certain to include specifics such as sampling procedures, basic research design utilized, and instruments needed. It may be helpful to organize your strategy in the form of a standard research report, using headings such as "review of related literature," "methodology," "results," and "discussion."

1. You are a therapeutic recreation specialist employed by an agency serving delinquent youth. This year you are initiating a model "wilderness survival program" to be run in a camp setting. You are interested in evaluating the long- and short-term effects of the program on the self-concepts, educational performance, and camping skills of the youths.

2. You are a therapeutic recreation educator in a university setting. You wish to determine if incoming students, majoring in therapeutic recreation, have attitudes toward disabled people which are different from college students in general or other students majoring in the allied health care professions.

3   You are a therapeutic recreation professional in a large nursing home. You are interested in determining whether a new "reality orientation through recreation" program you have instituted really results in less confusion, increased alertness, and improved motivation on the part of your clients.

4. You are a therapeutic recreation specialist working with mentally retarded children. You have been approached by an adapted-equipment sales person who has a line of special toys and games which are guaranteed to "increase socialization" and "improve communication skills." The salesperson offers to let you borrow some of the toys and games on a trial basis. You wish to determine if the equipment is significantly better than the toys you currently use to promote socialization and communication.

5. You are a therapeutic recreation specialist employed in a municipal recreation setting. Your supervisor has charged you with finding out from the community at large if there would be enough interest, support, and commitment on the part of disabled persons to justify starting a wheelchair sports program involving seasonal basketball, football, and track and containing at least three full teams in each sport.

6. You are interested in whether or not the adult mentally retarded citizens of a community really differ from their nonmentally retarded peers in terms of their patterns of leisure participation. Of particular interest to you are factors such as whether the mentally retarded population, as a whole, is more sedentary in its leisure and whether they prefer, as a group, noncompetitive sports.

7. You are a therapeutic recreation specialist in a psychiatric setting. You would like to determine what factors are most important in influencing individuals to participate (or not participate) in the recreational program you offer. The variables of age, sex, type of diagnosis (psychotic versus nonpsychotic), and possible previous hospitalization have been suggested as potential factors which could have an effect. You wish to determine if these variables do affect participation, and if so, which are the most important.

8. You are a therapeutic recreation sepcialist working with physically disabled adults. A fellow therapist has developed a leisure interest inventory instrument and claims it will "predict" whether or not a client will participate in community recreation acitivities upon discharge. Specifically, clients scoring above a certain standard score are more likely to take part in community recreation than those not achieving this score. You wish to determine its reliability (consistency across applications) and its validity (whether or not it will really do what has been claimed for it).

ANNOTATED BIBLIOGRAPHY

DIXON, JESSE T., and DANIEL L. DUSTIN, "Living up to the Name: Research Support for Therapeutic Recreation Service," in *Exetra Perspectives: Concepts in Therapeutic Recreation,* pp. 31–40, eds. Larry L. Neal and Christopher R. Edginton. Eugene, Oreg., University of Oregon, Center of Leisure Studies, 1982. Illustrates through examples the need for therapeutic recreation to substantiate the claims it makes for its programming efforts with special populations. The specific research investigation cited is a leisure education strategy for mentally retarded children, which is designed to impact on their intrinsic motivation. Features a summary discussion of the investigation's relevance for program justification and external funding.

ELLIOTT, CATHERINE, "Research and the Mentally Retarded: Their Rights," *Therapeutic Recreation Journal,* 10, no. 3 (1976), 91–93. Briefly reviews the American Association for Mental Deficiency's official position on research conducted with mentally retarded persons, focusing on two major points: the issue of consent and the question of benefits to be received. The author's major position is that therapeutic recreation specialists must be cognizant not only of the scientific judgment associated with the current body of knowledge, but also of the moralistic decisions inherent in certain types of research. Effective in generating discussion on means-versus-ends questions in research, in stimulating general debate on the ethical responsiblity of therapeutic recreation workers to their clients.

HAUN, PAUL, *Recreation: A Medical Viewpoint.* New York: Columbia University, Teachers College Press, 1971. Although the material in this book dates back to the 1940s, it is extremely provocative in its perception of research needs in therapeutic recreation. Statements such as the folllowing stimulate discussion on desirable research directions in the field.

We must eventually design research studies that will accurately compare field hockey as a treatment with other therapies. We will have to show, for example, that on balance it is 20 percent more effective than deep coma insulin, slightly less reliable than trichlor-promazine in the accepted dosage range, and not more than 50 percent as useful as enforced participation in mixed-team volleyball.

HERSEN, MICHAEL, and DAVID H. BARLOW. *Single-Case Experimental Designs: Strategies for Studying Behavior Change,* Elmsford, N.Y.: Pergamon Press, 1976. Describes research designs which assess behavioral change in individuals across time among others. Valuable in evaluating the effects of programming on individual participants for the many therapeutic recreation specialists conducting activities and programs to bring about improvements in physical, psychological, and social behaviors in clients. Enables readers to compare and contrast idiographic (single-case) research designs with the more traditional nomothetic (between-groups) approaches used in therapeutic recreation research.

LOCKE, LAWRENCE F., and WANEEN W. SPIRDUSO, *Proposals That Work.* New York: Columbia University, Teachers College Press, 1976. Provides a systematic approach to the development of research projects, using sample dissertation proposals of both valid and invalid designs. Useful in planning individual research endeavors and in critiquing other investigations.

NATIONAL THERAPEUTIC RECREATION SOCIETY, *Therapeutic Recreation Journal,* 14, no. 4 (1980). Devoted to assessment in therapeutic recreation, this issue deals with the current status of assessment in the field and also provides specific techniques for determining client needs and interests in a variety of settings. After this overview of the entire topic, individual or small-group study could focus on a particular type of assessment, such as mental health programs. Each article contains several useful references for further study.

ROBINSON, JOHN P., and PHILLIP R. SHAVER, *Measures of Social Psychological Attitudes.* Ann Arbor, Mich.: The University of Michigan, Institute for Social Research, 1973. For those engaged in therapeutic recreation research, an excellent comprehensive overview of the instruments available to investigators in the behavioral and social sciences today and a reference for evaluating current research that lists the strengths and limitations of each of the commonly used instruments.

SEAMAN, JANET A., "Effects of Municipal Recreation on the Social Self-Esteem of the Mentally Retarded," *Therapeutic Recreation Journal,* 9, no. 2 (1975), 75–78. Assesses the effects of a nine-week community recreation program on the self-esteem and social interaction patterns of two groups of mentally retarded children. Uncomplicated in design and procedures, the study is easily analyzed and discussed. Because it subjects the recreation integration process to empirical testing, it could also be used in conjunction with, or directly following, the chapter on normalization in this text.

CHAPTER NINE
THERAPEUTIC
TECHNIQUES: ISSUES
AND TRENDS

Earlier chapters in the text outlined the challenges inherent in defining therapeutic recreation as a discipline and provided insights into the current status of therapeutic recreation as a profession. In this discussion, therapeutic recreation was portrayed as an eclectic field, drawing on and recombining information from educational areas including the arts, the humanities, and the physical and social sciences. Reference was also made to the relationship of our field to other human service professions, particularly the allied health care occupations. This chapter focuses upon issues associated with the practice of therapeutic recreation on two planes.

First, it examines the fundamental question related to the *boundaries* of practice between our profession and related disciplines. This might be thought of as the "Who does What?" dilemma. To illustrate the basis for this controversy, selected literature from two related service areas, art, and occupational therapy, is reviewed with particular reference to areas of potential overlap. *Second*, the chapter deals with basic concerns related to the *appropriateness* or *desirability* of employing certain techniques and technologies. This conflict might be conceptualized as the "Should, When, and How?" controversy. In this section, several common practices used by therapeutic recreation personnel are discussed, and potential problems related to these practices are explored. The final portion of the chapter illustrates how both questions concerning territorial boundaries and concerns related to the propriety of practice have formed the basis for today's debate over the process termed *leisure counseling.*

THE QUESTION
OF BOUNDARIES

Considerable confusion exists concerning distinctions between practices employed by therapeutic recreation specialists and those trained in other therapeutic interventions utilizing a single-treatment modality such as music therapy, dance therapy, play therapy, art therapy, psychodrama, horticultural therapy, bibliotherapy, pet therapy, and even therapeutic horseback riding. When the variety of activity media used as treatments is examined, and the training and backgrounds of therapists employing these activities are considered, several questions immediately come to mind:

— Do all individual recreational media have an inherent "therapeutic" potential? Is the "therapeutic," potential of certain activities greater than others?
— Is it feasible to train (and employ) therapists who specialize in a wide variety of activity modalities in settings serving disabled persons? Specifically, can and should activity therapy departments be instituted in facilities, and should these organizational units be comprised of several activity specialists each concentrating on one particular intervention such as drama, dance, music?
— Can we expect a proliferation of therapists specializing in new mediums such as competitive sports, aerobics, and combatives?
— How much and what type of training should be required before an individual can utilize an activity as a specific therapeutic intervention? When does an activity cease to be diversional or purely recreational and become therapeutic? When does activity participation escalate from being therapeutic to becoming a therapy?
— If therapeutic recreation personnel are "generalists" using a variety of activity media on a daily basis, what should their role and relationship be relative to other "single-activity specialists?"

To illustrate areas of overlap and the potential confusion which may exist between the practice of therapeutic recreation and a related medium, the following passages were chosen from a recent article in the *American Journal of Art Therapy.* The first quote defines the field and nature of art therapy; the second provides a concrete example of its practice.

> . . . the definition of art therapy does not depend on the population with whom one works, any more than it is a function of the setting in which the work occurs. When art activities are made available to handicapped or disturbed individuals, they may well be educational or recreational in nature. When one is teaching or providing art for the purpose of constructively filling leisure time, that is *not* art therapy. The essence of art therapy is that it must partake of both parts of its name—it must involve art *and* therapy. The goal of the art activity therefore, must be primarily therapeutic. This might, of course, include diagnosis as well as treatment. . . . In order to be an effective *art* therapist, you must know a great deal about both components of this hybrid discipline, you must know *art*: the media and processes and their nature and potential. . . . You must also know *therapy*. You need to know about yourself and about others in terms of development, psychodynamics and interpersonal relations.

And you must know about the nature of the treatment relationship and the underlying mechanisms that help others to change.[1]

Anyone watching a family art evaluation would see an interesting exercise in which family members make things individually and jointly and then talk about them to one another. If they are relaxed about it, it might look like a pleasant recreational activity for the family. And yet, while they may have fun or learn new skills, the therapists's primary goal is understanding family dynamics through the symbolic medium of their art in the context of their behavior.[2]

Upon analysis of these statements and examples, some interesting parallels, overlaps, and paradoxes appear when art therapy and therapeutic recreation are compared. *First,* both art therapy and recent definitions of therapeutic recreation view these disciplines as being independent of setting and population. In other words, providing art or other activities to disabled persons per se does not constitute a "therapy." *Second,* both disciplines recognize that their activity(ies) may range from diversional to interventionist. Art therapy concedes that art can be recreational, educational, or therapeutic. As previously indicated, the field of therapeutic recreation has identified itself with the provision of *recreation,leisure education,* and *therapy* areas of service.

Concerning the hybrid nature of art and therapy, while the results of the recent NTRS poll indicated that the continuum-of-services position was favored as one which should represent the field, a significant proportion of respondents indicated that they were presently providing treatment or treatment and recreation. Strong similarities also exist between art therapy and therapeutic recreation in the terminology used to describe the process followed by each. Terms such as *diagnosis, treatment, evaluation, behavior, development, psychodynamics, interpersonal relations, treatment relationship,* and *change* are stressed in both fields. Similarly, the family art evaluation session strongly resembles the family recreation therapy approach advocated and practiced by therapeutic recreation specialists in many clinical settings today. To further assist the reader to reflect upon possible areas of overlap between therapeutic recreation and other activity modalities, the following examples and questions (again related to art as a medium) are provided.

STUDY GUIDE QUESTIONS

1. Do therapeutic recreation specialists have the background and training to provide basic instruction in the visual arts—painting, ceramics, sculpture, and the others? Are therapeutic recreation personnel qualified to conduct art appreciation and education sessions? Should this activity be left to other specialists?

2. Therapeutic recreation specialists frequently gather subjective assessment data by observing clients in artistic (and other) pursuits. For example, a therapeutic recreation professional might record information concerning the way clients approach an art activity, the way they manipulate objects and materials related to the activity, their

---

[1] Judith A. Rubin, "Art Therapy: What It Is and What It Is Not," *American Journal of Art Therapy,* 21, (January 1982), p. 57.

[2] *Ibid.,* p. 58.

affective and cognitive involvement during participation, and their future interest in art. Are these legitimate functions of the therapeutic recreation specialist? Where do our boundaries and limits lie in terms of using an art activity or product as a diagnostic tool?

3. If working on a treatment team with an art therapist, what should our role be concerning art activities? Should we refrain from utilizing this medium? Should we work only under the supervision and direction of the art specialist when employing this medium? Should we limit our activity offerings to diversional art projects?

4. Therapeutic recreation specialists frequently design treatment plans around arts and crafts sessions, which include behavioral objectives related to increasing socialization skills, self-esteem, independent leisure skills, and so forth. Does this constitute a form of art therapy? Can you distinguish between the therapeutic use of an art activity and using an art activity as therapy?

Although overlaps in the types of services provided by therapeutic recreation specialists and single-medium therapies such as art frequently occur, they are not as complex as those associated with disciplines employing multimedia interventions such as occupational therapy. The potential similarities which may occur in the provision of therapeutic recreation and occupational therapy service become apparent when the following definition of occupational therapy, proposed by the American Occupational Therapy Association (AOTA), is considered:

> The art and science of directing man's participation in selected activity to restore, reinforce and enhance performance, facilitate learning of those skills and functions essential for adaptation and productivity, diminish or correct pathology and to promote and maintain health.[3]

Professional preparation programs in therapeutic recreation and occupational therapy also reveal a significant degree of consistency in certain content areas. Table 9-1 shows a typical four-year undergraduate curriculum in occupational therapy and Table 9-2, two sample course descriptions. These provide insight into parallels in content areas and approaches to preservice education between the two fields.

Standards of practice for occupational therapy and therapeutic recreation also reveal a strong degree of consistency relative to program planning, evaluation and implementation, and assessment of client performance, as evidenced by the following practices and procedures which have been adopted by the AOTA:[4]

— Basic to the development of any program are its intended purposes. Objectives and applicable policies should be clearly outlined for each separate activity such as patient treatment (both groups and individual). . . .

— Objective permanent records of each aspect of the service program should (1) justify each type of treatment or service given by indicating an appropriate evaluation of need for it, (2) indicate that the treatment or activity was performed, and (3) provide results of the same. . . .

[3] H. Tristram Engelhardt, "Defining Occupational Therapy: The Meaning of Therapy and the Virtues of Occupation," *American Journal of Occupational Therapy*, 31, no. 10 (1977), 666.

[4] American Occupational Therapy Association, *Standards for Occupational Therapy Service Programs* (Reprinted from *American Journal of Occupational Therapy*, 23, no. 1 (1969), 81–82.

TABLE 9-1   Sample Occupational Therapy Four-Year Curriculum

PREREQUISITES FOR ADMISSION
(Taken within the first two years of study)

English .... 6 semester hours
Biological Sciences .... 12 semester hours
   Must include laboratory courses in human
   physiology and anatomy
Psychology .... 12 semester hours
   Must include developmental psychology and
   psychology of personality
Sociology .... 6 semester hours
   These are considered minimum requirements.
   Students are encouraged to pursue further
   study in biology, psychology, and sociology.

JUNIOR YEAR, FALL SEMESTER	SEMESTER HOURS	JUNIOR YEAR, SPRING SEMESTER	SEMESTER HOURS
Functional Human Anatomy ..	4	Neuroanatomy	3
Communications and Group Dynamics	3	Developmental Tasks and Occupational Roles II	1
Developmental Tasks and Occupational Roles I	1	Physical Dysfunction and Occupational Therapy II	3
Physical Dysfunction and Occupational Therapy I	3	Psychosocial Dysfunction and Occupational Therapy II	3
Psychosocial Dysfunction and Occupational Therapy I	3	Skills Laboratory II	2
Skills Laboratory I	2	History and Theory of Occupational Therapy	3
	16		15

SENIOR YEAR, FALL SEMESTER	SEMESTER HOURS	SENIOR YEAR, SPRING SEMESTER	SEMESTER HOURS
Developmental Tasks and Occupational Roles III	2	Administration and Supervision of Occupational Therapy Services	3
Physical Dysfunction and Occupational Therapy III ...	5	Research Methods in Occupational Therapy	3
Psychosocial Dysfunction and Occupational Therapy III ...	5	Occupational Therapy in Health Care	3
Skills Laboratory III	2	Special Topics in Occupational Therapy	3
Elective	3	Elective	3
	17		15

FIELD WORK SESSIONS	SEMESTER HOURS
Field Work	6–9
Field Work	6–9
Field Work (Optional)	6–9

DEVELOPMENTAL TASKS AND OCCUPATIONAL ROLES I. Semester course; 1 lecture hour, 1 credit. This course explores principles of growth and processes of developmental adaptation of the infant through the childhood years. Performance skills related to self-help tasks, play-and-leisure tasks, and school and work tasks, viewed as occupational roles, are the focus of this course.

DEVELOPMENTAL TASKS AND OCCUPATIONAL ROLES III. Semester course; 1 lecture and 3 laboratory hours, 2 credits. A study of adult ontogenesis and developmental tasks as they interrelate with adult occupational patterns. The course will examine work, productivity, leisure, retirement, and recreation in the adult years, with emphasis on the importance of occupational success and balance for adaptation in adulthood and old age.

— The occupational therapist shall accept responsibility for recording details of the client's program at regular intervals and when change has occurred in the client's status. . . .

— When appropriate, the client shall be involved in program planning. The occupational therapy program objectives shall include both long- and short-term goals. . . . The program plan shall outline those activities necessary to provide the client with opportunities to achieve the stated objectives. The plan should be developed in sufficient detail to allow other persons concerned with the client to understand the results expected of the occupational therapy program through those activities utilized. Assessment measures shall be incorporated into the plan to determine effectiveness of the program. . . .

— The therapist shall evaluate and document the client's goals, functional abilities, and deficits in occupational performance (activities of daily living): a. self-care skills, b. work skills, c. play/leisure skills. . . .

— The therapist shall evaluate and document the client's goals, functional abilities, and deficits in the following performance component areas: a. psychological/interpersonal skills, b. social/interpersonal skills, c. cognitive skills. . . .

The following viewpoints expressed in literature in the occupational therapy field illustrate the strong role which recreation and leisure have played in the evolution of that discipline:

A new step [in the evolution of the field of occupational therapy] was to arise from a freer conception of work, from a concept of free and pleasant and profitable *occupation—including recreation in any form of helpful enjoyment as the leading principle.*[5]

Concerning the above quotation:

This historical sketch of occupational therapy provides us with a picture of the profession as one that uses recreational activities and engagement in tasks as ways of promoting health.[6]

What Bockoven seems to identify in occupational therapy is a form of discipline in recreation. Recall here the etymology of recreation—from *recreate,* to create anew.

[5] A. Meyer, "The Philosophy of Occupation Therapy," *Archives of Occupational Therapy,* 1, (1922), p. 2.

[6] Engelhardt, "Defining Occupational Therapy," p. 669.

Occupational therapy aims at recreating the adaptation of individuals through engagement in tasks.[7]

Occupational therapy thus offers a meaning of therapy that accents the process of human adaptation through involvement in recreation and in physical and mental activities generally.[8]

The following statement, extracted from a recent occupational therapy text, provides additional insight into the jurisdictional overlap between recreational and occupational therapy which may occur in treatment settings:

Recreation plays an important part in everyone's life. For hospitalized and handicapped persons it is often necessary to provide special facilities. Recreation has always been used as one of the modalities of occupational therapy. In some cases, however, a separate department is established. When this is the case every effort should be made to ensure coordination.[9]

The manifold modalities identified by the field of occupational therapy as appropriate treatment interventions have apparently generated controversy from within the field and from other related disciplines, notably therapeutic recreation and physical therapy. In recent articles appearing in the *American Journal of Occupational Therapy*, practitioners have pointed out what they perceive to be inadequacies in the current definition of occupational therapy. These discussions have centered around the general means by which the field has identified its parameters and the wide variety of media through which it lays claim to professional competence. Urging a return to more traditional media such as handiwork, Shannon feels that "Occupational therapy cannot be defined descriptively (What it is) nor is there agreement on a normative definition (What it ought to be)."[10]

Other authors feel that the breadth of the current definition of occupational therapy excludes certain skills possessed by practitioners within the field, particularly those involved in the restorative areas of physical disabilities practice. Taking exception to what they feel is an ambiguous approach to defining the field of occupational therapy with the concept of *purposeful activity,* English and others stated:

Purposeful activity is a vague term that will be interpreted in many ways both inside and outside the profession by those who wish to limit our practice of physical disability occupational therapy. For instance, a case could be made for the fact that any direction or assignment given to a patient by a therapist should have a purpose, whether or not it achieves an end product.[11]

[7] *Ibid.*, p. 670.

[8] *Ibid.*, p. 672.

[9] Clare S. Spackman, "Occupational Therapy: Its Relation to Allied Medical Services," in *Occupational Therapy* (Philadelphia, Pa.: J.B. Lippincott Company, 1971), p. 9.

[10] Phillip D. Shannon, "The Derailment of Occupational Therapy," *American Journal of Occupational Therapy*, 31, no. 4 (1977), 230.

[11] Carroll English and others, "The Issue: On the Role of the Occupational Therapist in Physical Disabilities," *American Journal of Occupational Therapy*, 36, no. 3 (1982), 199.

Recognizing the natural overlaps between occupational and physical therapy, Spackman, an O.T.R. noted

> In the treatment of physical disabilities occupational and physical therapy have a similar ultimate goal, namely to contribute to the restoration of the physical function of the patient. Personnel from these fields must work together closely and must have a mutual understanding of the goals and the treatment methods employed by each. Their work often supplements or complements the other in the treatment of the individual patient. For example, for the patient who is able to use an injured part voluntarily but does not do so because of pain, the objective of the treatment given by the physical therapist may be solely to relieve pain and precedes the treatment given by the occupational therapist which encourages voluntary motion and works to maintain power and endurance.[12]

In summary, considerable overlap exists between the services provided by therapeutic recreation specialists; single-medium therapies such as art, drama, and dance; and multimedia interventions such as occupational therapy. Discussion and debate among representatives of these fields will likely occur over the next several years, as each discipline continues to develop. An immediate challenge to each health care profession would seem to be the establishment of a vehicle to facilitate positive interactions across disciplines. In this fashion, the ultimate goal of improved services to our clients can be met.

STUDY GUIDE QUESTIONS

1. React to each of the questions about boundaries posed near the beginning of the chapter. Try to provide concrete examples to support your answers.
2. Compare the definition of occupational therapy provided in the chapter to the second paragraph of the NTRS philosophical position statement. What similarities or overlaps are evident?
3. How does the sample occupational therapy curriculum provided earlier in this chapter compare with curricular offerings in bachelor's degree programs in therapeutic recreation? Which program of study offers more specialized training?
4. Compare some of the statements related to standards of practice in occupational therapy to the standards developed by our professional organization. What similarities and differences exist?
5. Four viewpoints expressing the historical relationship which recreation has to occupational therapy appear earlier in this chapter. How do these positions compare to our own view of the relationship of recreation to therapeutic recreation?
6. Identify several common techniques or practices employed by both therapeutic recreation specialists and occupational therapists. List several techniques which appear to be used exclusively by one field or the other.
7. Do you feel that overlap among the services provided by health care professionals is beneficial for consumers of these services?
8. There appears to be a trend toward the administrative grouping of several departments, such as recreation, occupational therapy, physical therapy, and dance, under the title *Activities Therapy* in large facilities. What pros and cons can you see to this organizational arrangement?

[12] Spackman, "Occupational Therapy," p. 8.

CONCERNS RELATED
TO SPECIFIC PRACTICES

The preceding section explored some possible areas of overlap between therapeutic recreation servics and other disciplines.[13] This portion of the chapter attempts to pose specific questions related to the appropriateness and desirability of employing certain practices and procedures in therapeutic recreation settings. To assist the reader in confronting and overcoming these potential dilemmas related to service provision, several problem-solving case study examples are provided.

Problem Area 1—Defining
Scope of Service

Exercise A. You have just been employed as the head of a small recreation therapy department in a large residential center for emotionally disturbed children and adolescents. In addition to your three recreation specialists, the center employs several counselors, teachers, two occupational therapists, and a physical education specialist. The director has recently completed a survey of other similar facilities, to determine the types of services they offer. The following programs appear to be commonplace in these settings:

Sex-education Groups in which information concerning human sexuality and knowledge related to human reproduction is provided.

Perceptual Motor Training in which batteries of diagnostic tests are administered to children and individualized perceptual motor training activities are prescribed and conducted.

Boredom Clinic in which feelings concerning free time are explored and leisure education takes place.

Relaxation Classes in which physiological and psychological processes leading to relaxation are discussed and relaxation training exercises are conducted.

Play Therapy in which play situations are used as a tool to diagnose and treat psychosocial disorders.

Assertiveness Training in which adolescents are taught to defend their rights without aggression.

Upon sharing the results of the survey with you, the director asks you to identify the role which your department would play in each of these services should they be initiated within the facility. Specifically, you are to identify which programs would come directly under the auspices of the recreation department, which programs you would make a significant staff commitment to but not assume primary responsibility for, and which activities you would not become involved in or provide minimal resources for. What would your response be to the director? Why would you distribute your resources in this fashion?

[13] Acknowledgement is given to graduate students Diane Hayes and Linda Love for assistance in developing this topic.

Exercise B.   You are a one-person recreation department in a newly constructed 200-bed extended care facility for adults needing skilled nursing care. Your
"staff" consists of six dedicated, but untrained, middle-aged volunteers of both
sexes. Upon conducting a survey of clients and staff concerning programming needs
in the facility, the following needs and program areas are identified:

> *A women's goup*—requested by the predominantly female population
>
> *A men's club*—requested by the male residents
>
> *An exercise group*—requested by all residents
>
> *A self-help skill-development group* (personal care, hygiene, dressing, etc.)—
> requested by residents
>
> *A crafts group*—suggested by residents
>
> *A cooking club*—suggested by residents
>
> *A family and residents' council*—suggested by residents and their families
>
> *A reality orientation program*—suggested by staff

Which of these program areas would you assign top priority to? Should all
these activities be the essential responsibility of your "department"? Would you
enlist the aid of other staff members in conducting these activities? If so, who would
you seek to involve?

Exercise C.   You are head of a four-person recreation department in a state-
operated center for youth administered by the department of corrections. Juvenile
offenders are sent to the center by the courts for an indeterminate period of time.
When judged "rehabilitated," the children are released back into their communities
under the supervision of a caseworker who works for the department of corrections.
High rates of recidivism for these youth are quite common. The director of the
center points out that there is little or no referral or follow-up predischarge and
postdischarge by community recreation agencies. Therefore, "the kids have no
knowledge of recreational opportunities in their neighborhoods, which predisposes
them to further delinquent acts." The director charges your department to take
direct responsibility for correcting this situation. You are asked to develop a *community referral system* which would help each child to identify and make contact
with community recreation agencies upon discharge. Remembering that you and
your staff are currently "spread thin" by having to program for large numbers of
children at the center, how would you respond to the director? Is this task, in fact,
the total responsibility of the recreation department? If not, who else should be
involved in this endeavor, and what tasks should they be assigned?

Problem Area 2—Determining
Appropriateness of Service

Exercise A.   You are a therapeutic recreation supervisor employed in a
large residential psychiatric facility. A new chief administrator of the institution has
scheduled a meeting with you and several other department heads to discuss some
new ideas for programming. The administrator has two proposals which would

directly impact on your program. The first suggestion is that recreation staff members be required to assist ward personnel in restraining unruly patients when necessary and in the transportation of residents to treatments such as electroconvulsive therapy and neurological testing. The director suggests that this would maximize the personnel resources of the facility and "establish more rapport" between the recreation personnel, ward staff, and residents. *Second*, "because of the expertise your staff has in the area of programming," the director suggests that your department be put in permanent charge of organizing and conducting special events in the agency including staff parties at holidays, special activities for the staff during National Nurses Week, and receptions for legislators and other public officials who may visit the facility on "special business." Your staff vocally rejects these proposals, taking the position that their responsibility is service to the residents. How would you respond to the director's ideas? Should the recreation department ultimately be responsible for all recreation programming within an agency? Where does one draw the line?

Exercise B.   You are in charge of a summer camp program for "predelinquent" disadvantaged youth. The camp advisory board has suggested that you and your staff implement a model wilderness survival program which they have read about. It involves a series of one-week trips to remote areas, stressing cooperative high-risk activities such as rock climbing, caving, and white-water canoeing. Advocates of such programs have made claims for the effectiveness of the intervention, ranging from its beneficial effect upon school performance to increased self-concept, to decreased participation in delinquent acts. Some of your staff members remain unconvinced, however. They state that such changes in delinquents have been isolated and short-lived. They point to the expense and risk associated with such a sophisticated program. Finally, they feel that because most of the campers come from disadvantaged urban areas, they would have little inclination and opportunity to participate in such pursuits when they return home. How could you collect data which would support or refute their arguments? What are your personal feelings regarding the efficacy of such programs? Do you feel activities and programs should be avoided which require equipment, materials, and supplies which would not be readily available to a client in his or her home environment?

Exercise C.   You are employed in a group-home setting for mentally retarded adults. The home has recently adopted a strong behavior modification approach aimed at developing and sustaining independent living skills. A basic premise of this program is that privileges must be purchased by obtaining points or tokens earned through the performance of daily chores and tasks. It has been suggested that participation in recreation, including evening activities in the home, outings, and even leisure snack foods be contingent upon earning a specified number of tokens by demonstrating proper grooming and hygiene, completing schoolwork, maintaining one's room in proper order, and other tasks. Due to the developmental level of certain clients, however, it appears that it could be days or even weeks before they would be eligible for recreation. Would you, as a therapeutic recreation specialist, support such a system? Should participation in regularly scheduled recreation programs be reserved as a reward for appropriate behavior or withdrawn as a consequence of inappropriate behavior?

Exercise D.   You are the coordinator of a play and recreation program in a medical-surgical hospital for children. One of your chief areas of programming is the operation of three playrooms where children are allowed to engage in supervised free play. Recently your staff members who oversee these areas have come to you with a complaint. They report that on several separate occasions, members of the nursing staff have entered the playrooms and performed medical procedures such as giving injections and drawing blood from children. The staff state that these procedures upset the children who received these treatments, as well as other children present. When your staff confronted the nurses they were told that these procedures were a necessary part of hospitalization, that the nursing staff was shorthanded, and that medical treatment took precedence over "fun and games." A regular weekly meeting of department heads is scheduled for tomorrow. Both you and the director of nursing will be in attendance. How would you approach this problem with the nursing director?

Exercise E.   You are a therapeutic recreation specialist working at a center for adults with varying degrees of cerebral palsy, ranging from mild to severe. Another staff member at the center (a self-confessed video-game addict) has approached you with an idea. The staff member suggests that the center purchase a programmable video-game machine which would allow adjustments to be made which could vary the degree of difficulty for each player. Specifically, the game could be slowed down for those with severe cases of cerebral palsy and speeded up for those with moderate and mild cases. In the opinion of the staff member, this procedure would result in fair and interesting competition between all players and would even allow members of the center to compete on an equal basis with non-disabled members of the community. Can you envision any potential problems which could occur from this "handicapping" procedure? To what extent is it desirable to modify games and competitive sports to achieve equal probability of success by disabled persons?

THE COUNSELING CONTROVERSY

— Leisure Counseling: More Rehetoric than Reality?
— Leisure Counseling: A Potential Danger
— Leisure Counseling: Recreators, Keep Out!
— Whose Role Leisure Education?
— Leisure Counseling or Leisure Quackery?
— State Licensing May Regulate Leisure Therapy/Counseling*

These provocative titles of current professional articles are indicative of the controversy which surrounds the process and practice of leisure counseling today.

*Complete references to these articles appear in footnotes 42, 28, 32, 25, 33, and 43.

Indeed, few issues have generated the interest, concern, and effort toward resolution that the ''counseling controversy'' has spawned. This interest has transcended the field of therapeutic recreation to the point where community recreation and park educators and practitioners have become thoroughly involved in the fray. Indeed, since 1976, this topic has been the focal point of a ''mini theme'' at a NRPA annual congress and of a national forum on leisure counseling sponsored by the U.S. Bureau of Education for the Handicapped. This sudden interest in leisure counseling has not been limited to the recreation and parks field. Indeed, respected publications like the *Wall Street Journal* and *Parade* magazine have featured articles on the subject.

The remainder of this chapter reviews the origin and history of the controversy surrounding leisure counseling by overviewing the major issues of concern to educators, practitioners, researchers, and consumers. To achieve this objective, five major areas of concern, based on the 1979 National Forum on Leisure Counseling, will be reviewed by examining extant literature.[14] A list of study guide questions will follow each of these areas of inquiry. This process will allow readers to internalize information and reflect upon the implications of each major problem for the field of recreation in general and therapeutic recreation in particular. In approaching this material, it is important to note the natural connections which exist between issues. For example, disagreement as to the fundamental nature of the counseling process would logically lead to discrepancies in terminology in identifying the field, concerns over professional disciplines and training, related ethics, and research needs.

Problem Area 1—What Human Needs Should Be Addressed Through the Medium of Leisure Counseling, and, Consequently, What Approaches and Techniques Should Be Employed in This Process?

Since its formal inception in psychiatric settings in the mid-1950s, leisure counseling has been employed in a variety of forms and settings with diverse groups of clients. Until the mid-1970s however, little reflection took place on issues related to what fundamental needs (if any) were (or could) be met through the counseling process. Consequently, the process took on forms and procedures as varied as the counselors, counselees, and settings in which it was practiced. Perhaps the following three orientations best illustrate the range of forms and processes which leisure counseling can assume:

[14] Fred Humphrey, Jerry D. Kelley, and Edward J. Hamilton, eds., *Facilitating Leisure Development for the Disabled: A Status Report on Leisure Counseling* (College Park, Md.: University of Maryland, 1980), p.v.

Leisure counseling as a leisure resource guidance service. This approach simply matches the interests or expressed desires of a client to existing leisure or recreation resources. It does not deal with underlying difficulties related to attitudes or values regarding leisure participation.

Leisure counseling as a life style developmental-educational service. This model assumes that the client is experiencing a "felt difficulty" related to his or her leisure. It focuses upon both internal and external barriers to leisure participation and is more comprehensive and structured than the resource guidance approach.

Leisure counseling as a therapeutic-remedial service. This model is intensive and assumes that the client has a fundamental lack of knowledge about leisure skills and attitudes. It is likely to take place in a "clinical" setting and is frequently of long duration.[15]

Beyond this relatively basic classification of leisure counseling approaches, "to date no nationally or universally accepted leisure counseling model or approach exists. The leisure counseling process differs from hospital to hospital, agency to agency, municipality to municipality and from hospital setting to hospital setting."[16]

Noting the proliferation of approaches, authors such as Neulinger have advocated an analysis of the theoretical basis of leisure counseling and issued a "Plea for Complexity."[17] Pointing to the fact that leisure counseling has emerged from the areas of education, counseling, and psychotherapy, Neulinger proposed three dimensions which should be addressed in designing any approach to leisure counseling. These include the orientation of the program, the nature of the problem, and the nature of the client.

Compton, Witt, and Sanchez echoed this concern over the development of a theoretical basis for leisure counseling:

> A . . . point which must be agreed on in order to build a theory or model of leisure counseling is to determine whether the intention is rehabilitation (as in problem solution) or education (as in ongoing personal development and growth). When these problems are added to the definitional and implicational nuances of terms like recreation and play, it is easy to see why leisure counseling is in a stage of relative infancy with regard to standardized theories and models.[18]

Other observers such as Sessoms pointed to a fundamental question which

[15] Chester F. McDowell, Jr., *Leisure Counseling: Selected Lifestyle Processes* (Eugene, Ore.: University of Oregon, Center of Leisure Studies, 1976).

[16] Peter A. Witt and Rhonda Groom, "Dangers and Problems Associated with Current Approaches to Developing Leisure Interest Finders," *Therapeutic Recreation Journal*, 13, no. 1 (1979), 19.

[17] John Neulinger, "Leisure Counseling: A Plea for Complexity," *Leisure Today*, (April 1977), pp. 3–4.

[18] David Compton, Peter A. Witt, and Barbara D. Sanchez, "Leisure Counseling," *Parks and Recreation Magazine*, 15, no. 8 (August 1980), 24.

may need to be answered before further insights are gained relative to the addressing of human needs and the development of theoretical approaches in leisure counseling.[19] Specifically, "Have we conceptually and operationally defined the ideal leisure state?" It would appear that until this basic question is answered, attempts at sound model building in the area of leisure counseling may be futile.

The lack of development of valid and reliable measuring tools and instruments, and, indeed, the entire process of assessment in leisure counseling, appear to be symptoms of our inability to generate leisure-state models. Indeed, we may be guilty of inappropriately adopting models from other fields in our counseling practices. Specifically,

> Many of the models developed in vocational education, psychiatry, vocational rehabilitation, guidance counseling and school psychology have been modified to fit our needs. We have encouraged our students to elect courses from these professions and disciplines to develop their competencies in the counseling process and are even now developing our own courses in counseling. But the effectiveness of these models is questionable. They may be reliable procedures and models in vocational rehabilitation or educational settings, but their validity in a recreation setting is unclear.[20]

Our inability to define the leisure state and the lack of consistent approaches to meeting human needs have manifested themselves in current criticisms of instruments in widespread use in leisure counseling settings. Leisure "interest finders" have become a primary focal point of controversy. Indeed, the criticisms related to their use epitomize the question of which human needs should (and can) be addressed by which approaches and techniques in the leisure counseling process. Witt and Groom raised several points of contention relative to the design and utilization of interest finders.[21] These may be summarized as follows:

— Substantial confusion exists as to the nature of the concept's needs, wants, and interests. Whereas needs appear to be innate, wants are learned. Interests, on the other hand, may be transformed into wants or needs. However, satiated interests may or may not be followed by reduced wants or needs.

— The construct *interest* is difficult to define. A counselor may be dealing with an *expressed*, *manifest*, or *tested* interest. Consequently, the validity and reliability of interest finders is in question.

— Notions such as *activity substitution,* or "whether commonalities can be found between activities so that counselors and clients can deal with a reduced list of activity types as opposed to an endless list of individual activities,"[22] have not been adequately addressed.

— Interest finders can, but should not be, used independently of values clarification, attitudinal exploration, decision making, or social skills development techniques.

[19] H. Douglas Sessoms, "Leisure Counseling: A Frank Analysis of the Issues," *Parks and Recreation Magazine*, 16, no. 1 (January 1981), 65.

[20] *Ibid.*, p. 68.

[21] Witt and Groom, "Dangers and Problems."

[22] *Ibid.*, p. 27.

STUDY GUIDE QUESTIONS

1. Make a list of basic human needs. Which of these needs do you feel can and should be addressed through the medium of leisure counseling?
2. To date, Gestalt, Transactional Analysis, Reality Therapy, Rational Emotive Therapy, Values Clarification, Assertiveness Training, Neurolinguistic Programming, and other metacommunication models have been adapted for use in leisure counseling. Do you think there is adequate theroretical justification for the application of each of these approaches to the area of leisure counseling? If so, which basic human needs, as developed in question 1, could best be met by each of these approaches?
3. Considering the fact that leisure counseling has been practiced since the 1950s, should we be concerned that "no nationally or universally accepted leisure counseling model or approach exists?"
4. It was suggested that leisure counseling programs reflect three factors: the orientation of the approach, the nature of the problem, and the nature of the client. What fundamental assumptions does each of the models of leisure counseling mentioned in question 2 make relative to each of these factors?
5. It has been suggested that conceptually and operationally defining the "ideal leisure-state" should be a high priority of the recreation and parks field. Do you feel that the ideal leisure state must be defined before truly valid leisure counseling models can be developed?
6. Do you agree with the criticisms of leisure interest finders, as raised by Witt and Groom? Are the problems associated with these instruments symptoms of fundamental weaknesses in our counseling models?

Problem Area 2—What Term(s) Should Be Used to Describe the Process of Leisure Counseling?

With fundamental disagreement concerning the basic nature of a leisure counseling model(s) widespread, it is little wonder that a lack of consensus exists regarding an appropriate term to describe this process. At various times, the following labels have appeared in the literature relative to this helping process:

— Leisure Counseling
— Leisure Education
— Recreation Counseling
— Activities Counseling
— Avocational Counseling

To further compound the problem, these terms have been used interchangeably, with little regard for the relationships between and among them. The distinction between leisure counseling and leisure education has been particularly nebulous. The dilemma which this situation can bring about was illustrated by Epperson as follows:

An equally serious problem is the lack of understanding of the relationship between leisure education and leisure counseling. It is reasonable to assume that a leisure counselor can help people choose leisure activities that would be of interest to them only if those people have some skill in or knowledge of the activities discussed.[23]

This same author, in reviewing his recent edited text *Leisure Counseling: An Aspect of Leisure Education* (Charles C Thomas, publisher) further illustrated this problem by the following critique:

> While it has a number of excellent articles by leisure counseling experts, most of them deal with techniques and approaches of leisure counseling with particular audiences. Little mention is made of the relationship of leisure counseling to leisure education and the need to educate our students as well as society in good leisure attitudes and skills.[24]

While few would argue that "leisure education is compatible with the current goals, programs and services of the profession, and would enable these to be expanded, reoriented and restructured to better facilitate the leisure development of people,"[25] the questions remain: What is leisure counseling? What is leisure education?

In an attempt to clarify basic nomenclature and the relationship of various terms, Chinn and Joswiak have proposed that leisure education be associated with the use of comprehensive models which relate to the overall educational process influencing the leisure life-style of an individual *and* with the use of any aspect of that approach. Leisure counseling would then be viewed as a subset of leisure education which " . . . facilitates the process of problem solving, decision-making, and conflict management regarding leisure interests, awareness, values and opportunities."[26]

Because it is essential to determine whether counseling techniques have been used, these authors noted:

> The term, recreation counseling, has purposely been deemphasized. This process is viewed as more appropriate under the "umbrella" of leisure counseling and utilizing that particular nomenclature. However, if one chooses to use the term recreation counseling, the same criteria concerning the use of counseling techniques should be applied.[27]

STUDY GUIDE QUESTIONS

1. What are basic differences in orientation connoted by the terms *leisure counseling, leisure education, recreation counseling, activities counseling,* and *avocational coun-*

---

[23] Arlin Epperson, "Educating Recreators for Leisure Counseling," *Leisure Today*, (April 1977), 15.

[24] *Ibid.*, p. 16.

[25] Jean Mundy, "Whose Role Leisure Education?" *Parks and Recreation Magazine*, 16, no. 3 (1981), 22.

[26] Karen A. Chinn and Kenneth F. Joswiak, "Leisure Education and Leisure Counseling," *Therapeutic Recreation Journal*, 15, no. 4 (1981), 6.

[27] *Ibid.*

seling? Are the terms *recreation counseling, activities counseling* and *avocational counseling* different from *leisure counseling*?

2. Is there a strong need for a single definition of leisure counseling at this stage of the processes development? Is it possible to arrive at such a definition?

3. Do you agree with Chinn and Joswiak's view that leisure counseling should be viewed as a subset of leisure education?

4. Do you feel that it is relatively easy to determine when one is functioning as a counselor as opposed to an educator?

5. What suggestions would you have for discriminating between leisure counseling techniques and leisure education techniques?

Problem Area 3—Which Discipline(s) Should Provide Leisure Counseling Services? What Training Should Take Place within These Disciplines?

The lack of agreement regarding the fundamental nature of leisure counseling in relation to client needs and confusion over counseling models, approaches, and terminology have manifested themselves in the current debate over the background and training required to function as a "leisure counselor." A recent *Parks and Recreation Magazine* editorial brought this issue to the fore when it inquired of college and university personnel "Are you training professional counselors or potentially dangerous opportunists?"[28] This question appears most appropriate, as institutions of higher learning have eagerly initiated leisure counseling instruction within their curricula. A 1977 study, for example, found that 58 percent of one hundred sample colleges and universities surveyed offered formal leisure counseling instruction.[29] Of these institutions, 28 percent offered a separate course on the topic and 72 percent included the material within existing courses.

In 1980 a follow-up study was undertaken to assess the impact of the leisure counseling movement over the past few years. In this investigation, a small number of universities, rehabilitation agencies, public recreation facilities, and commercial leisure counseling services were contacted to determine what effect the proliferation of course work in universities has had upon leisure counseling practice in rehabilitation and other fields. Although the investigators again found strong evidence for the "trend toward universal coverage of the leisure counseling subject"[30] in higher education, there appeared to be no formal specialization or concentration in this area in university programs, nor was there perceived to be such a need.

Other findings raise serious questions concerning the relationship between academic preparation in leisure counseling and the utilization of these skills in real-

[28] "Leisure Counseling: A Potential Danger," editorial in *Parks and Recreation Magazine*, 14, no. 3 (1979), 17.

[29] A. Weiner and W. Gilley, "The Instructional Status of Leisure Counseling," *Therapeutic Recreation Journal*, 11, no. 4 (1977), 148–55.

[30] Compton, Witt, and Sanchez, "Leisure Counseling," p. 26

world treatment settings. Specifically, rehabilitation personnel found that university graduates were generally lacking in both fundamental knowledge of human behavior and specific counseling processes. They recommended psychology, sociology, and human behavior courses as means to gain this competence, as well as extensive supervised practicums. Furthermore, these professionals felt that many university graduates with backgrounds in leisure counseling "lacked the basic conceptual skills to place leisure counseling into the rehabilitation framework."[31] The authors conclude that at present there are no efforts at establishing valid educational competencies in the area of leisure counseling, and, there is a dearth of preservice and inservice training in this process.

Other observers have argued that while professional preparation programs in the recreation and parks field could conceivably offer introductory courses in leisure counseling in subspecialities such as therapeutic recreation, these programs cannot produce full-fledged leisure counselors ready to serve clients. In their opinion, recreators:

> . . . are neither philosophically, socially, or professionally attuned to the requirements of counseling. They must use psychology in their work with others, of course. But they use it to spur others to action rather than into self-examination. They are basically action people, while counselors are basically contemplative people who emphasize self-awareness.[32]

Kinney and Dowling also questioned the appropriateness of including counseling instruction in recreation and parks university curricula. Taking the position that counseling qualities such as empathetic human skills are inherent, they, like others, urged recreators to reconsider assuming counseling roles. In their words "It is an opportune time for recreators to pursue status on their people-oriented strengths rather than seek credibility by association with pseudo-scientific techniques that bear the trappings of a medical or authoritarian model."[33]

This debate over the appropriateness of including leisure counseling instruction in professional preparation in recreation and parks (and consequently) therapeutic recreation curricula appears to stem from a fundamental disagreement as to the nature of leisure counseling. The various notions of what this process is (or should be) have been outlined by Sessoms, through the concept of *roles*:

> If leisure counseling is viewed as a single role set, then the training, credentialling, and legitimizing of that function will be quite different from our approach to leisure counseling as one of several roles performed within a general role set of the professional. Simply stated, is leisure counseling a profession in its own right, or is it a job

---

[31] *Ibid.*

[32] Patsy B. Edwards, "Leisure Counseling: Recreators, Keep Out," *Parks and Recreation Magazine*, 16, no. 6 (1981), 42.

[33] Walter Kinney and Dorothy Dowling, "Leisure Counseling or Leisure Quackery," *Parks and Recreation Magazine*, 16, no. 1 (1981), 106.

function, a set of tasks performed by most recreation professionals regardless of title?[34]

To resolve this controversy, Sessoms suggested that leisure counseling be conceptualized as a specialty area within the park and recreation field and that a "layering of specialized education" be added to a generalist education to train one as a leisure counselor.

Others such as Hayes have advocated in "in-depth, interdisciplinary approach" to the academic preparation of leisure counselors. Pointing to the fact that the field of recreation has by no means a monopoly on problems related to the leisure of individuals, he suggested that disciplines such as vocational counseling, social work, psychology, and psychiatry be represented in any program designed to train leisure counselors.[35]

In a preliminary attempt to define the competencies inherent in a body of knowledge associated with instruction in leisure counseling, a subgroup of a national forum identified the following areas in which counselors should possess skills. It would appear that many of these categories could best be addressed through an interdisciplinary effort, as previously described. These major areas include:

> . . . Knowledge of the sociological and psychological aspects of leisure behavior; life span development; abnormal development; community resource analysis and development; personality theory; knowledge of instrumentation and assessment; knowledge of group dynamics; communication skills (including perception of affective domain sensitivity, verbal and non-verbal communication, self-awareness and self-assessment); specific counseling theories, skills and techniques; philosophy of leisure; and perspectives of leisure counseling.[36]

STUDY GUIDE QUESTIONS

1. Concerning the previously cited 1980 study, do you feel that the concerns expressed by rehabilitation personnel relative to the background and training of recreation personnel in leisure counseling are justified?
2. Do you agree with Kinney and Dowling that leisure counseling may be a pseudoscientific process with the "trappings of a medical or authoritarian model"?
3. Sessoms suggested that leisure counseling may be viewed as a profession in its own right or as a set of tasks performed by most recreation professionals regardless of title. Which view do you feel most accurately reflects the state of the art of leisure counseling today?
4. It has been suggested that an interdisciplinary approach be taken to the training of those who will be performing leisure counseling duties. Do you favor such an orientation to professional training? If so, what disciplines should be represented?
5. Review the areas of competency identified by the national task force earlier in this

---

[34] Sessoms, "Leisure Counseling," p. 69.

[35] Gene A. Hayes, "Professional Preparation and Leisure Counseling," *Leisure Today*, (April 1977), p. 14.

[36] Humphrey, Kelley, and Hamilton, "Facilitating Leisure Development," pp. 103–4.

chapter. Do you agree that all of these are necessary prerequisites to performing leisure counseling?

6. Is leisure counseling (as a service or a process) an appropriate domain for all human-service professions, or is it exclusive to recreation, therapeutic recreation, or both? Should all recreation and parks professionals receive formal academic training in leisure counseling? Should only therapeutic recreation specialists be trained specifically as leisure counselors?

7. Do you feel that leisure counseling training should be offered as a separate program or discipline in institutions of higher education? Should people receive degrees specifically in leisure counseling?

8. In recreation and parks professional preparation curricula, should leisure counseling training for therapeutic recreation specialists take place at the undergraduate or graduate, or both levels? Design a course or series of courses which you feel would adequately prepare a therapeutic recreation specialist to perform leisure counseling in a variety of agency settings.

9. Should accreditation standards and procedures be developed to regulate training institutions which produce leisure counselors? If so, what form should these standards take?

10. What differences in training and academic preparation would exist in the preparation of individuals to provide leisure resource guidance, developmental and educational or therapeutic and remedial leisure counseling?

Problem Area 4—What Legal and Ethical Concerns Must Be Resolved Before the Practice of Leisure Counseling Can Be Legitimized?

The question of legal and ethical issues as outlined in the recent report of the National Forum on Leisure Counseling must be considered *in addition* to the previously discussed issue of professional preparation and training, or competence. The distinctions between professional competence, ethics, and law may be viewed as follows:

Competence relates to the requisite ability of the individual to deliver services in accordance with established standards.
Ethics refers to the moral conduct or behavior in relationship to standards.
Ethics are usually expressed in formal codes adopted by a professional organization to protect the client and professional.
Law transcends the questions of standards and competence and relates to rules of conduct which are formally recognized as binding or enforceable by controlling authority.[37]

The recent concern over ethical and legal questions which transcend issues of professional competencies is illustrated forcefully in the following statement: "With leisure counseling assuming a growing importance, it may necessitate development of leisure consumer organizations, quasi-political action and advocacy groups, or Ralph Nader Leisure Corps to protect the average citizen from public or private enterprise rip-offs!"[38]

[37] *Ibid.*, pp. 10–11.
[38] Compton, Witt, and Sanchez, "Leisure Counseling," p. 23.

In response to such fears, the following legal and ethical considerations were raised in a national mini conference on leisure counseling in 1977:

— Should there be licensing, registration, or certification policies governing leisure counseling personnel?
— What type of career ladders might be considered for leisure counseling personnel?
— Concerning confidentiality, privacy and constituent rights: To what extent is the leisure counseling relationship/process governed by the ethical concerns of other counseling relationships? To what extent should it be? What thought should be given to liability of personnel and agencies and institutions?[39]

Several discussions of legal and ethical questions relating to leisure counseling have followed this initial attempt to generate debate in this area. Authors such as Sessoms have pointed out that no clear guidelines exist as to what extent recreators should advise or influence behaviors or attitudes of clients.[40] He further observed that since no consensus has been reached concerning the ideal leisure state, it is unreasonable and perhaps dangerous to instill in others our perception of this frame of mind. Kinney and Dowling also reflected upon the danger inherent in practicing leisure counseling without a well-developed code of ethics. They felt that current definitions of this process imply omniscience on the part of the counselor, which may foster an unhealthy dependency relationship through a "pervasive aura of scientific expertise, authority, and mysticism."[41] Hunter noted that leisure counseling could, if used improperly, become a mechanism which "blames the victim" and promotes change in the client rather than in the environment. She felt that if leisure counseling is practiced in conjunction with the principles of normalization, it would "be recognized as a mechanism by which persons with a disability can assume the role of active consumer versus passive recipient."[42]

Although these and other ethical concerns have been raised and partially discussed, little information has been generated concerning the exact legal ramifications which may apply to those practicing leisure counseling, Kozlowski urged certain precautions. Specifically, because leisure counseling could conceivably be construed as the practice of psychology or a form of counseling (both of which are regulated in many states), potential leisure counselors should check the licensing requirements of individual states in both these areas. He further suggested that individuals and institutions of higher learning should ban together in an effort to define the parameters of leisure counseling in anticipation of approaching states and national organizations such as the American Psychological Association to resolve potential conflicts.[43]

[39] David M. Compton and Judith E. Goldstein, eds., *Perspectives of Leisure Counseling* (Arlington, Va.: National Recreation and Park Association, 1977), p. 168.

[40] Sessoms, "Leisure Counseling."

[41] Kinney and Dowling, "Leisure Counseling," p. 70.

[42] Jan Hunter, "Leisure Counseling: More Rhetoric Than Reality?" *Leisurability*, 9, no. 2 (Spring 1982), 5–12.

[43] Jim Kozlowski, "State Licensing May Regulate Leisure Therapy/Counseling," *Parks and Recreation Magazine*, 17, no. 1 (1982), 22, 25–26.

Until such ethical and legal questions and concerns are resolved, leisure counselors and potential recipients of leisure counseling services have little sound guidance when entering into a helping relationship related to leisure guidance. Perhaps the best available advice can be obtained from an existing draft of a leisure counselor's "consumer guide"[44] which was developed by a subgroup on ethics of the National Forum on Leisure Counseling, led by Gerald Fain.

Consumer Guide to Assessing Leisure Counselors:

1. Leisure Counselors should convey a philosophy as it relates to higher personal leisure well being.

2. Leisure Counselors must use reliable and valid instrumentation in assessing a client's leisure well being.

3. The consumer should assess the Leisure Counselor's awareness of the problems and expect the counselor to demonstrate a sensitivity to the external (environmental) barriers and internal (personal) barriers that limit leisure functions/opportunities.

4. The consumer should investigate the Leisure Counselor's fee structure prior to the initial session and should expect fees/charges to be commensurate with other allied health fields.

5. Consumers should ask about the types of services available from Leisure Counselors (disclosure of services, truth in advertising); for example, assessment methods and procedures, evaluation methods and techniques.

6. The Leisure Counselor should possess a healthy leisure state (modeling) while personally progressing toward the leisure ideal.

7. After the initial session, the Leisure Counselor should give the consumer some notion as to the anticipated length of treatment.

8. The consumer should investigate the types of approaches, strategies, techniques, and methodologies of the Leisure Counselor and should fully expect the Leisure Counselor to identify and discuss the above concerns so that the consumer can make a choice based on his/her own needs.

9. The consumer has the right to expect the Leisure Counselor to interpret in terms understandable to the client the assessment procedures and results. The Counselor should also be expected to inform the consumer when treatment appears to be ineffective in improving his leisure well being.

10. The consumer should have the right to investigate the Leisure Counselor's "history" before submitting to counseling, i.e., educational training, special training related to assessment tools, experience, successes with other clients/consumers.

STUDY GUIDE QUESTIONS

1. In response to the questions raised at the previously mentioned mini conference on leisure counseling, would you favor licensing, registration, or certification plans to govern the practice of leisure counseling? If so, who should be responsible for implementing such procedures?

2. What difference(s), if any, exists between the provision of leisure counseling to a client in a therapeutic recreation setting and the rendering of leisure counseling services to the general public? What, if any, ethical or legal differences exist in the provision of service in these two different areas?

[44] Humphrey, Kelley, and Hamilton, "Facilitating Leisure Development," pp. 112–13.

3. Do you agree with several of the previously cited authors that leisure counseling has the potential to foster dependency on the part of the client and instill values and attitudes that are really part of the counselor's personality?

4. Research current licensure practices in your state concerning fields such as psychology, vocational counseling, career counseling, and marriage or family counseling. How do these regulations impact on the area of leisure counseling?

5. Review the proposed guidelines for consumers of leisure counseling. What additions or revisions would you make to this document?

Problem Area 5—What Research Needs to Be Conducted Related to Leisure Counseling? How Should Research Areas Be Prioritized?

It is obvious that research efforts must be centered around the resolution of the four previously outlined problem areas. Yet, defining and prioritizing our research efforts vis à vis leisure counseling is in itself a challenge. To date, the research questions which have been suggested can largely be grouped into the broad categories of problems related to the counseling process itself and topics related to the delivery of leisure counseling within the larger leisure delivery system. The following statement is illustrative of the concern which has manifested itself relative to the *process* of leisure counseling:

> In general, research and empirical evidence regarding the effectiveness of these procedures is lacking. . . . Failure to generate appropriate theories and models makes it difficult to know what to test. The failure is aggravated by problems of terminology, procedures and focus. Few attempts have been made to measure actual gains made by participants in leisure counseling programs and what efforts have been made suffer from small samples, subjectivity of data, and limited depth of dependent variable used.[45]

To truly understand the nature of the counseling process, it may be necessary to address the following questions suggsted by Witt and Bishop:

— Which personality characteristics are important to consider in assessing a person's leisure needs?

— What are existing methods of describing or categorizing leisure activities?

— What are the important ways in which adjustment or psychological well-being have been measured?

— To what extent are expressed leisure interests, current activity choices, and perhaps personality needs themselves confounded by situational constraints, learned habits, and resource availability (real or imagined)?

[45] Compton, Witt, and Sanchez, "Leisure Counseling," p. 24.

— To what extent should leisure counseling incorporate information about other aspects of life, e.g. work and personal care?

— What are current methods of counseling (behavior modification, directive versus non-directive, group versus individual, testing based versus clinical, etc.) and what impacts do they have on client awareness, behavior change, and, ultimately, need satisfaction?[46]

More recently, attention to research needs in leisure counseling has shifted beyond the process itself to questions related to the provision of counseling services within the broader context of the leisure service delivery system. The following topics for investigation in this area were generated by a subgroup on research of the National Forum on Leisure Counseling, led by David Compton:

— What is the responsibility of the leisure service delivery system in facilitating leisure development?

— What are the roles and functions of leisure service deliveries in facilitating opportunities?

— What delivery models exist that affect leisure delivery and the effect of each on consumerism?

— What models ars most appropriate for facilitation of various levels of leisure development?

— What are the competencies, roles and functions (of leisure service personnel) in facilitating leisure development?[47]

STUDY GUIDE QUESTIONS

1. Should research questions related to the process of leisure counseling be given less, equal, or more priority than topics concerning leisure counseling in the larger context of leisure service delivery? Can (and should) these two major areas of research be investigated simultaneously?

2. Prioritize the topics suggested by Witt and Bishop and the subgroup led by Compton. Defend your rank ordering of each set of questions.

3. Is the number of current journals and other research dissemination vehicles in therapeutic recreation and the parks and recreation field adequate to report new information on leisure counseling? Should new research organs be developed for this purpose?

ANNOTATED BIBLIOGRAPHY

APPLEBAUM, STEPHEN A., "The Quest for Identity of Adjunctive Therapists," *Bulletin of the Menninger Clinic*, 32, no. 5 (1968), 271–79. The classic description of the search for professional identity of occupational, music, art, educational, and recreational therapists, written by the Senior Staff Psychologist of the Menninger Foundation and delivered as a presentation in April, 1968. Pointing out that the term *adjunctive*

---

[46] Peter A. Witt and Doyle Bishop, "Needed Research in Leisure Counseling," in *Leisure Counseling: An Aspect of Leisure Education*, eds. Arlin Epperson, Peter A. Witt, and Gerald Hitzhusen (Springfield, Ill.: Charles C Thomas, 1977), pp. 354–61.

[47] Humphrey, Kelley, and Hamilton, "Facilitating Leisure Development," pp. 109–10.

therapist was not the name of a discipline or a profession, but rather a classification for employment, Applebaum describes major barriers to achieving identity under this administrative arrangement. Challenges recreators in clinical settings to choose between roles as "therapists" or providers of a "steady benevolent atmosphere."

ARMSTRONG, BARBARA, "The Creative Art Therapists: Struggling for Recognition," *Hospital and Community Psychiatry*, 30, no. 12 (1979), 845–47. Chronicles the efforts of the American Art Therapy Association, the American Dance Therapy Association, the American Society of Group Psychotherapy and Psychodrama, and the National Association for Music Therapy to win recognition as autonomous mental-health professionals. Each of these professional organizations experienced growth in the 1970s (as did the NTRS), and they are currently working to "professionalize their disciplines, establish criteria for training and credentialling, to build a literature and to develop a set of professional standards and ethics." Many of the challenges faced in professionalizing these fields are identical to the issues facing therapeutic recreation specialists.

BRILL, NORMAN Q., "Delineating the Role of the Psychiatrist on the Psychiatric Treatment Team," *Hospital and Community Psychiatry*, 28, no. 7 (1977), 542–44. This brief position paper outlines the resistance which many nonmedical mental-health professionals feel toward working under the direct supervision of psychiatrists, particularly the current reluctance of these professionals to embrace the medical model. Complements the writings of Rusalem ("An Alternative to the Therapeutic Model in Therapeutic Recreation") in classroom discussions.

DAY, H.I., "A Role for Recreation in Vocational Rehabilitation," *Leisurability*, 1, no. 2 (April 1974), 29–36. Criticizes many vocational rehabilitation programs for providing only job skill training and not education for leisure and examines the relationship among work, play, and the work ethic especially for disadvantaged individuals.

HUBER, HERMAN, "The Psychiatrists' Role as Team Leader: What About the Other Professionals?" *Hospital and Community Psychiatry*, 28, no. 12 (1977), 918. Rebuts Brill's position that a psychiatrist should be "the captain of the treatment team" in mental health settings, pointing out that no one mental health professional can possess all the skills and abilities necessary to provide comprehensive care.

KIESLER, CHARLES A., "The Training of Psychiatrists and Psychologists," *American Psychologist*, 32, no. 2 (1977), 107–8. A reaction by the American Psychological Association to a recent suggestion of the American Psychiatric Association that only psychiatrists be considered qualified to receive national health insurance reimbursement. Outlines the differences in training of each of these mental-health professionals, exemplifying the competition which exists among health care professionals for third-party payments.

LOWE, JANE ISAACS, and MARJATTA HERRANEN, "Conflict in Teamwork: Understanding Roles and Relationships," *Social Work in Health Care*, 3, no. 3 (1978), 323–330. Details the conflicts which can arise between professional members of a renal failure treatment team, utilizing constructs from sociology, psychology, and group theory, to analyze decision-making mechanisms. Alerts therapeutic recreation specialists to potential areas of conflict with other professions and suggests techniques and processes for resolving these difficulties.

LYNCH, BONNIE L., "Team Building: Will It Work in Health Care?" *Journal of Allied Health*, 10, no. 4 (1981), 240–47. Describes the concept of a team, the process of team development, and the characteristics of an effective team, especially for health care professionals and organizations. Points up the veritable lack of consistency between the way a profession defines its roles and the way it is perceived by others, particularly when "high-status" professions define roles for "lower-status" professions. Offers concrete suggestions for team building which have particular application in therapeutic recreation settings.

PLUCKHAN, MARGARET L., "Professional Territory: A Problem Affecting the Delivery of

Health Care," *Nursing Forum*, 11, no. 3 (1972), 300–310. Drawing parallels between Ardrey's concept of territoriality and the overprotectiveness of health care professionals, this position paper outlines several problems which arise when health team members' tasks are not aligned in appropriate fashion. Stressing "the need for logical boundaries," the author argues that patient needs and overall objectives must transcend issues of status and control between and among health team members.

RAE-GRANT, A.F. QUENTIN, and DONALD J. MARCUSE, "The Hazards of Teamwork," *American Journal of Orthopsychiatry*, 38, no. 1 (1968), 4–8. Covers potential misuses and abuses of "therapeutic" teamwork, arguing that instead of benefiting individual clients, clinical teams are likely to engage in "emotional buckpassing," "reciprocal alibiing," and "over-differentiation of roles." Useful for discussions of the strengths and weaknesses of the team approach practiced by therapeutic recreation specialists and other allied health care professionals in clinical settings.

RULLMAN, LEE, "Adapted Activities and the Handicapped," *Leisurability*, 1, no. 1 (1974), 15–19. Illustrates with case study examples several principles for adapting activities without compromising the abilities of physically disabled persons.

SCHINDLER, FRED E., MICHAEL R. BERREN, and ALLAN BEIGEL, "A Study of the Causes of Conflict between Psychiatrists and Psychologists," *Hospital and Community Psychiatry*, 32, no. 4 (1981), 263–66. This investigation asked four groups of mental-health professionals to evaluate the degree to which psychiatrists and psychologists performed certain everyday activities in mental-health settings and how competent they were in performing these duties. This approach would seem to be a valuable one for determining the perceived competencies and responsibilities of therapeutic recreation specialists versus other allied health care fields such as occupational therapy.

TANNER, LIBBY A., and ETHEL J. SOULARY, "Interprofessional Student Health Teams," *Nursing Outlook*, 20, no. 2 (1972), 111–15. Depicts a demonstration project in which ten health teams composed of a medical, a nursing, and a social-work student provided comprehensive health care to one family over a seven-month period. Although not problem-free, the experience appeared to help students "appreciate and relate to each other's discipline." This process appears to be applicable and valuable in the academic preparation of therapeutic recreation students and personnel from other related disciplines.

VOGT, MOLLY T., and ALEX J. DUCANIS, "Conflict and Cooperation in the Allied Health Professions: An Analysis of the Sources of Conflict and Recommendations for Its Management," *Journal of Allied Health*, 6, no. 1 (1977), 23–30. Explores specific sources of conflict within the allied health care field including issues in higher education and PSROs and HSA regulations. Makes several recommendations for reducing competition between health care professionals of which administrators of therapeutic recreation programs should be aware.

ZWERLING, ISRAEL, "The Creative Arts Therapies as Real Therapies," *Hospital and Community Psychiatry*, 30, no. 12 (1979), 841–44. Takes strong exception to the notion that creative arts therapies (i.e., art, movement, music therapy, psychodrama, and poetry therapy) are "adjunctive" in nature. Extends the position that such interventions are "real therapies" and not auxiliary subordinates of psychiatry. Stimulating for discussions on the status of therapeutic recreation in mental-health and other settings.

CHAPTER TEN
EPILOGUE

Throughout this text it has been emphasized that the field of therapeutic recreation has made inroads in resolving some of the issues which face it as an emerging and rapidly developing profession. Naturally, the force behind this movement has been the work undertaken by the profession's chief representative organization, the NTRS. Indeed, the efforts of this body are chiefly responsible for defining the dimensions of each of the issues described within the preceeding pages. Therefore, to provide the reader with an accurate perspective of each issue and an insight into future measures and directions related to its resolution, it is necessary to overview some of the current activities of the NTRS. The following pages represent a summary of the charges and relevant actions reported by various task forces and subcommittees at a recent board meeting of this organization, with additional comments by the authors.[1] This information has been organized generally and presented to correspond with the topical chapters within the text.

NTRS PHILOSOPHICAL STATEMENT TASK FORCE

The development of any profession naturally requires clarity about the nature of that profession. In 1982 a philosophical position statement was adopted. In the same

---

[1] National Therapeutic Recreation Society, *Minutes of the Board of Directors Meeting*, Anaheim, California, February 9–13, 1983.

year the Philosophical Issues Task Force was charged with the responsiblity "to document historical and conceptual issues related to the adopted philosophical position statement, prepare a paper on current status of membership opinion and current interpretations of the position statement, and to recommend future directions for the dissemination and review of the position."[2]

In carrying out this charge, the committee distributed a questionnaire to members of the organization concerning the acceptability, strengths and weaknesses, and interpretations of the philosophical position statement. If the responses to the selected questions on the seventy-two returned questionnaires are representative of the views of therapeutic recreation professionals in general, it would appear that the current position statement has a high degree of acceptability and perceived applicability to the practice of therapeutic recreation service. However, the question raised by the authors, resulting from a review of the responses to the questionnaire, is not only whether the adopted philosophical statement is a true reflection of therapeutic recreation at this stage of professional development, but also whether the statement has been developed with sufficient precision to suggest educational objectives. The statement needs to seek these objectives that are broadly desirable for preparing therapeutic recreation practitioners in a changing profession to carry out tasks required of them in the present as well as the foreseeable future.

All helping professions subscribe to the view that a human being must be seen as a whole. However, both the complexity of human functioning and the increase of scientific specialization have made it necessary for each profession to take one aspect of human functioning as the primary focus of its activities. This does not imply that a person can be divided into separate compartments or that there is not a great deal of overlapping among activities of the several helping professions.

The ultimate goal of therapeutic recreation is seen as the enhancement of leisure experiences, whenever the need for such enhancement is individually or socially perceived. The functions of therapeutic recreation are of three kinds: (1) restoration of impaired capacity through leisure experiences, (2) enhancement of individual leisure attitudes and skills, and (3) enhancement or restoration of independent leisure functioning. Therapeutic recreation as a profession is viewed as having an obligation to intervene at any point in the light of an assessment of the individual and social factors involved. Such professional activity will consequently result in improved leisure functioning. The method of achievement of leisure functioning has been noted earlier, but requires repeating: assessment of the problem, planning for a solution to the problem, implementing the plan, and evaluating the outcome.

In sum, therapeutic recreation as a profession has both a perspective and a distinctive focus of activity. This perspective is a conception which views leisure functioning as important in humanity's environment. The focus of activity is professional intervention in that aspect of human functioning which lies in the realm of leisure behavior. The focus on leisure is suggested as the *distinguishing characteristic* of the therapeutic recreation profession.

---

[2] National Therapeutic Recreation Society (NTRS) Minutes, February 9–13, 1983, *Philosophical Statement Task Force Report*, January 15, 1983, p. 1.

LICENSURE TASK FORCE

The immediate concerns of this committee are to "develop a position paper on therapeutic recreation licensure" and to establish a "resource center for those needing information on occupational therapy licensure bills."[3] A major objective of this committee over the past year has been to assist state therapeutic recreation organizations to negotiate with occupational therapy groups concerning the provisions of occupational therapy licensure bills which have been introduced in state legislatures.

Licensure was originally created in the public interest for the protection of the public from incompetent practitioners. Today, however, with the proliferation of many new categories of health personnel, there has been a scramble to delineate the parameters of practice of the emerging and existing groups of health care workers. There is no doubt that reform will take place within the credentialling system of health care personnel. The question is whether the initiative for such reform will be assumed by the professions or imposed by society.

The activities of this body also reflect the previously discussed concerns found in Chapter 9 over territorial boundaries of service which exist between, but are not limited to, occupational therapy and therapeutic recreation. In all probability, questions related to the purview of services of all allied health care professions will increase sharply over the next several years.

Currently, there are federal and state pressures for interprofessional service endeavors in health care delivery. Although this goal may appear commendable from an economic viewpoint, several issues and problems are evident. One of the critical issues is the complexity and diversity of some disciplines and of interdisciplinary endeavors and the limited conceptualization of core elements to be integrated across interdisciplinary lines. There appears to be much talk, but the authors are unaware of any hard evidence of interprofessional core content. Further, a quick review of the literature indicates little systematic and critical examination of interdisciplinary core content in the health field.

Another critical problem is the limited number of therapeutic recreation practitioners who are prepared to work in interdisciplinary service. Such practitioners who have been involved in interdisciplinary service realize the tremendous importance of imploring colleagues' interpretations and perceptions of interdisciplinary programs. Not only is basic knowledge of the philosophy and theory of other disciplines needed, but basic terms such as *interdisciplinary cooperation, collaborative practices, captain of the team, in charge, team control,* and *assistants* need to be understood thoroughly at the outset, or management difficulties occur in a short time.

Therapeutic recreation practitioners involved in interdisciplinary designs must not only be strong and knowledgeable, but also be able to raise critical questions,

---

[3] NTRS Minutes, *Licensure Task Force Report*, February 1983, p. 1.

remain a bit suspicious (yes, it is permissible), and develop ways to reach therapeutic recreation objectives through the skills of other disciplines.

CONTINUING PROFESSIONAL DEVELOPMENT REVIEW BOARD

The purpose of this body is "To revise, update and monitor operational/administrative procedures for continuing professional development; to review applications for endorsement by NTRS; to work in conjunction with the National Council on Therapeutic Recreation Certification."[4]

It is currently in the process of establishing specific evaluation guidelines which will govern the approval of proposed programs requesting endorsement by the NTRS. It is also actively seeking alternatives to awarding Continuing Education Units for validating professional development. Finally, it is engaged in an active dialogue with the National Council on Therapeutic Recreation Certification concerning the current and future role and function of continuing professional development.

The notion of continuing professional education and training appears to be widely embraced by therapeutic recreation practitioners and educators. As noted in Chapter 4, however, there appears to be little national consensus within and outside of our profession. A review of the available literature on the efficacy of continuing education (CE) leaves one with a sense of uncertainty. On one hand, the results of various CE research projects lead mostly to confusion, whereas, on the other hand, there are studies which promote and support the argument that an effective means of increasing practitioner competence is through CE courses.[5] Although no resolution concerning this matter is foreseen in the near future,[6] the health insurance industry is extremely concerned about continued competence because it has a direct relationship to quality and cost of health care services. The extent of this concern is reflected in the Health Insurance Association of America's working with the National Commission for Health Certifying Agencies on the issue of the continuing competence of health care personnel.[7]

---

[4] NTRS Minutes, *Continuing Professional Development Review Board Report*, February 1983, p. 1.

[5] Peggy McCarberg, "The Efficacy of Continuing Education," in *To Assure Continuing Competence*. Report of the National Commission for Health Certifying Agencies, DHHS Publication No. (HRA) 81–5. (Washington, D.C.: U.S. Government Printing Office, April 1981), pp. 90–91.

[6] *Ibid.*, p. 94.

[7] Daniel R. Thomas, "Continuing Competence from a Health Insurance Industrial Perspective," in *To Assure Continuing Competence*. Report of the National Commission for Health Certifying Agencies, DHHS Publication No. (HRA) 81–5. (Washington, D.C.: U.S. Government Printing Office, April 1981), pp. 85–88.

ARTICULATION WITH
HEALTH SERVICE
MONITORING AGENCIES

In recent years significant effort has been devoted to communicating with organizations who monitor health care related servcies to clients in a variety of agencies. At least four separate bodies have been established within NTRS for this purpose. These committees and their central functions are listed next:

Committee	Purposes
NTRS Third Party Reimbursement Committee	**To develop strategies to educate third-party reimbursers about therapeutic recreation service.**
	To provide resources and information to NTRS members about third-party reimbursement for therapeutic recreation service.[8]
Joint Commission on Accreditation of Hospitals Standards Subcommittee	**To provide ongoing communication between NTRS and JCAH to improve the quality of services to clients in JCAH accredited facilities.[9]**
Long Term Care Standards, Joint Commission on Accreditation of Hospitals	**To develop a relationship with the Long Term Care Accreditation Program of JCAH.[10]**
Commission on Accreditation of Rehabilitation Facilities, Subcommittee of Program Standards Committee	**To provide professional guidance and consultation services to CARF in order to upgrade therapeutic recreation services in the rehabilitation facility movement and improve quality of services provided to the disabled and disadvantaged.[11]**

A partial list of the objectives and accomplishments of these groups to date includes:

— Initiating dialogue with Medicare program policy officials to determine their understanding of therapeutic recreation service and appropriate methods to influence Medicare operations so that decisions about coverage of therapeutic recreation service are consistent throughout the Medicare system.

[8] NTRS Minutes, *Third Party Reimbursement Committee Report*, February 1983, p. 1.

[9] NTRS Minutes, *Joint Commission on Accreditation of Hospitals Standards Subcommittee Report*, February 1983, p. 1.

[10] NTRS Minutes, *Long Term Care Standards–Joint Commission on Accreditation of Hospitals Committee Report*, February 1983, p. 1.

[11] NTRS Minutes, *Commission on Accreditation of Rehabilitation Facilities–Subcommittee of the Program Standards Committee Report*, February 1983, p. 1.

— Developing and distributing a brochure designed to educate third-party payers about therapeutic recreation services.

— Developing guidelines and determining resources to be used by therapeutic recreation professionals when seeking reimbursement for therapeutic recreation service.

— Drafting a NTRS position statement which examines and explains the distinctions between therapeutic recreation and occupational, physical, art, music and dance therapy.

— Creating a NTRS committee charged with the task of further defining the standards of practice document including: assessment procedures, treatment goals/objectives, treatment methodologies and evaluation procedures for various settings, hospital service areas and disabilities.

— Publishing a list of selected research literature documenting the value of therapeutic recreation services for various disabilities and service settings.

— Drafting a NTRS position statement explaining operationally how therapeutic recreation service can contribute to quality care and treatment.

— Reviewing the *Accreditation Manual for Hospitals* and Consolidated Standards of the Joint Commission on Accreditation of Hospitals.

— Pursuing the possibility of obtaining at least one position on the Joint Commission on Accreditation of Hospitals Review Board for Long Term Health Care Standards.

— Adding the definition of ''therapeutic recreation specialist'' to the *Standards Manual,* (glossary of terms section) of the Commission on Accreditation of Rehabilitation Facilities and including therapeutic recreation in the aggregate of services along with physical therapy, occupational therapy, rehabilitation nursing, social work, psychology, and speech and language services.[12]

The impetus for these efforts has been a strong realization that the field of therapeutic recreation must continue to seek recognition from agencies who directly monitor client health care services. But to seek recognition requires the need to identify therapeutic recreation's unique contribution to health care and service in order to justify its existence among other health workers who are seeking to carve their own niche in the expanding and, for some, profitable health care field. In order to avoid playing the role of dog in the manger, therapeutic recreation must carefully examine its role and determine how well it meets the health care needs of society.

Therapeutic recreation has to some extent contributed to its problems of recognition because it has failed to develop an autonomously effective practice that is recognized as worthwhile by either the public or other professionals. Therapeutic recreation needs to identify, to describe, and to categorize its practice so that the public, as well as other professionals, will know what it is. By the same token, therapeutic recreation practitioners must be more assertive in identifying autonomous therapeutic recreation practice and in setting and communicating standards in whatever agency they practice. The authority for setting the standards must derive from the effectiveness of the therapeutic recreation care and service plan, not from administrative acquiescence or through pseudomedical or paramedical competence.

[12] *Ibid.*

Recognition of the existence of such factors as society and its deep concern over the problems of health care and service, patients and their concern for a more equitable standard of care and service, agency philosophy and purpose including its resources to achieve goals, and other health providers and their impact should provide therapeutic recreation practitioners with cues to the action they must take, either individually or collectively, to improve the quality of therapeutic recreation service. In the final analysis, however, it is the individual practitioner who determines the acceptance of therapeutic recreation. The practitioner must have the self-image of an autonomous professional practitioner and the knowledge, skills, and assertiveness necessary for the role.

LEGISLATIVE ACTION COMMITTEE

The functions of this body are threefold: (1) "To identify and monitor all federal legislation (appropriations and regulations) relevant to the profession of therapeutic recreation;" (2) "To develop appropriate responses to said legislation" and; (3) "To keep members informed of developments, positions, and responses."[13]

This active committee responded to five issues which had strong implications for therapeutic recreation professionals over the past year. The following is a summary of each situation which called for a response on the part of this body:

1. Working closely with the NRPA's Office of Public Affairs, this committee developed testimony in opposition to proposed changes in the implementation of PL 94–142, which would have eliminated the definition of recreation as a related service. This testimony was given by NTRS members at the national level throughout the country.

2. Legislators were contacted and urged to support the continued full-funding of Section 316 of the Vocational Rehabilitation Act. This piece of legislation appropriates funds for the provision of direct service, demonstration, recreation projects to promote the independence and full functioning of disabled persons. In the past, these services have been provided in hospital, university, and community settings.

3. Revisions to Section 504 of the Rehabilitation Act, proposed by the Department of Justice through the Regulatory Task Force of the Office of Management and Budget, were monitored by this committee and various other consumer groups of disabled persons. These revisions, which could have weakened prohibitions designed to prevent discrimination against disabled persons in the provision of programs and services in agencies receiving federal financial assistance, were not implemented.

4. A statement and questions were developed for the confirmation hearing of a new Assistant Secretary for Special Education and Rehabilitative Services.

5. A "legislative alert" was issued to therapeutic recreation professionals in response to a study being undertaken by the Department of Health and Human Services relative to Medicare reimbursement. Under this plan, recreation services would be included in the research related to Diagnostic Related Groups (DRGs). However, recreation would not be mentioned as a service in rehabilitation units and hospitals, children's hospitals, or long-term hospitals. This situation could preclude recreation being built into room-rate

[13] NTRS Minutes, *Legislative Action Committee Report*, February 1983, p. 1.

reimbursements in these facilities. At this writing, the committee is cautiously optimistic that recreation will be included in the study presently being undertaken.

The preceding activities are indicative of the many ways in which therapeutic recreation service may be impacted by federal legislation. It is obvious that the profession of therapeutic recreation must continue its vigilance of the legislative docket and expand its political influence as it matures. These actions indicate increasing sophistication about the sources and uses of political power. Political clout can help therapeutic recreation obtain desirable, even essential, health legislation for the public, encourage support for therapeutic recreation education, and influence regulatory legislation in the direction of desirable standards of therpeutic recreation service.

EDUCATIONAL COMMITTEES

Two committees deal directly with matters pertaining to the education and training of therapeutic recreation specialists: the Therapeutic Recreation Curriculum Development and Standards Committee and the NTRS Paraprofessional Accreditation Board/Committee. Their purposes, respectively, are "To act as a liaison between NTRS, the Accreditation Council, and the National Council for Therapeutic Recreation Certification on matters related to curriculum and professional preparation in therapeutic recreation"[14] and to provide technical assistance and information to individuals and schools requesting such; and "to serve as the accrediting body for the NTRS 750-Hour Curriculum for therapeutic recreation assistants and coordinate paraprofessional education activities, issues, and concerns in therapeutic recreation."[15]

Both committees respond frequently to requests by individuals and institutions of higher education for information on certification procedures or for permission to provide training programs. A recent special task undertaken by the Curriculum Development and Standards Committee was working with the Office of Personnel Management to improve the review process for persons with masters degrees in therapeutic recreation in relation to the GS 638 series. Activities undertaken by the Paraprofessional Accreditation Board Committee included revision of the Accreditation process, interfacing with the Society for Park and Recreation Educators, National Recreation and Park Association's Accreditation programs, conducting a survey on the relevance of various course objectives within the 750-Hour Curriculum, and developing a reaccreditation procedure.

The activities of these committees indicate that curriculum development in therapeutic recreation is a continuous process, as we constantly strive toward improved professional training and direct client services. On the other hand,

[14] NTRS Minutes, *Therapeutic Recreation Curriculum Development and Standards Committee Report*, February 1983, p. 1.

[15] NTRS Minutes, *Paraprofessional Accreditation Committee Report*, February 1983, p. 1.

however, many issues continue to plague curriculum development, for example; Does therapeutic recreation possess a systematic body of knowledge, skills, and attitudes which can be applied to the various areas of therapeutic recreation practice? Is the content of therapeutic recreation education sufficiently well developed that it can be transmitted?

Progress toward answering these questions was made by the adoption of the NTRS Philosophical Position Statement,[16] but further study is needed. Therapeutic recreation education has also to face other educational issues:

— How best can it educate for professional practice still in the process of rapid change and development? Can it be broad enough in scope to enable therapeutic recreators to function in areas already established, as well as those which may emerge in the future?[17] Will breadth of education to encompass all areas of professional practice result in dilution of competence for specific areas?

— Should undergraduate education serve primarily entry level positions or as a basis for graduate training?

Answers to these questions, plus those which might emerge from additional discussion, would be obtained by focusing upon fundamental questions of curriculum planning and not giving piece-meal consideration to the specific questions posed or to others which might arise. In education for therapeutic recreation, as for other professions, the fundamental considerations in curriculum planning apply.

— What are the desirable educational objectives for professional education?

— What learning experiences should be selected and devised, and how organized to realize these objectives?

— What are the effective means of evaluating whether the objectives have been attained?

Without a clear formulation of the objectives of therapeutic recreation education, that is, the knowledge, skills, and values students are expected to acquire, it becomes impossible to plan the learning experiences or to evaluate their success. Therefore, both committees need to single out as their major task the identification of desirable objectives of therapeutic recreation education. Further, the educational objectives need to be framed in terms of both the *content* to be covered and the kind and quality of *behavior* to be expected from the student in relation to the content.

RESEARCH COMMITTEE

The stated purpose of this committee is "To identify current progress and professional concerns in therapeutic recreation research; to develop a plan for monitoring research activities and dissemination of research priorities."[18]

[16] National Therapeutic Recreation Society, *Philosophical Position Statement of the National Therapeutic Recreation Society* (Alexandria, Va.: National Recreation and Park Association, May 1982).

[17] See Gerald L. Hitzhusen, "Therapeutic Recreation–2000," in *Leisure 2000: Scenarios for the Future*, ed. Glenn A. Gillespie (Columbia, Mo.: University of Missouri, College of Public and Community Services, Department of Recreation and Park Administration, 1983), p. 148, for projected future roles.

[18] NTRS Minutes, *Research Committee Report*, February 1983, p. 1.

A major project undertaken by this committee was the planning of a national survey of research needs in the field. This survey will have four major thrusts. *First,* therapeutic recreation professionals, both NTRS members and nonmembers, will be polled as to their perceived research needs related to practice in addition to research progress in the field. *Second,* current faculty and graduate student research projects in therapeutic recreation curricula will be identified throughout the country. *Third,* research investigations from related fields will be examined. *Finally,* an open dialogue on research concerns and progress will be created by establishing communication with the readers of the NTRS newsletter.

The above-mentioned activities represent critical first steps in transposing research efforts in therapeutic recreation from random and isolated fact-gathering expeditions to systematic investigations aimed at progressively contributing to the body of knowledge upon which therapeutic recreation service is based. On the other hand, however, while the authors have no quarrel with the second and third points above, there is a question about the research efforts that might be produced from points one and four because therapeutic recreation practitioners on the whole have been found wanting, both in the practitioners' own research methods and in their relationship to research.

The role of the therapeutic recreation practitioner can be divided into four service areas; namely, providing service to the consumer, or the specific performance of the individual practitioner on the job; functioning as a staff member of the agency; acting as a member of one's profession; and participating in research. It would seem advisable, in light of our earlier professional-preparation discussion, that curriculum objectives and learning experiences be arranged to prepare future practitioners to have a more "research orientation." Although these roles are not mutually exclusive and do not necessarily require different curriculum objectives, they do provide stable points around which to structure capacities and define curriculum objectives.

One cannot help but feel that there is a definite and growing need for the practitioner to have research awareness as part of one who renders service. This view is apparently supported by twenty-seven practitioners and educators who responded to a recent open-ended survey concerning the future of therapeutic recreation.[19] The tasks most frequently performed by practitioners are those most clearly related to the practitioner's knowledge and skill in his or her own methods. However, it is questionable to what extent the practitioner may be adequately prepared within either the bachelor's or master's curriculum to perform such tasks as apply logical and orderly thinking to problems presented in one's own practice, apply an attitude of scientific inquiry toward one's own practice; adapt service skills to the needs of research, and apply research findings in practice. It is not the purpose of the authors to encourage or to discourage the need for more research courses or such related courses at either academic level, but rather to promote the need for effective curriculum planning which will enable the practitioner to accomplish the professional role more effectively and at the same time prepare the practitioner in

[19] Hitzhusen, "Therapeutic Recreation–2000," p. 145.

the process and principles of problem solving, applying an attitude of critical thinking.

SUGGESTED STRATEGIES
FOR UPDATING THE
MATERIAL IN THIS TEXT

This brief overview of important events taking place in the field of therapeutic recreation at the national level should create in the reader an urgency to become knowledgeable and remain abreast of current developments in the field. In this regard, for example, what is going to be the purpose and function of the proposed American Therapeutic Recreation Association as opposed to the NTRS? Similarly, it is hoped that therapeutic recreation professionals wil be further motivated to become involved in local, state, and national affairs influencing the practice of therapeutic recreation service. Fortunately, many vehicles exist to facilitate this process.

Naturally, maintaining an active membership in the NRPA's NTRS branch is a fundamental step in securing information. A current publication of this organization providing much needed material to the therapeutic recreation professional is the *Therapeutic Recreation Journal.* It contains scholarly articles in the areas of basic and applied research, program development and implementation, professional development, and other topics of interest to practitioners and educators alike. Three other publications of the NRPA frequently contain information of interest to those in the field of therapeutic recreation. *Dateline,* a monthly publication, contains much information, particularly of a legislative nature, which has relevance to the profession. *Parks and Recreation Magazine*, the general publication of NRPA frequently features articles pertaining to the provision of leisure service to disabled persons, primarily in community settings. It too provides briefs on legal and legislative developments which could impact on the practice of therapeutic recreation service. A third publication of another NRPA branch, the *Society for Park and Recreation Educators Newsletter,* highlights developments in the areas of curriculum development, credentialling, and standards which will directly influence professional preparation in the field.

The NTRS maintains a State and Regional Advisory Council which exists solely to facilitate communication between and among members of the profession. This body is an excellent vehicle for expressing concerns and transmitting information related to current developments in the field. As always, the office of the Branch Liaison of the NTRS remains a primary source of information and documentation relative to matters of professional preparation, credentialling procedures, standards of practice for service, and codes of ethical practice. Additionally, many states employ full-time therapeutic recreation consultants under a variety of administrative and organizational arrangements. These individuals can frequently provide technical assistance in the areas of grant writing and program evaluation and usually possess information related to the employment status of therapeutic recreation professionals within the state.

In addition to the publications of NTRS, several other periodicals exist which should be frequent reading for the practicing therapeutic recreation specialist. It is impossible to describe or even mention all of these sources, but the following few will be outlined. Additionally, the reader is referred to the annotated bibliographies which appear at the end of each chapter. The *Journal of Leisure Research* and *Leisure Sciences* are both sources of basic research related to the leisure pursuits of disabled persons. As mentioned before, the Canadian publication *Leisurability* is devoted to several topics including leisure, which impact upon the lives of disabled and disadvantaged persons. *Programming Trends*, a magazine published at Texas Woman's University, deals specifically with innovative practices in the direct provision of leisure services to clients in a variety of clinical and community settings. At the time of this writing, a new journal entitled the *Adapted Physical Activity Quarterly* is nearing print. Multidisciplinary in nature, it will contain various data-based investigations and position papers related to the broad area of adapted activity for a variety of disabled populations. Lastly, the reader is urged to obtain the publications of state recreation organizations and papers which are printed in various local, state, regional, and national conference proceedings.

SUMMARY
AND CONCLUSIONS

This text has provided an extensive overview of the most critical issues which may ever confront our field. It traced the origins of these trends and problems, presented the positions of noted professionals on these topics, and furnished numerous instructional references. Nevertheless, it cannot extend definitive answers to these complex points of inquiry. Rather, it serves as a gauntlet thrown down, and an invitation to embark upon courses of future deliberation and constructive action. Used in this fashion, it can be a vital force to assist us in meeting the challenges now facing our profession.

APPENDIX A

The National Council for Therapeutic Recreation Certification is an independently administered body of the National Recreation and Park Association. It is a self-financing, not-for-profit, non-governmental body.

The purpose of the National Council for Therapeutic Recreation Certification is to: (1) establish national evaluation standards for the certification and re-certification of individuals who possess the competencies of the therapeutic recreation profession; (2) grant recognition to individuals who voluntarily apply and meet the established standards; and (3) monitor adherence to the standards by certified therapeutic recreation personnel.

Professional Level—
Therapeutic Recreation
Specialist
(minimum requirements)

A. Baccalaureate degree or higher from an accredited college or university with a major in therapeutic recreation or a major in and an option in therapeutic recreation. Degree must be verified by an official transcript sent from the registrar. A student's copy is not acceptable.

OR

B. Baccalaureate degree or higher from an accredited college or university with a major in recreation *and* two years of full-time paid experience in a clinical, residential, or community-based therapeutic recreation program. Degree must be verified by an official transcript from the registrar. A student's copy is not acceptable.

Professional Provisional— Therapeutic Recreation Specialist (Non-Renewable) (minimum requirements)

C. Baccalaureate degree or higher from an accredited college or university with a major in recreation. Degree must be verified by an official transcript from the registrar. A student's copy is not acceptable.

This alternative permits temporary certification while a person acquires the two years of full-time paid experience in a clinical, residential, or community-based therapeutic recreation program necessary for renewal of certification as a professional.

Professional Equivalency Process—Therapeutic Recreation Specialist (minimum requirements)

D. Baccalaureate degree or higher from an accredited college or university in one of the related or allied health fields *plus* five years of full-time paid experience in a clinical, residential, or community-based therapeutic recreation program *plus* 18 semester or 27 quarter hours of upper division credits in recreation/therapeutic recreation competencies. Degree must be verified by an official transcript from the registrar. A student's copy is not acceptable.

Para-Professional— Therapeutic Recreation Assistant (minimum requirements)

A. Associate of Arts degree from an accredited educational institution with a major in recreation or a major in recreation and an option* in therapeutic recreation. Degree must be verified by an official transcript from the registrar. A student's copy is not acceptable.

OR

B. Associate of Arts degree from an accredited educational institution with a major in recreation *plus* one year of full-time paid experience in a clinical, residential, or community-based therapeutic recreation program. Degree must be verified by an official transcript from the registrar. A student's copy is not acceptable.

OR

C. Associate of Arts degree or higher from an accredited educational institution with a major in one of the skill areas (arts, crafts, dance, drama, music, physical education) and one year of full-time paid experience in a clinical, residential, or community-based therapeutic recreation program. Degree must be verified by an official transcript from the registrar. A student's copy is not acceptable.

OR

D. Completion of the NTRS 750-Hour Training Program for therapeutic recreation personnel, with verification by an official certificate of completion.

OR

E. Four years of full-time paid experience in a clinical, residential, or community-based therapeutic recreation program.

*Professional Option

The *professional option* includes:
a. A minimum of three courses dealing exclusively with therapeutic recreation content, and
b. Completion of a 400 hour field placement experience in a clinical, residential, or community-based therapeutic recreation program, and
c. Completion of supportive coursework to include a minimum of 18 semester or 27 quarter units from 4 of these 6 areas:

psychology

sociology

physical/biological science

special education

human services

adapted physical education

**Para-Professional Option

The *paraprofessional* option includes:
a. A minimum of two courses dealing exclusively with therapeutic recreation content, and
b. Completion of a 400 hour field placement experience in a clinical, residential, or community-based therapeutic recreation program, and
c. Completion of supportive coursework to include a minimum of 12 semester or 18 quarter units selected from psychology, sociology, physical/biological sciences, human services, and physical education activity classes.

NAME INDEX

Peterson, C. A., 25, 49, 50, 51, 52, 58, 125, 128, 130, 131, 133, 138, 139, 141, 175
Phillips, B. E., 16
Pumphrey, M. W., 30
Pumphrey, R. E., 30

Raths, L., 11
Rawson, H. E., 157
Reynolds, R. P., 60, 138, 139, 142, 160, 176
Robb, G., 21, 45, 46, 52, 129
Rokeach, M., 111
Roos, P., 157
Rosen, E., 39
Rowthorn, A. W., 45
Rubin, J. A., 201
Rusalem, H., 21, 43, 44, 45, 51
Rusk, H. A., 39

Sanchez, B. D., 212, 216, 219, 222
Schlicke, R. S., 98
Schulberg, H. C., 106
Scully, D. G., 142
Selden, W. K., 64
Sessoms, H. D., 13, 137, 212, 213, 217, 218
Shannon, P. D., 47, 48, 51, 205
Shapiro, I. G., 65
Shephard, W., 10
Shimberg, B., 67
Shirreffs, J. H., 90
Shivers, J. S., 43, 46
Silson, J. E., 17
Simon, S. R., 111
Sirgrist, H. E., 109
Smith, B. L., 102
Smith, S. H., 128, 129, 141

Spackman, C. S., 205, 206
Stein, T. A., 13, 125
Stewart, M. W., 125
Stillman, A. T., 41
Sylvester, C. D., 114

Taylor, J. L., 181
Theodorson, A., 134
Theodorson, G., 134
Thomas, D. R., 229
Thomas, J. B., 8
Tyler, R. W., 121

Van Andel, G. E., 101, 102, 103, 105
Vaughan, J., 24, 58, 102
Volger, E. W., 157
Vollmer, H. M., 10
Vosburgh, P., 16

Wehman, P., 157
Weiner, A., 159, 216
Weintraub, F. J., 94
Wheeler, J., 60
Wilensky, H. L., 9, 10, 28, 83, 108, 134
Williams, A., 14
Willner, A., 106
Wilson, P. A., 11
Winslow, R., 24, 102
Witt, P. A., 13, 21, 45, 46, 47, 51, 144, 212, 213, 216, 219, 222
Wolfensberger, W., 151, 152, 153, 154, 156
Wolffe, J. B., 16
Wyatt, W. J., 159

Zusman, J., 107

SUBJECT INDEX

Accreditation, 63-66
  Committee Report (NTRS), 25
  Council for Facilities for the Mentally Retarded, 98
  Council for Psychiatric Facilities, 98
  Council for Services for Mentally Retarded and Other Developmental Disabilities, 98, 102
  defined, 63
  historical development, 63-64
  institutional, 64
  pros and cons of, 73-74
  purpose, 65
  specialization, 64-65
  types of, 64
Accreditation Committee Report (NTRS), 25
Accreditation Manual for Hospitals, 231
Accreditation Manual for Psychiatric Facilities, 102
Activity, 200, 201, 202, 205, 227
Adapted Physical Activity Quarterly, 237
Advisory Council, 96
Alternative Positions and Their Implication to Professionalism (NTRS), 29
American Alliance for Health, Physical Education, Recreation, and Dance, 20
American Association for Health, Physical Education, and Recreation, 20, 126
  Recreation Therapy Section of, 20, 38
American Association for Leisure and Recreation, 130
American College of Physicians, 63, 64
American College of Surgeons, 64, 98
American Correctional Association, 19
American Hospital Association, 63, 99
Ameriplan of, 78
American Journal of Art Therapy, 200
American Journal of Occupational Therapy, 47, 205
American Medical Association:
  acknowledgement of recreation services, 16
  code of ethics, 109
  Committee on Allied Health Education and Accreditation of, 64
American National Standards Institute, 95
  Specifications for Making Buildings and Facilities Accessible to, and Usable by, the Physically Handicapped of, 95
American Nursing Home Association, 22
American Occupational Therapy Association, 202
American Park and Recreation Society, 23, 24
American Psychiatric Association, 16
American Recreation Society, 65
  Hospital Recreation Section of, 16, 19, 38
American Red Cross, 13
  controversy (TR), 37-38
American Therapeutic Recreation Association, 26, 28
Art Therapy, 200-202

Assessment
  in research, 175
Attributes, 122-126
  and body of knowledge, 122
  and continued of learning, 124
  of profession, 11, 28
  and professional education, 122
  and research, 124

Ball's Service Continuum Model (*figure*), 43
Basic Concepts of Hospital Recreation, 19
Bibliotherapy, 200
Blue Cross, 100
  Association, 99
  plan, 99
Bureau of Education for the Handicapped, U. S., 126, 127, 128, 130, 211
  research priorities of, 179

Canada:
  therapeutic recreation, 44
Certification, 122
  boards, 67
  definition and purpose, 66
  historical development, 66, 67
  levels of, 68
  pros and cons of, 75-76
Children's Bureau, 101
Civil Rights Act, 96
Civil War, 69, 70
Code of ethics, 11, 83
  concept of, 108, 110-13
  in curricula, 113-16
  historical development, 109
  of National Recreation and Park Association, 109
  of National Therapeutic Recreation Society, 109
  and practitioners, 108
  profession, 108
  and professionalization, 108
  purpose, 108
  and service ideal, 108
Commission on Accreditation of Rehabilitation Facilities, 99, 231
Committee on Accreditations, 65 (*See also* National Recreation and Park Association; National Commission on Accreditation)
Committee on Licensure, U. S., 79, 80
Committees (NTRS):
  education, 233-24
    curriculum development and standards, 233-34
    paraprofessional accreditation board, 233-34
    commission on accreditation of rehabilitation facilities,